Voices of Vermont Nurses

Voices of Vermont Nurses

Nursing in Vermont, 1941–1996

VERMONT STATE NURSES' ASSOCIATION

2000

Funded through private contributions to the Vermont State Nurses' Foundation

Printed at *Sharp Offset Printing, Inc.*, Rutland, Vermont
Editing and composition by *Asterisk Typographics*, Barre, Vermont
Designed by *Asterisk Typographics*
Cover design by Peter Holm, *Sterling Hill Productions*

This book is printed on acid-free paper.

On the cover
Front: Red Cross volunteer, 1943 (courtesy of Vermont State Archives, Office of the Secretary of State, Montpelier, Vermont).
Back: Portrait of Florence Nightingale (courtesy of Anita F. Ristau).

Dedication

These green hills and silver waters are my home,
*they belong to me!**

THE EARLY SETTLERS of Vermont gave to future generations those unique characteristics that define Vermonters. From the time of Ethan Allen and the Green Mountain Boys, Vermonters have displayed a fierce determination to preserve that which makes Vermont a special place: respect for the environment, dedication to the ideals established by the founders of Vermont and the United States, respect for the individual, and a sense of common purpose defined by shared community values and actions.

Vermont nurses, whether born in Vermont, or drawn to Vermont by love of these special qualities, have amply demonstrated their devotion to upholding the basic principles which Vermonters treasure. This history depicts Vermont nurses answering the call of duty to serve the United States during times of military conflict, from World War II to the Gulf War. It tells the stories, often in their own words, of Vermont nurses who were drawn to the practice of nursing by their desire to care for the individual in humane and sensitive ways. It gives many examples of nurses who have participated in promoting the common good as defined by the larger community: preserving the environment, caring for those unable to care for themselves, seeking ways to better use limited resources. Vermont nurses have achieved these goals in one of the most rural states in the nation where winters are long and harsh, and where in the past cows were more numerous than people. Just as Vermont can contribute to a sense of isolation for some of its citizens, so illness can create the same feeling of loneliness and separation. Whether in the hospital or out in the community, nurses in their daily work strive to allay fears and to dispel that sense of isolation. It is to these nurses, whose voices are heard on these pages, that we dedicate this book.

---

* "These Green Mountains," composed by Diane Martin, arranged by Rita Buglass, 1999. Chosen from 107 entries, this was adopted as the Vermont State Song by the 1999–2000 legislative session, effective July 1, 2000.

Table of Contents

SECTION TWO
Nursing Practice

SECTION THREE
Nursing Organizations

SECTION FOUR
Vermont State Board of Nursing

Preface

IN 1941, the Vermont State Nurses' Association (VSNA) published *We Who Serve: A Story of Nursing in Vermont.* In a ten-year undertaking, members of the History of Nursing Committee of the VSNA documented nurses and nursing activities from the earliest records available through 1940, and described the book as a "contribution to Vermont's Sesquicentennial Celebration." Since then, this compilation of valuable material has been the source providing the baseline for countless nursing papers and reports.

In 1964, on the occasion of the VSNA's fiftieth anniversary, its members, under the leadership of VSNA President Jean Milligan and VSNA Historian Mary Thompson, published *Fifty Years of Progress: Past/Prospective.* This thirty-two page publication "pays homage to two pioneers in modern nursing . . . Linda Richards and Ada Stewart Markolf," and briefly updates the history of Vermont nursing to 1964. Mary Thompson's introduction describes the brochure as commemorative, and not a detailed historical account.

In 1996, the VSNA Board of Directors created a Historical Task Force to update and trace the growth and development of nursing in Vermont through the latter half of the twentieth century. As was the case with those who preceded us, this publication, *Voices of Vermont Nurses*, represents the efforts of many Vermont nurses, working together, through the Vermont State Nurses' Association. It is financed by private contributions to the Vermont State Nurses' Foundation. The content reflects changes in nursing education, nursing practice, and organizational development which have occurred in the past fifty-five years, 1941–1996. *Voices of Vermont Nurses* is a compilation of historical material written by nurses throughout the state, and by some who now reside outside Vermont but spent their working years serving Vermonters. It is also a collection of the personal experiences of many nurses.

Another component of this effort to record the history of nursing in Vermont is an oral history consisting of forty-five taped interviews with Vermont nurses that were a rich source of material for contributing writers, as well as a valuable collection for posterity. This collection of tapes is a part of the VSNA Special Collection at the Library Research Annex, The University of Vermont, Burlington.

Voices of Vermont Nurses is only a beginning in recording the role of nursing in Vermont health care over the past fifty-five years, and is not inclusive of all areas of nursing. It is our fervent hope that this beginning will motivate others to pick up where we have left off, and that it may act as a stimulus for additional research and writing about the history of nursing in Vermont.

VSNA Historical Task Force

Priscilla (Pat) Allen and Audrey Larrow, *Co-Chairs*

Jane Campbell
Lynne Ann Dapice
Jean Milligan
Anita Ristau
Bonnie Stiles
Joan Smidutz

Acknowledgments

Voices of Vermont Nurses is the product of the combined efforts of many Vermont nurses over the past five years. These are nurses who gave up their limited free time to attend meetings, contact potential writers and interviewees, write letters, develop policy statements and plans, search for funding, and finally, to write manuscripts.

The VSNA Historical Task Force wishes to acknowledge and to thank the following people and groups of people who have made this publication possible:

—The Vermont State Nurses Foundation, for the grant of funds to support printing and associated publishing costs.

—Asterisk Typographics, who came to our rescue when the task force attempted to produce "camera ready" material! Leslie Sanborn and her dedicated staff provided all the editing, composition, and technical preparation for the printer. They took the rough drafts of our nursing experiences and polished them into this professional publication.

—Faye Parsons, for her careful and excellent work. She patiently endured our constant revisions in text, converting them into useable materials, ready for Asterisk to work its magic.

—All those nurse specialists who spent hours carefully reviewing and editing manuscripts for technical nursing content.

—Representatives of Vermont schools of nursing and specialty nursing organizations who generously responded to our requests for historical information.

—Archivists Gregory Sanford and Christie Carter and their staff at the Secretary of State's Office, and David Blow and Sylvia Bugbee of the Library Research Annex at The University of Vermont; these individuals gave generously of their time in support of this publication.

—The Board of Directors and the staff of the Vermont State Nurses' Association, especially Faith Brothers and Pam Perkins who helped with so many mailings and other support activities that moved this publication forward.

—Judy Cohen of The University of Vermont nursing faculty and the students in her class who interviewed and recorded the voices of twenty-six nurses who were practicing in Vermont.

—We are especially grateful to the authors whose willingness to share their personal experiences is the very heart and soul of *Voices of Vermont Nurses*, and to the nurses who diligently researched and wrote the more didactic historical accounts. These are the voices of Vermont nurses!

ONE

Nursing Education

History of Nursing Education in Vermont

In the early 1940s there were 1,279 registered nurses in the state of Vermont[1] and nursing schools were responding to the war effort by initiating training programs under the U.S. Cadet Nurse Corps, established by the Nurse Training Act of 1943 (called the Bolton Act). Vermont had to meet a quota of 49 nurses before January 1, 1945 and the majority of nurses to be recruited were new and recent graduates.[2] Schools of Nursing based at Mary Fletcher, Bishop DeGoesbriand, Barre City, Fanny Allen, Heaton, St. Albans, and Rutland Hospitals participated in this national initiative.* By 1945, at the end of the war, the Cadet Program was phased out.

Many universities across the country were beginning to offer undergraduate degrees in nursing. By 1943, a new five-year program offering Vermont's first baccalaureate nursing degree was established at The University of Vermont (UVM) under the leadership of Faye Crabbe.†

Practical nursing education in Vermont had been provided by the Thompson School for Practical Nurses in Brattleboro since 1907.‡ The regulation of practical nurses became an item of interest for the Vermont State Nurses' Association (VSNA) in 1944, about the same time that the state's second school of practical nursing, the Putnam Memorial School of Practical Nursing, was being organized in Bennington. Several bills pertaining to practical nurse licensure were introduced in the Legislature in the mid-1940s and failed. The VSNA newsletter, *Vermont Registered Nurse* (*VRN*) reported that "Physicians were frequently opposed because such licensed people would consider themselves too good to do what was needed to be done, laundry, cooking, etc."[3]

Using the argument that licensure of practical nurses would deprive rural areas of Vermont of "domestic nurses," Senator Asa Bloomer, R-Rutland, opposed legislation because he feared "that this motherly lady who is trained in the field of this experience would be eliminated by the

* For more on Vermonters in the U.S. Cadet Nurse Corps, see "Vermont Nurses in the Military" pp. 286–312.

† See "The University of Vermont School of Nursing," pp. 25–37.

‡ See "Practical Nursing Programs," pp. 72–74.

passage of this act and this type of nursing would disappear."[4] It would take until March 1951 to formalize the licensure of practical nurses.

Diploma education was alive and well in the early 1940s, with many small hospitals offering three-year nursing programs. Eleven programs were in operation in 1940 in the following hospitals:[5]

	Opened	*Closed*
Mary Fletcher (Burlington)	1882	1971
Rutland	1896	1950
Heaton (Montpelier)	1896	1962
Brightlook (St. Johnsbury)	1898	1948
Fanny Allen (Winooski)	1899	Merged 1953*
St. Albans	1890	1948
Brattleboro Memorial	1904	1945
Barre City	1907	1956
Gifford (Randolph)	1903	1959
Rockingham (Bellows Falls)	1913	1942
Bishop DeGoesbriand	1907	Merged 1953*

The popularity and the stability of diploma education would be shaken by the 1948 report "Nursing for the Future," written by Dr. Esther Lucille Brown and published by the Russell Sage Foundation. Dr. Brown described a new era for nursing and nursing education. She pointed to the authoritarianism in hospitals, charging that most hospitals operated nursing schools to avail themselves of the services of the students. Brown advocated that schools of nursing be located in universities and colleges, and that diploma schools, smaller schools in particular, be phased out.[6]

It appeared that Vermont was listening. By the end of the decade, seven diploma schools remained of the eleven in existence in 1940. Five more would close in the next decade.

The 1950s and 1960s: Beginning of Associate Degree Education

In 1956, the number of hospital beds was increasing and nursing schools were closing. A nursing shortage was predicted. In response to this diminishing availability of diploma nurses, a dozen organizations met for three days in April 1956 to discuss Vermont's increasing needs for nursing care. This discussion culminated in the formation of the Vermont Conference on Nursing Education. The first reference to associate degree educa-

* Merged into Jeanne Mance School of Nursing in 1953, which closed in 1971.

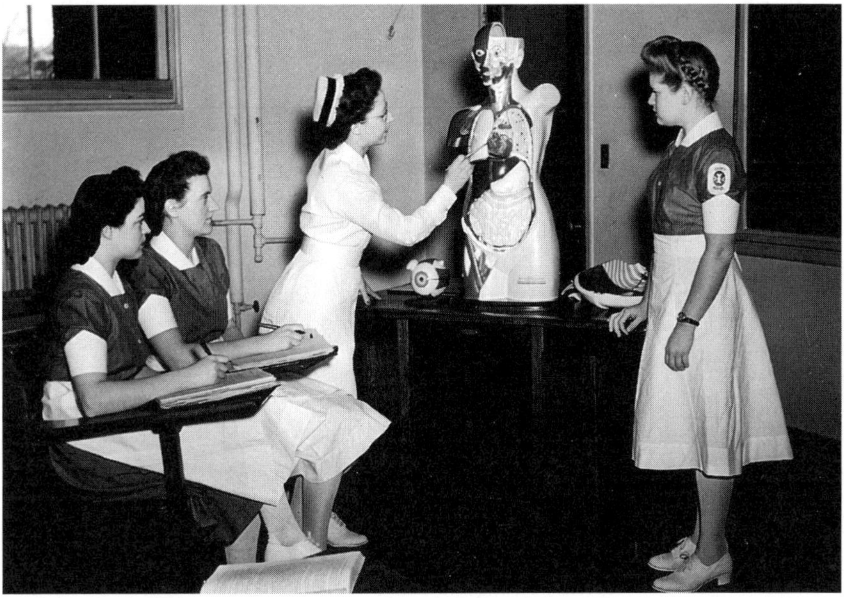

Courtesy Central Vermont Medical Center

Eleanor Dyke, RN, instructing beginning nursing students in human anatomy, Barre City Hospital, 1945. Dyke was also a member of the State Board of Registration of Nurses.

tion occurred at this conference when Dr. Marvin Buechel, consultant to the National League for Nursing (NLN) in the Associate of Arts Research Project at Columbia University, proposed placing education of registered nurses in junior college settings.

The conference participants were intrigued and the suggestion was included in their final report. The following recommendations were also adopted by the conference participants:

1. UVM explore the establishment of a Master's level program on a regional basis
2. UVM explore the establishment of a Baccalaureate program for diploma nurses
3. UVM remove the School of Nursing from the College of Education and create a separate College
4. Investigate the possibility and encourage Vermont Junior College in the establishment of an Associate Degree Program
5. Continue practical nursing programs in Brattleboro and Bennington
6. State appropriations for vocational education be increased and more funds be used for practical nurse education

> 7. Executive committee of the conference initiate a study of the quantity and quality of nursing care
>
> 8. State appropriations for nurse scholarships be increased.[7]

The Vermont Legislature became involved in 1957 when it named an Interim Commission on Nursing. Representing the Vermont Senate and House of Representatives, Vermont State Nurses' Association, Vermont Hospital Association, Vermont League for Nursing, Vermont State Medical Society, and Vermont Practical Nurses Association, members appointed were Dr. Benjamin Clark (chair); Representative Bernice Bromley; Grace Buttoph, RN; M. Ferry Chastney, RN; Gertrude Mallory, RN; Gladys Pike; and Clara Roitero, LPN.

This Commission concluded that there was a shortage of nurses in Vermont, particularly professional nurses in hospitals. In their report, published in 1958, they wrote:

> The professional nurses are not well distributed through out the state. There is a heavy concentration of nurses in the counties of Chittenden and Rutland. By counties, the distribution of active nurses ranges from 2 to 513.
>
> Severe shortages exist in rural areas and in the small hospitals. . . .
>
> . . . Many married nurses are working short shifts or part-time weeks. One hospital told the commission that 23 of 32 professional nurses on general duty were on such a program.[8]

The Commission concluded that the reasons for the nursing shortage were many and varied. Contributing factors included

> 1. The shift to a 40 hour week in most hospitals has resulted in a minimum increase of 20% of the number of nurses needed.
>
> 2. There has been an increase in the number of hospital beds, as hospitals have been enlarged and new hospitals built.
>
> 3. Nurses were doing many things which doctors used to do. Nursing itself has become more skilled than it was in the past, and more of the nurses' time was required for administration of complicated medical procedures and techniques.
>
> 4. The armed forces are employing many nurses who would formerly have been available for work.
>
> 5. Salaries are, in general, not as high as those in other occupations requiring a comparable educational preparation. Policies with regard to salary increases, paid holidays, educational leave, group insurance and other fringe benefits are not consistent between hospitals and in some institutions are unsatisfactory, and in some institutions, ill defined.
>
> 6. The percentage of nurses who are married and therefore likely to retire from nursing for personal reasons has increased from 1 out of 5 in 1930 to 4 out of 5 in 1956.

7. The concentration of most of the schools for professional nurses in Burlington* has accentuated the problem of nurses distribution.[9]

The Commission made thirteen recommendations. Increases in scholarships, loans, appropriations, nursing recruitment, and salaries were suggested as ways to increase the nursing supply. Other proposals included the establishment of refresher programs and increased utilization of practical nurses.

It appears that very few of the more far-reaching recommendations from the Conference on Education, such as master's degree education and a baccalaureate program for diploma nurses, were given much credence or support. The major recommendation which the Commission did wholeheartedly endorse was the creation of an Associate Degree Nursing Program.

> The commission believes that nursing occupies a position comparable to that of teaching in relation to society as a whole. It therefore believes that the burden of the major responsibility for nursing education must increasingly be borne by society as a whole rather than primarily, as at present, by patients in hospitals.
>
> Therefore, the Commission recommends that legislation be introduced in the 1959 General Assembly to establish a two year school of nursing at Vermont College in Montpelier, leading to the associate in arts degree in nursing and that an appropriation of $50,000 per year be made to Vermont College for the operation of the school.[10]

When Senator Bernice Bromley from Windsor County proposed such legislation in 1959, there was opposition from organized groups of nurses in Springfield, Rutland, and Brattleboro. Nurses from the southern part of the state questioned the standards of nursing training that would be offered in a two-year or eighteen-month program. Gifford Memorial Hospital, which had recently discontinued its diploma program, joined the opposition.[11]

Mrs. Robert Chastney, administrator of Heaton Hospital, supported the proposal and responded by saying, "There are no bargain basements in our hospitals—we are dealing with lives—and for hospitals to operate efficiently we must have adequate nurses. We are getting very meager care

---

* By 1959, Vermont's hospital diploma schools had dwindled to Heaton Hospital (Montpelier) School of Nursing (which would close in 1962), Mary Fletcher Hospital School of Nursing, and Jeanne Mance School of Nursing, (which had replaced Fanny Allen and Bishop DeGoesbriand Schools of Nursing). Practical nursing schools in Brattleboro, Bennington, and the recently-opened (1957) Fanny Allen Memorial School in Burlington, combined with the degree program at UVM, all added up to a concentration of nursing education programs (four of seven) in Burlington.

in smaller hospitals. There is a real shortage of nurses in central and northern Vermont."[12]

Dr. Benjamin Clark urged the passage of the bill. He testified that "There were 91 RNs (graduates) in the state in 1957, down from 110 in 1946." He added, "Hospital admissions increased from 36,000 to 46,000 during the same period." Dr. Clark was supported by the Vermont Hospital Association, Vermont State Nurses' Association, and the Vermont League for Nursing.[13]

But opposition persisted against the proposed two-year program in Montpelier. Ruby Carr, who would later become the first Director of the Vermont College Nursing Program, noted in a letter to the editor of a local paper that the NLN had accredited five associate degree programs in the country.

> It would seem that the Associate in Arts Degree in Junior College Programs has indeed passed beyond the experimental phase in nursing education. It would seem that hospitals can no longer meet the costs of qualified faculty in hospital schools of nursing. Economic pressures prevent ill patients from being able to pay the cost of nursing education today.[14]

Carr called the two-year program "not the traditional pattern of the diploma nursing program but a new look at nursing education carefully based on research which has resulted in a change in nursing education with a purposeful design and direction."[15]

Opposition was unrelenting, however, particularly regarding the location of the program. Dr. Richard Dundas, president of Castleton State Teachers College, questioned why one of the teachers colleges was not considered as a possible site. He argued that Castleton could educate a nursing student at half the cost anticipated at Vermont College.

Senator Bromley, beset by the opposing forces, "buried" the bill in the Senate Appropriations Committee. One June 8, 1959, she admonished nurses: "The real distressing aspect to me is that it appears to divide your profession at a time when nurses and the public should be solidly behind a move to improve nursing services."[16]

A compromise solution suggested by Senator Bromley in January 1960: that two schools of nursing be established to solve the critical shortage of nurses, one school in Montpelier and one in Castleton.*

Now the battle focused on accreditation. The Vermont State Board of Nursing's requirement for licensure stipulated that the applicant must be

---

* See "Vermont College/Norwich University Nursing Programs," pp. 54–58; and "Castleton State College Nursing Program," pp. 42–49.

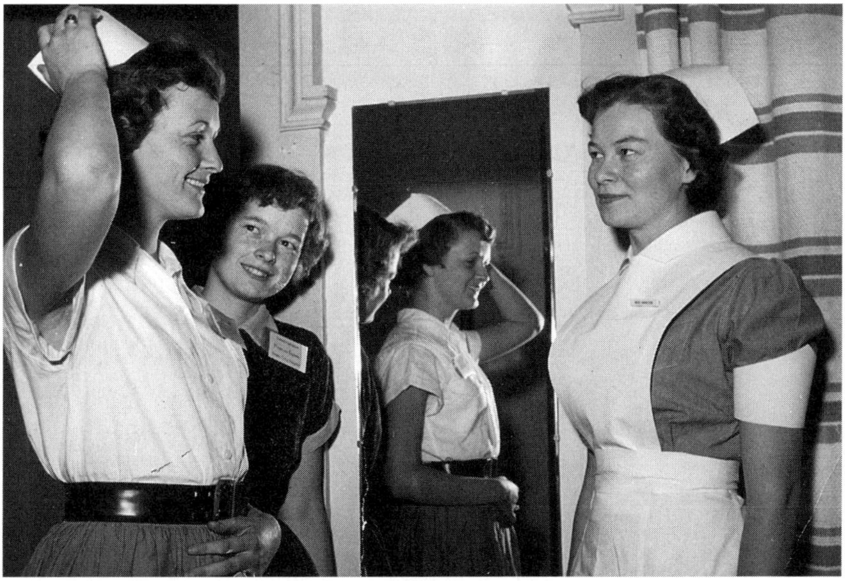

Courtesy Central Vermont Medical Center

Doris Hamilton, right, a first-year nursing student at Barre City Hospital School of Nursing, shares experiences with young women considering admission, 1954.

a graduate of an accredited school. Vermont College was accredited by the New England Association of Colleges and Secondary Schools. Castleton State Teachers College was not accredited.

The Hospital Association supported the Commission's recommendation that the education of nurses should be the state's responsibility, but because the state teacher colleges were not accredited the Association supported the Vermont College site.

By the end of January 1960, the legislative proposal was known as "Bromley's Boondoggle" and reporter Bob Smith wrote in the *Montpelier Graphic* on January 22, 1960, "The nursing school bill has as much chance of passage during the adjourned session as a snowball in Hades."

Laura Dustan, professor of nursing at The University of Vermont, editorialized:

> We must pinpoint the issue on what is best for the citizens of Vermont, not only for those in need of care but for the prospective students who will enroll in such a program. Further, we must devise ways to make employment within our state so satisfying that the nurses we educate will wish to remain here. It will cost a little money but it will be worth it. Smallness of size and exchequer does not excuse smallness of vision and action.[17]

On a 16 to 12 roll call vote, the Senate offered its own solution, passing a bill on January 29, 1960, calling for the creation of a two-year school of nursing at Castleton while amending the title of the measure requiring the school to award an associate of science degree.

On the same day, an editorial in the *Rutland Herald* said,

> The intensity of feeling stirred up by the nurses training bill in the legislature is more than a little difficult to understand. The bill, which was dead, except for the last rites at the end of the last session, was brought to new life in the Senate—because of the sectional factor the amount of interest in it has been multiplied several fold.[18]

Supporters of the measure provided figures to give further evidence of a nursing shortage, and support the need for the creation of new nursing programs. H. Claire Chaffe, Secretary of the Board of Nursing, reported there were 226 students enrolled in 3 professional nursing schools, 76 in 3 schools of practical nursing, and 138 at The University of Vermont on February 1, 1960.[19]

But on February 6, 1960, the *Burlington Free Press* reported that the bill was being talked "into oblivion." Senator Hector Marcoux, of Burlington, diagnosed with a viral infection, left his bed at Heaton Hospital to be on hand for what he thought was a critical vote. Despite his dramatic gesture, the bill was killed on the floor.

In an editorial in the *The Times Argus* on July 15, a summary of the legislation was described as "in again out again actions." The Senate acted first on the measure to underwrite the program at Vermont College. It then amended the bill and switched the location to Castleton, the bill next went to the House, the location switched back to Montpelier and then, primarily due to the pressure exerted by the Rutland delegation, the measure was killed. The *Times Argus* editorial writer declared this issue the most hotly contested issue of the adjourned session.

The seesaw action of the Legislature did not deter Dr. Ralph Noble, president of Vermont College. In what was considered a major educational breakthrough, he announced in July 1960 that Vermont College would initiate an associate degree nursing program independent of the Legislature. With this action, Vermont College became the first educational institution in Vermont to offer a two-year nursing program, and in September 1961 the first students enrolled.*

Following Dr. Noble's announcement, the Legislature geared up to resurrect the proposal to offer a two-year program at Castleton. That col-

---

* How this program alleviated the shortage of nurses in Vermont was questionable: In a survey of Vermont College's first graduating class, only six chose to work in Vermont of the twenty-two that graduated in 1963.

lege was now accredited, and with the initiation of a nursing school in Montpelier, no "sectional" bias was anticipated.

A December editorial in *The Times Argus* supported the second program in Castleton and predicted that there was still a need for nurses. The editorial supported scholarships that could be used for any approved school of nursing.

> Many Vermont girls go into nursing for one or two reasons to which the legislators ought to give serious attention. Either their family does not have the financial means to send them to college for four years or their high school marks are not in the top bracket which earns scholarships for expensive college careers. Those young women can fill a much needed want in the state by taking up nursing rather than teaching or some other profession that requires four years or more of formal college education.[20]

In 1961, the General State Assembly approved the establishment of a nursing program at Castleton State Teachers College, and in January 1962 the trustees of the Vermont State College system agreed that they would offer the nursing program at the newly named Castleton State College. In 1962, nineteen students enrolled in the first associate degree program in the state college system.

With two associate degree programs now firmly established in Vermont, the 1965 American Nurses' Association (ANA) Position Paper on Education for Nursing rocked the nursing community with this statement:

> The education for all those licensed to practice nursing should take place in institutions of higher learning; the minimum preparation for beginning professional nursing practice should be a baccalaureate degree; the minimum preparation for beginning technical nursing should be an associate degree in nursing; and education for assistants in health service occupations should be short, intensive preservice programs in vocational education rather than on-the-job training.[21]

In 1969, The University of Vermont followed the recommendation of the ANA's Position Paper by establishing a Department of Technical Nursing. The two-year program would be headed by Doctor Virginia Allen, a nationally known associate degree educator.

UVM also had moved ahead in the area of continuing education by offering noncredit educational courses to nurses throughout the state. UVM's commitment to lifelong learning for nurses seemed validated by the establishment in 1966 of a fulltime continuing education program for nurses under the direction of Mary Beam. A three-year grant funded by the American Nurses Foundation (1963–66) developed a demonstration project for such a program.

Efforts were also made at UVM to aid the RN in obtaining a BSN degree. RNs in 1968 were admitted directly into the baccalaureate program and offered advanced placement based on the successful completion of challenge examinations in nursing and selected courses and transfer credit.

The 1970s and 1980s: Growth of Career Mobility

The 1970s were a time of educational change and growth. The remainder of the diploma programs closed. Mary Fletcher Hospital School of Nursing, which had offered quality nursing education since 1882, closed its program in 1971. Fifty students were enrolled at Mary Fletcher at the time of the announcement. Miss Grace Buttolph, Director of the program wrote to the school's alumni,

> This decision was made because the University of Vermont will be admitting students to a new Associate Degree Program in Nursing in September 1969. We have been active in promoting the development of this new program as we believe that the preparation of nurse practitioners is a responsibility of institutions of higher learning as soon as adequate resources in these institutions can be developed. The University of Vermont will be offering both a baccalaureate (4 year) and an associate degree program (2 year) in nursing utilizing the clinical facilities of the Medical Center Hospital of Vermont.[22]

Jeanne Mance School of Nursing, which was the name given to the school after the merger of Bishop DeGoesbriand and Fanny Allen Schools of Nursing, also closed its doors in 1971. Administrators of Jeanne Mance were equally supportive of its closing in light of the introduction of a new program at UVM. At the time, both diploma programs were based at The Medical Center Hospital of Vermont.

Thus, in 1971 Vermont had no diploma schools and was educating all nursing students in three associate degree programs and one baccalaureate program.

UVM discontinued its continuing education program in 1972 due to financial difficulties, but embarked on a new venture in 1973 by offering an Adult Nurse Clinician Certificate Program in cooperation with the Burlington Visiting Nurse Association. This endeavor was supported by funding from the Northeastern Regional Medical Program to educate nurses to function in an expanded role in the care of adults in ambulatory care.

A family nurse practitioner program was funded in 1974 through a federal grant which offered twelve month on-the-job continuing education. Upon completion, the nurses were awarded a certificate and were able to function as primary care providers in rural settings. This program was offered at UVM from 1974–77 and 1978–81. Ninety-three nurses completed the program.

UVM reinstituted a continuing education program in 1974 by offering selected programs. A fulltime program was funded by a three-year grant (1978–81) from the Division of Nursing, U.S. Department of Health, Education, and Welfare. After the grant expired, the School of Nursing continued the program until 1987, when it was no longer feasible financially.

Elsewhere in the state, by 1976 Shirley Belock, chair of the Castleton Nursing Program, had developed the first baccalaureate program especially designed for RNs. Although the program was never nationally accredited, it operated for twelve years, and was popular with RNs because it recognized their previous education and was geared to adults. This endeavor would spearhead other programs to offer similar educational opportunities for RNs.

In 1979, Vermont College launched an Upper Division Baccalaureate Program also geared to RNs. Anita Ristau, chair of the Vermont College Nursing Program, justified the need for the program by citing the increasing numbers of RNs interested in extending their education, and the ANA's emphasis on increasing career mobility programs in nursing. Vermont College's program was accredited in 1982.

Entry Into Practice

The ANA 1978 resolutions formalized the 1965 position statements on entry into practice, and this time there seemed to be a momentum for change. The Vermont State Nurses' Association responded to the position statements, establishing a task force "to study and make recommendations as to the qualifications necessary for professional nurses to practice in Vermont."[23]

The goals of the task force were (1) to study the issue of preparation for entry into professional nursing practice as it affects the state of Vermont, and (2) to make recommendations to the VSNA Board of Trustees regarding a position for VSNA on the issue of entry into professional practice. The members of the committee were Doris Adams (chair), Michele Hadeka, Mary Wright, and Virginia Allen.

The task force presented the following position statement to the VSNA Board of Trustees with the intent that it be submitted to the 1978 convention. It recommended:

> 1. that the VSNA develop a plan for establishing the baccalaureate degree in nursing as a requirement for licensure as a registered professional nurse

> 2. that the second category of nurse be identified, titled and established
>
> 3. that this effort provide through grandfather clauses and/or other appropriate means, full protection of all practice privileges, titles and status of all individuals licensed prior to the implementation of this position
>
> 4. that the VSNA support efforts to increase the accessibility of flexible high quality educational programs for Vermont individuals seeking baccalaureate degrees in nursing.[24]

At the 1978 VSNA fall convention, the recommendations were accepted with one change. An amendment was approved which read: "A second category of nurse prepared with an associate degree be established and titled." This amendment reflected strong lobbying from associate degree educators and support for associate degree education in Vermont.[25]

In March 1979, the VSNA established a task force to plan the implementation of the VSNA's resolutions on entry into practice. Barbara Beeker was named chair. A second task force was established at the same time to increase accessibility of educational programs for Vermont nurses seeking baccalaureate degrees in nursing, with Michele Hadeka appointed as chair. Both task forces agreed that their main priority was to educate all nurses in Vermont on issues related to entry, current actions on the national level relevant to entry, and educational programs available to those nurses seeking a BSN.

The entry issues were controversial on both the state and national levels and it seemed that there was a concerted effort to approach the recommended changes slowly. Little action occurred until 1984, when another task force was established by the VSNA to define competencies of graduates of associate and baccalaureate degree programs. Members of the task force were Kathleen Smith (chair), Barbara Beeker, Anita Ristau, Ann E. Logsden, and Sherri Bathgate.

The task force was interrupted in its charge of developing competencies by the ANA mandate for immediate response to titling and licensure.

In April 1985, Kathleen Smith wrote: "Our task force objected strongly to the ANA's subcommittee proposal that an individual who practices professional nursing be called *nurse* and the individual who practices technical nursing be called *practical nurse*."[26] The ANA later rescinded its recommendation due to the outcry of its constituents, and recommended instead that the BSN graduate be called *registered nurse* (RN) and the associate degree nurse be called *registered technical nurse* (RTN).

The recommended titles were never implemented and the titling issue is not resolved to this day on either the state or national level.

The task force did meet its mandate to address competencies and to differentiate associate degree and baccalaureate nursing practice. A list of assumptions noted in the document prepared by the task force and approved by the VSNA read as follows.

> Regarding the graduates of both associate degree and baccalaureate nursing programs:
> – Recognizes own role in the nursing care system and within the institutional health care system.
> – Will function within the legal boundaries and ethical frameworks consistent with the scope of own practice.
> – Is responsible and accountable for defined scope of nursing practice.
> – Assumes responsibility for continued learning as a means of growth and development and maintenance of competence within the scope of own practice.
>
> Regarding the graduate of an associate degree nursing program:
> – Provides nursing care to individual clients with common, well defined health problems who are experiencing acute or chronic illnesses with predictable outcomes.
> – Practices in any structured care setting but primarily within acute and extended care facilities.
>
> Regarding the graduate of a baccalaureate degree nursing program:
> – Provides nursing care to individuals, families, and communities with basic and complex health needs.
> – Practices in diverse settings (structured and unstructured) in a variety of roles which reflect responsibility and autonomy.[27]

The competencies were defined using the nursing process as the organizing framework and were accepted at the 1985 VSNA convention. The two categories of nurses, to this day, pose problems in terms of differentation.

In 1987, the ANA revised its Scope of Practice and identified a single scope of clinical nursing practice. Ruth Blauer, chair of the Castleton Nursing Program, described the ANA's position:

> The revised Scope of Practice for Nursing identifies the core essence of clinical nursing practice as the nursing diagnosis and treatment of human responses to health and illness.
>
> The extent to which the individual nurse engages in the total scope of clinical nursing practice depends on the knowledge base, the role of the nurse, and the nature of the patient population within the practice environment. There is a clear qualitative and quantitative differentiation between the knowledge base for professional and technical nursing practice.[28]

The ANA reiterated its position that education for professional nursing occur at the baccalaureate level, but now added the statement ". . . or graduate degree with a major in nursing level." This change incorporated those nurses bypassing a baccalaureate nursing degree for a generic master's degree. The ANA stood firm on its position that education for technical practice of nursing occurs on an associate degree level.

This Scope of Practice statement represented twenty years of discussion, debate, and dissent on the entry issue. It continues to this day.

More Educational Options

While the entry issue was looming, Vermont schools continued to address the changes in nursing practice. In 1981, UVM's Department of Professional Nursing formalized the alternate track leading to a BSN with a major in nursing for RNs. This program allowed RNs the opportunity to complete all but one semester on a parttime basis.

Elsewhere in the state, Southern Vermont College, a small independent college located in Bennington, established the first associate degree nursing program geared exclusively for LPNs in 1984.* It was offered over three semesters or one calendar year, and credit was given for the LPN's educational experience.

In 1982, Vermont College was awarded a three-year grant to establish a satellite program in rural areas of Vermont. The first two sites were set up in Springfield and St. Johnsbury. This program provided videotaped campus lectures, allowing students to stay in their communities and receive their clinical experiences in the local hospitals and health care agencies. Vermont was indeed responding to the ANA's mandate to provide accessibility for continued education for nurses.

With four associate degree nursing programs now established in the state, the associate degree educators, in 1982, organized the Vermont Council of Associate Degree Programs Inc. Its purpose was primarily to promote general and professional understanding and active participation in the support of sound associate degree programs, and to promote appropriate studies and research in nursing education in AD programs.[29]

By 1987, according to a VSNA survey, 43% of all nurses had attended a diploma program. Other educational preparation was 27% BSN, 25% ADN, and 4% MSN. Of all the nurses surveyed, it was discouraging to learn that 69% had no plans to further their education. Nurses felt that opportunities were available but only "if one is willing to travel a

---

* See "Southern Vermont College Nursing Programs," pp. 51–53.

significant distance." Others voiced concern about expense and limited return for the time and money necessary to complete a program.[30]

A milestone in the history of nursing education in Vermont occurred in 1988 when UVM launched a graduate nursing program in the state after many years of intensive study and earlier proposals. Dr. Rosemary Dale, Dean of the School of Nursing, was instrumental in implementing a master's degree program that had been discussed and studied for many years. The master's program provided a track in adult health, community health, and later a primary care nurse practitioner track. It was accredited by the NLN in 1993.

The Beginning of the 1990s: Change Continues

Growth of nursing programs continued in the early nineties but the emphasis was now on baccalaureate programs. Southern Vermont College launched its baccalaureate program for RNs claiming it was "flexibly designed for the working RN." The program started in the fall of 1989 and was accredited by the NLN in 1996.

Norwich University, which already had an Upper Division Baccalaureate Program, made the decision in 1995 to add a generic BSN program. The reasons given were the NLN's support of baccalaureate degree nursing as the entry level into practice, and the "greater influence of contemporary health care trends that dictate that nurses be in leadership roles as managers of care."[31] The baccalaureate program, located in a military college, also aspired to prepare students for leadership roles in the military as well as "civilian service."

While the baccalaureate programs were growing, associate degree programs were beginning to phase out. In 1994, UVM made the decision to terminate its technical nursing program. Lorraine Clark, chair of the Associate Degree Program, wrote in a letter to the students:

> The direction for undergraduate emphasis should be away from associate degree education. The Associate Degree program should admit its last class in Fall 1994 and graduate its last class in 1996.
>
> . . . The landscape before us seems to be in a state of constant change—the impact of a new economic and health care environment has resulted in strategic planning that will shape nursing education for the next decade.

In the early nineties there was an identified need for primary care providers. Thus the faculty at UVM made a commitment to develop an emphasis on graduate nursing education, particularly the nurse practitioner program.

The shift away from associate degree education was now becoming evident. Norwich University began to consider terminating its associate degree program, and by 1995 the consideration became a solid plan. By 1995, baccalaureate programs, both generic and upper division programs for RNs, were the dominant mode of nursing education.

Summary

A review of history indicates that there has been a dramatic evolution in the public and political perception of nursing in Vermont since the 1940s, when LPNs were described as "domestic nurses" and RNs were described as not bright enough to earn scholarships to expensive four-year colleges.

Today nurses are regarded as professionals, central to health care delivery. There is also a conventionally accepted contemporary notion that nursing education is a vital segment of that health delivery system.

—ANITA F. RISTAU, RN, MS

NOTES

1. "Overview of History of Vermont State Nurses' Association, Part II," *Vermont Registered Nurse* (newsletter of the Vermont State Nurses' Association), 56, no. 3, 17.
2. *Burlington (Vermont) Free Press*, August 1944.
3. "Overview of History."
4. Ibid.
5. Vermont State Nurses' Association, *We Who Serve: A Story of Nursing in Vermont* (Winooski, Vt.: Vermont State Nurses' Association, 1941), 64–65.
6. P. A. Kalisch and B. J. Kalisch, *The Advance of American Nursing* (Boston: Little, Brown and Co., 1986).
7. "Junior College Nurse Program Gets Support," *Barre (Vermont) Times*, 27 April 1956.
8. *Report of the Interim Commission on Nursing in Vermont*, 1 November 1958. Norwich University Archives, Northfield, Vermont.
9. Ibid.
10. Ibid.
11. "Proposed Nursing School Runs into Opposition," *Burlington Free Press*, 17 April 1959.
12. "Nurses Fail to Agree on VC Nurse School," *Evening Argus* (Montpelier, Vermont), 17 April 1959.
13. "Number of Registered Nurses Drops," *Burlington Free Press*, 18 April 1959.
14. Editorial, *Burlington Free Press*, 10 April 1959.
15. Ibid.
16. "Two Year Nursing School at Vt. College Dead Issue for Present, Says Sen. Bromley, " *Burlington Free Press*, 8 June 1959.

17. Laura Dustan, The People's Forum, *Burlington Free Press*, 23 January 1960.
18. Editorial, *Rutland (Vermont) Herald*, 29 January 1960.
19. "Vermont Board May Survey Nurse Education Need," *The Times Argus* (Barre, Vermont), 1 February 1960.
20. "Nursing Scholarships Needed," *The Times Argus*, 23 December 1960.
21. "American Nurses' Assoc. First Position on Education for Nursing," *American Journal of Nursing*, 66 (March 1966): 515–17.
22. Muriel Palmer Campbell, *The Heritage: A History of the Mary Fletcher Hospital School of Nursing, 1882–1971* (Burlington, Vt.: Medical Center Hospital of Vermont, 1971).
23. Doris Adams, "An Update from the VSNA's Task Force on Entry Into Practice," *Vermont Registered Nurse* (April 1978): 3–5.
24. Doris Adams, "Task Force on Entry Into Practice," *Vermont Registered Nurse* (July 1978): 28–29.
25. "Report of Business Meeting," *Vermont Registered Nurse* (November 1978): 8.
26. Kathleen Smith, "Entry Into Practice," *Vermont Registered Nurse* 51, no. 2 (April 1985): 10.
27. "Task Force Entry Into Practice, Competencies of Graduates of Associate Degree or Baccalaureate Degree Programs," *Vermont Registered Nurse* 51, no. 4 (September 1985): 9–12.
28. R. E. Blauer, "Defining the Scope of Practice," *Vermont Registered Nurse* 53, no. 4 (September 1987).
29. "Vermont College of Norwich University Nursing Department News," *Vermont Registered Nurse* (December 1982): 10.
30. "Profile of the Vermont Registered Nurse, 1987," *Vermont Registered Nurse* 53, no. 3 (June–July 1987): 3–4.
31. Norwich University Self Study Report, 1955, available at the Vermont State Board of Nursing, Montpelier, Vermont.

Memories of a Diploma Nurse

A Personal Account

I WAS A STUDENT at Judevine Memorial High School in the early 1940s, actually 1941–44. Our small country high school was decimated by World War II—all the boys eligible for military service volunteered and left long before graduation. Those of us left behind determined that we would enter the effort in some way.

One of my neighbors was an extremely attractive young nurse; she looked like the model on those wartime posters recruiting nurses for the armed forces. While her husband was overseas at war, she lived with her elderly mother-in-law. I, and some of my classmates, were fascinated by her neat white uniform and the attractive navy blue cape with its bright red lining and her name embroidered in gold; but mostly we were impressed by her support of the war effort in her practice at the local hospital (St. Johnsbury, Vermont). Maxine was such a special role model, and I became determined to enter nursing school just as soon as I graduated, particularly since the local hospital was offering membership in the Cadet Nurse Corps. I was so excited; but, not so fast! The first interview with hospital personnel revealed that I was lacking in science courses, I was too young, and I was not eligible for admission to the nursing program. But the hospital was experiencing a severe shortage of nurses; in fact, they admitted three separate classes in 1944, one each in January, June, and October. The nurse director secured permission from the Vermont Board of Registration of Nurses to admit students at less than the required 18 years of age. Our high school principal tutored me throughout the summer of 1944 in biology and general science in exchange for "sitting" his young children.

I made it into Brightlook Hospital's October 1944 nursing class one whole week late—a communication problem with the nurse director! This made me most unpopular with the two primary nursing instructors; this plus the fact that I was "too young"! I soon learned that there would be no Cadet Nurse Corps at Brightlook Hospital School of Nursing; arently the school did not meet qualifying criteria. It was a "rocky" nning and it never really changed.

I suspect we were almost as regimented as our male classmates in military service. We had to stand at attention (no salutes tho'!) whenever a nursing instructor or senior nurse entered or passed through a room where we, the lowly "probie," might be. We were taught (indoctrinated) that we must always stand whenever a physician entered the room or approached the nurses' station desk.

We worked long hours, 7 AM to 7 PM. This included two hours off for personal time that sometimes included classtime; if assigned to night duty, one tended to doze off in the latter. (I lived to regret missing Dr. Crampton's lectures on the eye.) If you were not "on duty" at the hospital, evenings were for study, then early to bed. There was a designated "lights out" time that I seem to have repressed; it was monitored by instructors and favored senior students.

The food was spectacular; we were all certain that the cook, a delightful motherly type, had a not-so-secret goal: add thirty pounds to every new student. I came to look very pudgy in my blue-and-white-checked dress and white apron.

Time away from Brightlook on affiliation in Jersey City was a much anticipated experience. Obstetrical nursing was studied and practiced at the Margaret Hague Maternity Hospital, a facility of outstanding repute at that time. During our time there my roommate and I were privileged to be involved, though not directly, in the nursing care of Frank Sinatra's wife and baby. Upon completion of the three-year program at Brightlook, a number of our graduates accepted positions at "The Hague." Brightlook graduates had an established reputation for excellence in nursing practice, and were sought after by the affiliating schools.

My memories of the pediatric experience at Jersey City Medical Center are somewhat different. I recall my assignment to the Boarders Unit. Poor, sad, disturbed children were placed in this facility by law enforcement and social service agencies following terrible family disruptions; and these children did act out. One day, my last one on that unit, I hung out a five story window for what seemed like hours while two of these kids discussed whether to drop me off or pull me in. It was the Grace of God that saved me, certainly NOT my nursing skills! My classmate, assigned to night duty on the same unit, was literally "flooded out." Some of these children pulled the sinks off the wall and flooded the unit. Unable to get help, the situation was discovered at 7 AM by the unfortunate on-coming staff nurses—as the elevator door opened, they were met by lots of water and a distraught student nurse.

In spite of these harrowing experiences, we did have good learning experiences in pediatrics and obstetrics. I believe each was a six-month assignment, but for some reason, it seemed like a year. Except for those who found other more important interests, we were all glad to return to St. Johnsbury. My close friend and classmate throughout high school and nursing school met and married a wonderful young man from Jersey City; and my roommate was secretly married while we were there. We did enjoy the Jersey and New York City social life!

Throughout the three-year diploma nursing program we worked hard, we became good nurses, and we learned a lot about life. Upon completion of the program I was not yet 21 years old—too young to be licensed even though I had taken and passed state board examinations. We went to Montpelier to take "boards," and the members of the State Board of Registration of Nurses, including a physician, personally administered the examination from the well of the House of Representatives at the State Capitol. The examination took two days to complete and I recall that we wrote answers to essay questions as well as responding to a variety of other types of questions.

That was fifty years ago.

—Pat Allen, RN, MSN
Brightlook Hospital Class of 1947

Life as a Student Nurse, Circa 1948

A Personal Account

FROM THE EARLIEST DAYS of my childhood, I played hospital in our bedrooms at home instead of playing house. I role played being nurse, and the dolls were sick or injured. I do not remember performing surgery on my doll patients, but I do remember asking my father to "fix" the broken dolls (maybe a precursor of a life working with male doctors).

We had to meet certain requirements to get into nursing school. This included two years of one language and three years of another. I chose Latin and French. Latin was very helpful to me as a nurse, i.e., naming diseases, drugs, etc. Chemistry and biology were also required. During my senior year in high school, after meeting all requirements, I applied to nursing school in Vermont. Tuition at that time was $500 for a three-year program, including books and uniforms.

As students we worked or went to classes 6½ days a week and had two weeks off during the summer. Our uniform was a blue-and-white-striped short-sleeved dress with a stiff white collar and cuffs. Over the dress we wore a white bib and apron, and we wore white stockings and shoes. Every morning we had to stand for inspection for length-of-dress (over the knees), shoes (shined), and hairnet at proper length (just below the ears).

Our hospital and nursing school was run by nuns. The Sisters were very strict (always checking up on you) but were basically honest and fair. We never considered it as discipline, merely part of the daily routine. Doctors were deities in 1948. You did what you were told, or else—including standing up when doctors were at the nurses' station or in patients' rooms. They always got on an elevator first!

Our hours on the floor were 7 AM to 7 PM, with three hours off during the work day. In those three hours we had classes in nursing arts, drugs and solutions, anatomy, psychology, and microbiology. Our floor assignments were divided between medical, surgical (post-op), obstetrics and gynecology, operating room, delivery room, or the nursery. Our hospital was small, so our psychiatric and pediatric services were in larger hospitals in Connecticut and New York City.

A TYPICAL DAY. Following "inspection" I would go to my assigned floor/service (usually three-month assignments). On days I was on an obstetrical floor taking care of new mothers, I would check my specific assignment, listen to reports, and review patient charts. At that time mothers stayed in bed for seven to ten days. We were generally assigned four to six mothers to look after. First we would bring them their tray and (after breakfast) water for bathing, which was followed by a back rub and change of linen including draw sheet and rubber pad. We checked bleeding and made sure they had voided and exercised. Exercises started with first day head raises, second day arm raises, etc.

If the assignment involved dispensing medications, it took considerable time, especially since all narcotics were counted before and after each shift. Narcotics like morphine came in tablets that had to be mixed with distilled water over a small alcohol lamp with spoon attached. When mixed, the solution was drawn off into a syringe and given to the patient. (Note: Dosages were checked three times before being administered.)

When the patient was comfortable we cleaned the room, checked water pitchers, and changed flowers before it was time for the babies to come. A different nurse was in the nursery. She brought in the babies while we did our "charting." By then it was time for lunch, then classes from 1:00 to 4:00, then back to the floor for afternoon care: back rubs, supper, bells to answer (bed pans, etc.), before babies were again brought to their mothers, and charts updated once again. By then it was 7 PM and back to the dorm to change out of our uniform, study for an hour or so, and possibly go for a walk before going to bed. "Lights out" was at 9:30 PM.

When assigned to the delivery or operating rooms, we were usually on call day and night. In the delivery room we stayed with our patients during labor, monitoring the time between contractions/labor pain and the babies' heart beat, along with seeing to the general well-being and comfort of the mother (fluids, back rubs, etc).

My rewards were many, for instance: an eight-year-old boy asking me to give him his shots, the smile on a mother's face when viewing and holding her baby for the first time, and coming to realize that small kindness (a glass of water, smile, or encouragement) really helped the process of healing. Truly, at the end of each day, I was thankful for my being a part of the nursing profession.

—MARY QUINN O'BRIEN, RN

The University of Vermont School of Nursing

FACULTY BEGIN the academic year at The University of Vermont (UVM) the week prior to the beginning of classes. It is a good week, with colleagues refreshed from summer activities and ready to greet students. The first faculty meeting of the School of Nursing is held during this week. Currently, the meeting is held in the largest school conference room, on the second floor of the Rowell building. Upon entering this conference room, one notices the portraits of five women lining a wall of the room. These are portraits of the women who have provided leadership to the school through the fifty-seven years of its existence. The stories of these leaders, Faye Crabbe, Norma Woodruff, Jean Milligan, Rosemary Dale, and Marie McGrath, hallmark the history of the UVM School of Nursing. The history of the School of Nursing is an important one because it frames a picture of nursing education from the perspective of the only public university in Vermont.

Establishing the Department of Nursing

The first portrait is that of Faye Crabbe. She had a reputation as a gracious and persuasive person who was well respected by colleagues and administrators. In 1943, Faye Crabbe was appointed chairman of the department of nursing in the College of Arts and Sciences. The department became a part of the College of Education (which later became the College of Education and Nursing) in 1945. Her challenge was to develop baccalaureate nursing education at UVM. She had consultation from the committee that had recommended the program, and the support of Mary Jean Simpson, the dean of women, who was a strong advocate.

Faye Crabbe was equal to the challenge—professionally and personally. She had earned bachelor's and master's degrees at Columbia University and had a sound background in nursing education, having taught at several schools of nursing. She was a determined and dedicated leader of the school for seventeen years, with vision and emphasis on quality. She retired in 1960, at which time a university award was established in her honor.

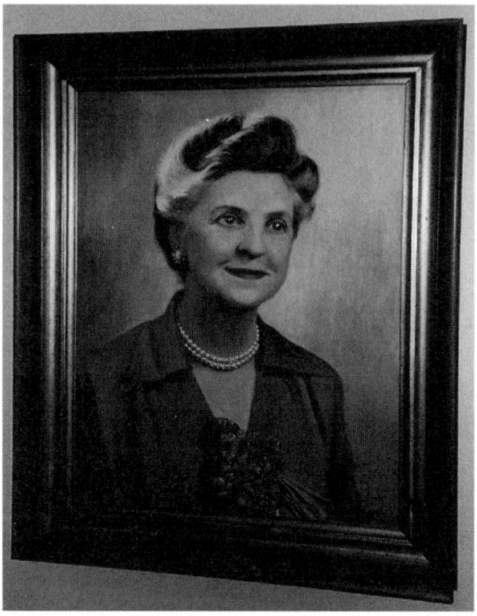

Faye Crabbe, Chairman
UVM Department of Nursing, 1943 to 1960
Portrait in the Rowell building, UVM

Gratitude for her contributions to nursing was also shown by an honorary membership in the Vermont State Nurses' Association. In 1963, the University again recognized her contributions by awarding her an honorary degree.

The initial baccalaureate program was five calendar years in length, with students required to take 120 credits in liberal arts courses in addition to nursing, for which no academic credit was given. In the beginning, students had medical-surgical nursing classes and clinical experiences with students enrolled at the Mary Fletcher Hospital School of Nursing, and other nursing courses in medical centers in New York City, Providence, Philadelphia, and Boston. The first class had five transfer students, with two continuing into the second year and graduating in 1947. The next class also began the program in 1943, with five graduating in 1948.

Many changes were made to strengthen the program of study. The length of the program was adjusted to four-and-a-half calendar years, and then to four calendar years, resulting in two graduating classes in 1957. Gradually, the clinical nursing courses were taught by UVM nursing faculty. By 1965, all nursing courses were taught by university faculty. Required science courses that had been taught by nursing faculty and medical college faculty were transferred to undergraduate science departments. During all these revisions there was continued emphasis on the liberal arts component of the curriculum. The National League for Nursing (NLN) has accredited the program continuously since 1956.

In the early years of the nursing program, Faye Crabbe demonstrated her understanding of the needs of nurses by designing programs to help them improve their practice. Nurses were admitted to an expanded baccalaureate program that provided advanced nursing courses, leading to a bachelor's in nursing education. Several of these students had served in World War II in the military nurse corps, and had support for their continued education through the GI Bill. The first two nurses were awarded degrees in 1946. Through the period 1946 to 1955, fifty-five nurses graduated from this program.

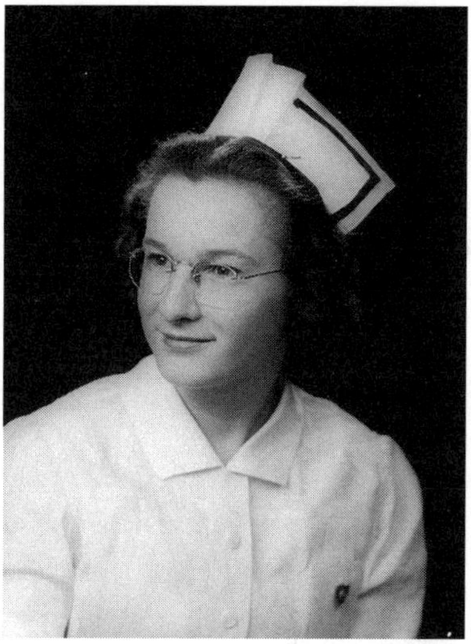

Courtesy The University of Vermont School of Nursing

Barbara Tennien Murphy, one of the first two graduates from The University of Vermont's baccalaureate nursing program, 1947.

I'm a good nurse . . . I got a lot of that from UVM, especially from Faye Crabbe. I took with me the idea of doing the best I could as a nurse and letting that be its own reward, and I've tried to follow that.[1]

Not only did Faye Crabbe and the faculty in the Department of Nursing teach on campus, they also traveled the state teaching nurses in their home settings. Such outreach efforts became the precursor for the later program in continuing education for nurses.

The UVM faculty also taught a pre-clinical program for students in several diploma programs. Lee Oakley, a faculty member appointed in 1947, was instrumental in developing the pre-clinical program. As its director, she served as teacher, advisor, housing coordinator, and administrator until her retirement in 1960. She was a very perceptive person with strong convictions and a progressive view of nursing as a profession.

Mary Patricia Lodge was chairman of the Department of Nursing between 1960 and 1962.*

Moving from a Department to a School of Nursing

Norma Woodruff's tenure at UVM represents another story of visionary leadership. She responded to the need for changes in academic programs precipitated by a knowledge explosion in the health sciences. A native Vermonter, Woodruff was also an alumnus of Columbia University where she earned both her master's and doctoral degrees.† She was appointed as chairman of the Department of Nursing in 1962.

---

* Portrait unavailable.

† It was at this time that the profession had established the doctorate as the terminal degree for administrators of nursing education programs.

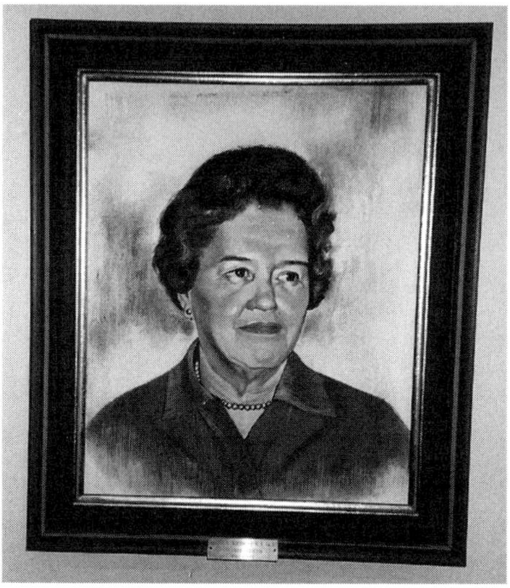

Norma Woodruff, Director
UVM School of Nursing, 1962 to 1974
Portrait in the Rowell building, UVM

Norma Woodruff was the director of the School of Nursing and chairman of the Department of Professional Nursing until January 1974. The landmarks of her leadership were the initiation of a program in continuing education in 1966, the establishment of the School of Nursing with two undergraduate nursing programs in 1968, the growth of the baccalaureate program stimulated by federal capitation funding, and the development of a certificate program for family nurse practitioners.

The continuing education program, initially funded by the American Nurses' Foundation in 1963 as a demonstration project, provided nurses with the opportunity to take brief noncredit courses to keep abreast of the knowledge explosion in the health sciences. At the end of the grant, the School of Nursing funded the program until 1972, when budget constraints necessitated the elimination of a faculty position. Great efforts were made to bring pertinent, high quality educational offerings to nurses throughout the state.

In 1968, the consolidation of new and existing health science programs changed the organizational structure of nursing from that of a department to a school. The new structure, the Division of Health Sciences, was the organizational home for the School of Nursing, the School of Allied Health Sciences, and the College of Medicine. The School of Nursing had two departments, the Department of Professional Nursing and the Department of Technical Nursing. The School was relocated to the newly constructed Rowell Building in 1972. Faculty offices, well-equipped classrooms, and colleagues from the professional programs in the School of Allied Health Sciences and the College of Medicine, gave the School a new sense of identity.

The development of the two-year associate degree nursing program—its first class graduating in 1971—coincided with the closure of Vermont's last hospital schools, Mary Fletcher School of Nursing and the Jeanne Mance School of Nursing. Grace Buttolph, the last director of the Mary Fletcher School of Nursing, recalled the momentous years leading up to the graduation of the hospital school's last class. She called the transition a testimony to the commitment to move nursing education into institutions of higher education without jeopardizing the supply of new graduates to provide Vermonters with quality nursing care.[2]

Virginia Allen was the founding chairman of the Department of Technical Nursing. She came to the University in 1968. While she was a student at Columbia University, Allen was greatly influenced by Dr. Mildred Montag, the developer of associate degree nursing education, from whom she acquired a clear vision about the nature of associate degree nursing education. Dr. Allen provided exemplary leadership to faculty who were themselves learning the distinction between technical nursing and professional nursing. She supported faculty in their development of a number of educational innovations including audiovisual tutorial laboratories, self-paced learning, and planned transitional learning experiences for students moving from student to the graduate nurse role.

Most students applying to the associate degree nursing program were adult men and women seeking career entry while working and supporting themselves and their families. Two-year education was the means to satisfy their desire to enter a health care field where they could make a significant contribution in their communities. Differences in the curriculum between the two- and four-year programs stimulated some lively discussion among faculty in the two departments. The parallel development of associate degree and baccalaureate degree programs, however, gave each program distinct goals and objectives.

The associate degree program was accredited by the NLN in 1973, and retroactively granted accreditation for the first two years of the program. The program continuously held NLN accreditation until the program closed in 1996.

In 1968, an alternative track program for registered nurses seeking the baccalaureate degree in nursing was introduced. Advanced placement was possible through transfer credit and examinations in both general education and nursing courses. At the same time, the first male students were admitted, with the first graduating in 1971.

The Family Nurse Practitioner program (initiated in 1973 as the Adult Nurse Clinician Certificate Program) provided education in primary care. In 1974, the program was continued with funding through a three-year grant from the Division of Nursing, U.S. Department of Health, Education, and Welfare. It was a program particularly needed in this rural state. Eventually, applicants to the program were required to have a baccalaureate degree in nursing, although a few graduates with associate degrees in nursing and a baccalaureate degree in another field were admitted. At the completion of the program, a certificate was awarded and the graduates were eligible to take the national certification exam.

Naming the First Dean of the School of Nursing

Third in the line of portraits in the UVM School of Nursing conference room is that of Jean Milligan. She earned her doctorate at Columbia University, and served as a member of the faculty, chairman of the Department of Nursing (1963–64), then as Associate Director of the School of Nursing. She was appointed Director in November 1974, having served as Interim Director since January. Later, this position was changed to Dean of the School of Nursing. Dr. Milligan's challenges were to lead through several difficult years, while maintaining the high quality of the educational programs and attending to the political viability of the school.

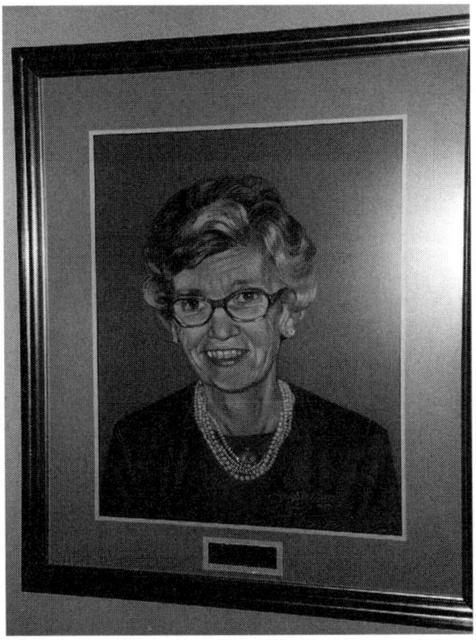

Jean Milligan, Dean
UVM School of Nursing, 1974 to 1987
Portrait in the Rowell building, UVM

The first challenge facing the School of Nursing in 1974 was precipitated by UVM budget problems. The administration recommended to the trustees the elimination of the associate degree nursing program, elimination of the football program, and cuts in faculty positions throughout the university. A campaign was organized to oppose the recommendation to eliminate the associate degree program. Statewide support for the continuation of the program came from nursing organizations, faculty in other schools of nursing, hospital administrators, directors of nursing, and many individuals (students, nurses, graduates, consumers, and professional colleagues). In a major triumph for the school, the trustees did not approve the recommendation to phase out the nursing program.

After a two-and-a-half-year national search, Dr. Barbara Beeker was appointed chairman of the Department of Professional Nursing in 1977. The appointment of a highly qualified, doctorally prepared chairman provided needed stability for the department, which had been served by two interim chairs during the search process. Dr. Beeker was an excellent administrator, teacher, and mentor for faculty, and an active participant in school and university affairs. She resigned in 1987 to serve as a dean for a school of nursing in New Jersey.

Judy Gray was the acting chairperson for the associate degree program while Virginia Allen was on sabbatical leave from 1977 to 1978. Professor Gray served again in 1979 to 1980 when Dr. Allen left UVM to become a dean at another academic institution. In 1980, Lorraine Clarke Welch was appointed chairwoman of the department and served in this position until 1996.

During these years, the associate degree nursing program continued to serve Vermont men and women who were nontraditional students but also emphasized career mobility for licensed practical nurses (LPNs). Career advising was provided to LPNs throughout the state of Vermont. Dr. Welch advised potential students about courses, which could be taken at the state colleges and then transferred to UVM for academic credit. Advanced placement exams translated practical nursing education into college credit. LPN students took a summer nursing course designed specifically to assist them in preparing for entry into the second year of the associate degree program.

Another event to adversely affect schools of nursing was a change in federal funding. Income from capitation grants provided funding for each full-time student enrolled in nursing. Since nursing education has the expense of clinical training, tuition does not provide sufficient revenues to cover such costs. Consequently, the loss of federal capitation monies helped to put nursing programs "in the red" on institution budgets. Funding to support programs became much more competitive, with many schools competing for the same small amount of funding that was available.

In the 1970s and early 1980s, admission to the two programs was very competitive, with many UVM students seeking transfer in addition to external applicants. Waiting lists became common, and in some years admission was denied to qualified applicants. By the mid 1980s, applications (and in turn, enrollments) had declined. Fewer high school graduates, wider career opportunities for women, and rising tuition dropped the number of applicants to nursing programs. Competition for students sent all the school's administrators on recruitment activities, either in conjunction with admission counselors or independently. Marketing to stimulate student interest in nursing on campus or in the community was typically on the calendar of the dean.

A third challenge for Dean Milligan was to help faculty realign the concept of their role in a university setting. In a practice discipline such as nursing, teaching encompasses both classroom and clinical instruction.

Teaching effort therefore takes many hours each week, but the university faculty role has additional requirements—namely scholarship and service. Faculty in nursing were often weighed down by teaching and service responsibilities. Scholarship and, in particular, research needed more faculty attention. Clearly, faculty would need to be doctorally prepared in order to be productive researchers. The shift to the doctorate as the terminal degree for faculty continued through the 1980s.

In addition to facing the many challenges of her administration, Jean Milligan added several new initiatives for the school. She was convinced that there was a need for closer contact with alumni of the school, and assisted in organizing an alumni association after a survey indicated strong interest. The association published a periodic newsletter, held an annual meeting, and established a scholarship. The association continues to be active.

The continuing education program was reinstated in 1974, first offering one to three sessions per year. A three-year grant was secured in 1978 to fully support a full-time continuing education program to meet the needs of nurses throughout the state. After expiration of the grant, the program was maintained for several years by the school. As the number of providers of continuing education increased, it was difficult to fund the program, resulting in its eventual closure in 1987.

A second three-year grant was awarded to continue the Family Nurse Practitioner program (1977–81). In 1981, additional external funding for the program was not sought because faculty believed that nurse practitioners should be prepared at the master's level (this was consistent with a national trend). The Family Nurse Practitioner certificate program provided an important cohort of nurses to serve Vermonters.

A Nursing Honor Society was organized in the school in the early 1980s in preparation for establishing a chapter of Sigma Theta Tau International, the honor society for nursing. The first induction ceremony for the Honor Society was held in December 1984, with the Kappa Tau chapter's installation in May 1988. This achievement was largely due to the efforts and perseverance of Hollace Reed, chairman of the committee and then faculty member in the School of Nursing.

As the challenges were addressed through careful budgeting and enrollment management, Dr. Milligan attempted to bring graduate nursing education to Vermont. Lack of institutional support (primarily due to budgetary constraints) prevented implementation of the proposal for a graduate program.

Jean Milligan's tenure as dean left a legacy for the school marked by a determination to maintain quality in those programs it could support, close programs that did not have sufficient resources, move toward a new era of scholarship, and set the stage for graduate education in nursing.

Bringing Nursing Service and Nursing Education Together

A conundrum for the UVM School of Nursing has been the direction of its alliances. Is nursing's major affiliation with medicine or with academia? The individual leader of the School of Nursing defines these affiliations according to her beliefs and values. These values in turn shape the relationships the school has with medical or other academic units. Clearly, the dean of the Division of Health Sciences and College of Medicine, when selecting an interim dean for the School of Nursing with the retirement of Jean Milligan in 1987, wanted closer affiliations between nursing and medicine. Dr. Rosemary Dale, vice president for Patient Care Services at the Medical Center Hospital of Vermont, was approved by faculty as the interim dean (1987–89) for the School of Nursing, then appointed dean in 1989. She served as dean and as vice president for Patient Care Services from 1989 to 1994. Dean Dale deployed her resources to accomplish some very innovative programs.

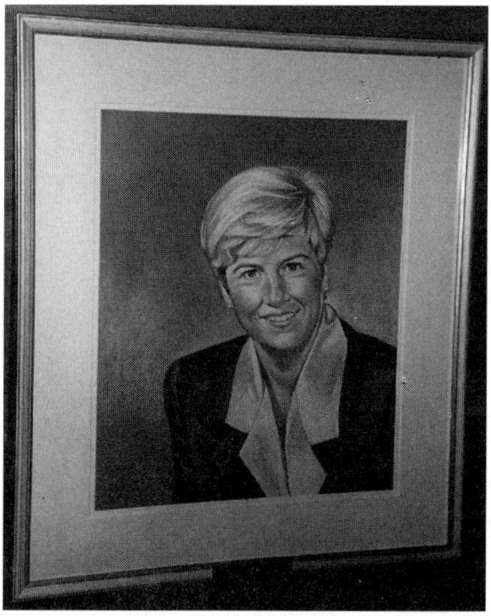

Rosemary Dale, Dean
UVM School of Nursing, 1987 to 1994
Portrait in the Rowell building, UVM

Dr. Dale began her tenure with a resolve to establish a master's program. She had support from the University to go forward and seek external funding. Vermont was the only state without graduate nursing education, so the proposal was enthusiastically received at the federal level. The initial proposal was revised on the advice of the funding source for a single track in adult health nursing. Later, a second track in community health was added. There was also considerable demand for a master's program to prepare nurse practitioners. Dean Dale determined that a post-master's certificate program would be an effective way to prepare a cadre of nurse practitioners to respond to the immediate need. She, then, supported the development of a grant to prepare primary care providers at the master's level. The proposal to add a primary care track to the master's program was funded, in part, because of the support it received from Vermont's congressional delegation.

There were critical nursing shortages during the late 1980s. The dean and Dr. Welch, chair of the associate degree program, devised a way to deliver the associate degree nursing program to licensed practical nurses in the southern part of Vermont. LPN students took science and general education course work at the Community College of Vermont. With support of a grant from the State of Vermont, summer and second-year nursing courses were delivered via Vermont Interactive Television. The faculty-supervised clinical practicum for these students was held at Mary Hitchcock Hospital of Dartmouth Medical Center. The educational partnerships created for the career mobility of LPNs demonstrated a then-unique approach to resource utilization. This educational outreach approach also put the School of Nursing in the forefront of distance education at UVM.

Rosemary Dale met with individuals from the Vermont State Colleges system and began a dialogue which led to the development of a statewide plan for public nursing education. It had already been decided that the practical nurse programs would no longer be under the jurisdiction of the Department of Education; they would be under the authority of the state college system and would evolve into "one plus one" programs. The first year would provide practical nurse preparation; the second year a completion of the associate degree requirements, qualifying these graduates for registered nurse licensure. The focus of education for the UVM School of Nursing would be on baccalaureate education for generic students, baccalaureate education for registered nurses with associate degrees or diplomas in nursing, and graduate nurse education.

Planning for Change

The portrait of Marie McGrath captures her quick smile that presents a playfulness that is refreshing. Dr. McGrath came to The University of Vermont in 1989 as the chair of the Department of Professional Nursing. She had administrative responsibilities for the baccalaureate program as well as the new master's program. She was the consummate educator. Her extensive background in higher education served the School of Nursing well. With the departure of Dean Dale, Marie McGrath was the person with the knowledge and experience to become the interim dean. In the three years (1994–97) of this interim position she firmly believed that one needed to think as a dean, not an interim dean. She negotiated well with the interim provost and moved forward the strategic plan developed by

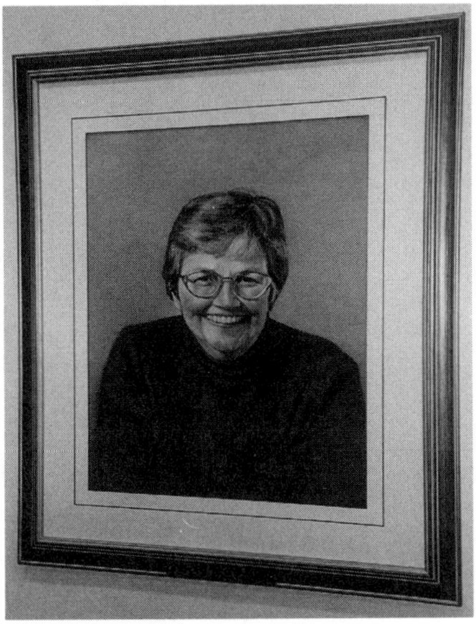

Marie McGrath, Dean
UVM School of Nursing, 1994 to 1997
Portrait in the Rowell building, UVM

faculty. The plan adopted, in part, from recommendations from the faculty of the associate degree nursing program, stipulated the phasing out of the two-year nursing curriculum, the redesign of the educational track for the returning RN student, and revisions to the baccalaureate nursing curriculum. The class of 1996 was the last to graduate nurses with the associate in science degree from The University of Vermont.

The associate degree program faculty at UVM had recommended the phasing out of the program in 1994. The decision was a timely one because of the state-wide plan for nursing education in public institutions. The practical nurse programs were placed at Vermont Technical College. In this way, it was now possible for practical nursing students to earn academic credit for their course of study. An optional second year of study at Vermont Technical College would complete the associate degree requirements. In the state plan, UVM would offer a new option for registered nurses wishing to complete their baccalaureate degree. The UVM faculty developed an accelerated master's degree program, allowing registered nurses to earn a baccalaureate degree. This course of study included two required graduate nursing courses that were accepted for credit in both the baccalaureate and the master's degree programs. If the student chose to pursue the master's degree, admission to the program occurred prior to taking graduate courses.

The revision of the baccalaureate curriculum focused on the changing health care environment, with greater attention to caring for healthy clients in addition to those with acute and chronic health problems. The faculty developed a contemporary program of study that would strengthen the practice of holistic nursing care that could be delivered to clients in any setting. The program was carefully built around the vision that nursing as a part of the health care system makes a unique contribution to the well-being of individuals, families, and communities.

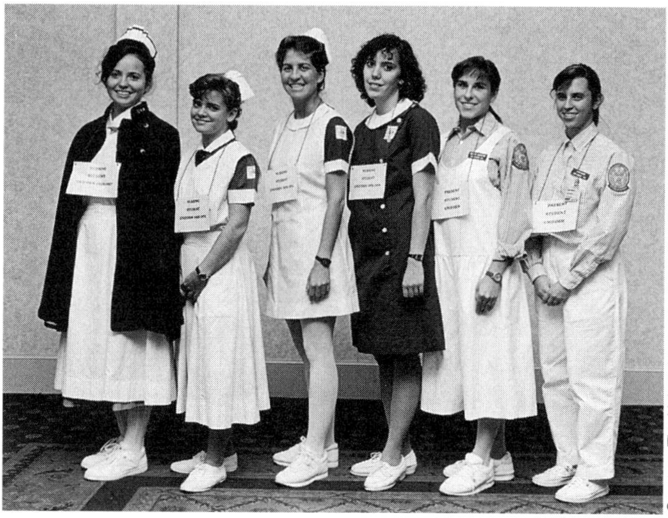

Courtesy The University of Vermont School of Nursing

Nursing students modeling student uniforms from 1943 through 1993, at the fiftieth anniversary celebration, The University of Vermont School of Nursing, 1993.

The Portraits Not Yet Painted

This is a story of several critical events in the history of the UVM School of Nursing. History, however, is happening as the words are written. Dr. Patricia Winstead-Fry is currently serving as the interim dean of the School of Nursing, and has served in that position for the past three years (1997–2000). During this same period of time, Dr. Mary Botter has served as the interim associate dean. The six year period (1994–2000) of interim leadership in the School of Nursing will end on July 1, 2000. Dr. Betty Rambur will begin her position as dean of the School of Nursing and the dean of the School of Allied Health Sciences.

In the past few years, UVM has experienced a tremendous change in leadership with a new president, a new provost, and several new deans in the eight schools and colleges. As the newest appointee, Dr. Rambur will provide leadership at a time of significant university evolution. New leadership brings with it new opportunities. The opportunity to build interdisciplinary health education and the continued development of strong academic programs that address the health care needs of our citizens in this new millennium awaits this new dean.

—Lorraine M. Welch, RN, EdD
with contributions from
Jean Milligan, RN, EdD
Diane Sande, RN, MS

NOTES

1. Scott Sutherland, "Nursing Celebrates 50 Years," *UVM Record*, September 24–October 7, 1993, 8.
2. Muriel Palmer Campbell, *The Heritage: A History of the Mary Fletcher Hospital School of Nursing, 1882–1971* (Burlington, Vt.: Medical Center Hospital of Vermont, 1971).

Memories of a Baccalaureate Student Nurse

A Personal Account

My first memory as a nursing student at The University of Vermont (UVM) is the uniform—a washed blue dress with very starched, detachable, cuffs and collars, black necktie, and a starched long white apron. The cuffs and collars would leave chafe marks on my neck and arms, but I loved to walk down the hall hearing the swish-swish of the apron. I never could understand why we had to wear the black tie, but I told everyone who asked that it was for emergency births in case we had to tie off the umbilical cord! The cap was another mystery. It came to us as a very starched doily and we put it together with paper clips—so many we didn't dare to go by a magnet. It had a green stripe (very different from the conventional black stripe that most schools had) and it had three folded peaks. I told those who weren't Vermonters that it represented the green mountains of Vermont. I guess I had a vivid imagination then.

When I entered nursing in 1955, UVM had a four-year program which included every summer. In our second year we all moved into the Mary Fletcher Nursing Residence. We cared for patients from 8:00 to 10:45 AM and then literally ran clear across campus to the Waterman building for our general psychology course. Professor Chaplin hated the nurses because, as you can imagine, we were always late for class.

In our junior year we affiliated to Cornell Medical Center in New York City for six months for pediatrics and maternity, and then we went to Boston for three months for pysch., and ended up in Rutland Heights, Mass. for six weeks caring for TB patients.

Miss Crabbe vowed to change this practice, for she told us "learning how to pack a suitcase was not one of the school's objectives." But I loved it. For a small-town Proctor girl it was an education in itself—living in the big cities and going to the theaters, the concerts, and the museums.

Returning to UVM for our last year we were told that there were not enough rooms on campus, and because the nurses were proven to be very responsible we were the first females to rent apartments off campus. We also had our community experience in that year and my roommate and I were sent to Bethel, Vermont. We were given our own rental car to make family visits. (The school didn't know that I had just received my driver's license!)

What wonderful memories!

—Anita Fregosi Ristau, RN, MS
UVM Class of 1959

My Life As a Student Nurse

A Personal Account

THE YEAR WAS 1972 when I decided to change my career. I applied for admission to the School of Nursing at The University of Vermont (UVM). After being out of school for three years, I was scared to death, and I asked myself what am I getting myself into. I knew at the time that I was entering a field that was predominantly made up of women. But I was not going to let that stop me from entering a career that I knew would be both rewarding and fulfilling. My goal was to take care of sick people and help them get well—nothing was going to stop me from fulfilling my dream!

My first year at school was OK, as I was mixed in with both female and male students. This first year was a transition period. I was not able to enter the School of Nursing, for the Associates Degree program had been filled. All of the nursing classes began in the fall. I entered the school to get some of my electives out of the way, and actually began my nursing career the next fall.

On my first day of class, we had orientation and at that time I realized that I was one of five male students in a class of approximately sixty. I was apprehensive that I would not be accepted into this health care profession. To my surprise, all the women and the professors welcomed me. From that day forward, the tension was off and I was happy to be part of the group. As time went on, two of the men dropped out, and the class was left with three male students.

I enjoyed my two years as a nursing student. The nursing classes were divided up into five modules. Each module covered the essentials of nursing. Maternity, pediatrics, psychiatric, medical, and surgical care were the areas that we focused on the most, and these studies made us the nurses that we are today. Working in the labs was a lot of fun, but when we went into the hospital we were apprehensive, as we were now going to care for people who were sick and needed our skills to help get them better. Our teachers were wonderful. They were always available to help with our assignments. Before we were allowed to care for the patients, we went over the nursing care plan for the day. This helped us to individually plan each person's care. Also, we students helped each other. We shared our knowledge and were proud to be a part of the health care team.

For me, the two most enjoyable modules were pediatrics and my surgical rotation. Caring for sick children and watching them get well was most gratifying. The surgical rotation was my best rotation. I was fortunate to work in the step down unit, which was a four-bed unit where patients would come after surgery. They would spend four days in this area until they were able to return to the surgical floor. It was here—and the four-week rotation that I did in the summer on orthopedics—where I learned most of my skills. Those eight weeks of training helped me to prepare myself to provide the care that was needed for patients when I entered the job world in a hospital setting.

Being a student wasn't all exciting. During those three years my life changed. I lived off campus for the first year in a one-room apartment. I had cooking privileges but I chose to eat on campus when I could. I had to leave my family, friends, and my girlfriend. My way of life changed dramatically. I worked summers on a golf course and in the winter I worked at a ski area. This was my only source of income for three years. During my second year of school I got married, moved to Duxbury, and commuted to school. Some of the time I was able to carpool and that saved us some money. My wife shared this college life with me, helping type my papers on a SmithCorona. I sure wish that I had a computer back then with a spellchecker! For those three years I was devoted to school. My social life was on hold. My nursing career was to be my future.

When I look back at those years, I would not change a thing. The years that I spent as a student were fun, hard work, and rewarding. Most of my classmates were like me, career and goal oriented with only one thing in mind. We were a team and we knew what we wanted to do with the rest of our lives and that was to be a nurse and give back to life what life had given to us. The most rewarding thing about my career as a student was to see the patients get better. You always knew that you had given good care because patients would thank you for making them comfortable. The praise would come after you gave them that special back rub. In your heart you knew that you were giving good skin care, but to the patient it was compassion that you were giving them, and time they may have needed just to talk to someone.

I was worried that I had made the wrong decision by entering the health field, and especially nursing. Now that I have been practicing nursing for twenty-five years, I am glad that I chose this field. It has been right for me. The reward for providing care to the sick and seeing them get well far exceeds any other job that I could have chosen.

—Bob Green, RN
UVM Class of 1975

Castleton State College Nursing Program

The 1950s would prove to be a turning point in nursing education in Vermont. As the decade evolved, most of Vermont's diploma schools of nursing closed their doors.* Vermont hospitals, on the other hand, were increasing the number of beds. The expansion of hospitals, coupled with the decrease of schools, it was feared, would lead to a critical nursing shortage in Vermont. This potential crisis needed to be addressed.

The Legislature responded in June 1957 by creating an Interim Commission on Nursing to explore ways to combat the nursing shortage. The Commission favored an Associate Degree Nursing Program concept and recommended that legislation be introduced in the 1959 General Assembly, "to establish a two year school of nursing at Vermont College in Montpelier, leading to the associate in arts degree in nursing and that an appropriation of $50,000 per year be made to Vermont College for the operation of the school."† These recommendations were strongly supported by the Vermont League for Nursing and the Vermont State Medical Society.

Dr. Richard Dundas, president of Castleton State Teachers College, questioned why one of the teachers' colleges was not considered as a possible site for the new nursing program. He argued that Castleton could educate a nursing student at half the cost anticipated at Vermont College. He had experience with both hospital and collegiate schools of nursing and was interested in establishing the nursing program at Castleton. The reason the teachers' colleges had not been considered as possible sites for a program was the lack of accreditation. Dr. Dundas' dogged pursuit of the program culminated in the Legislature permitting Castleton to offer a two-year program of liberal arts education, pending approval of the State Board of Education. The program was to be implemented in September of 1960. The liberal arts program would permit the implementation of the nursing program. Both the liberal arts program and the nursing program at Castleton were strongly supported by the Rutland Chamber of Commerce, headed by Elbert G. Moulton, Jr., and Rutland County legis-

---

* See "History of Nursing Education in Vermont," pp. 4–19.

† *Report of the Interim Commission on Nursing in Vermont*, 1 November 1958. Norwich University Archives, Northfield, Vermont.

lators. There was strong feeling in the community that the school of nursing be located in the southern part of the state and not in a private institution in the north, where most of the schools for professional nurses were located. The Rutland Hospital Board and its chief executive officer also supported a Castleton nursing program.

In 1959, Senator Bernice Bromley of Windsor County introduced bill S-56 for the establishment of a School of Nursing at Vermont College. It was tabled until the 1960 Legislature convened. The College Study Committee of the Rutland Chamber of Commerce, chaired by attorney Arthur E. Crowley, Jr., asked Senator Bromley if the bill could be amended to specify Castleton rather than Vermont College as the site of the new nursing program. The amended bill also decreased the amount to be appropriated from $50,000 to $25,000. There was much debate over the bill, and in the end it was defeated. In the interval, Dr. Dundas continued to correspond with various associations such as Vermont Hospital Association and Vermont State Medical Society to promote the idea of the school at Castleton. It wasn't until August 1961 that the General Assembly approved the establishment of the school at Castleton and appropriated $32,000 to defray the cost. In January of 1962, the Board of Trustees of the Vermont State Colleges approved the motion to establish a School of Nursing at Castleton with an appropriation of $32,000.*

In preparation, Dr. Dundas had been corresponding extensively with the Vermont State Board of Nursing, the American Nurses' Association, and the National League for Nursing (NLN). The first class of students was to be admitted in September of 1962. This gave the college only nine months to find faculty and to prepare a curriculum. A master's-prepared nurse with teaching experience, Fay Bennett, was hired as a consultant to help establish entrance requirements and a tentative curriculum plan. Lorraine Fisher was hired to be director of the program.

Castleton State College had received regional accreditation as a college and initial approval from the Vermont State Board of Nursing (July, 1962) and the NLN. Rutland Hospital, which was to be used as the clinical facility, also received approval by NLN. The first class consisted of nineteen students ranging in age from seventeen to forty years. The course included a four-week summer session. The uniform was light blue, and the cap for graduates was designed by student Grace Dennehy. The first years (1962–65) were full of difficulties, due in part to the short amount of time that was given to preparing the program, the community, and the facilities. The Board of Nursing expressed concern with the quality and

---

* At the same meeting, the Board voted to drop the word "Teachers" from state college names.

production of the program. The faculty continued with careful planning for program development. Although hindered by the lack of continuity of faculty and inadequate facilities, the staff accomplished much in a limited period of time. During this time, the nursing offices were on the third floor of the Leavenworth Building and consisted of two large rooms partitioned into small units. There were no telephones or secretarial help. The lecture hall was on the second floor and the student infirmary was used for a college nursing laboratory.

The year 1965 saw major changes in faculty and administration and a major undertaking to redevelop the program. Because of this, the Board of Nursing granted the new faculty one year to make needed changes and adjustments. Reasonable assurance of accreditation by NLN was made in 1966, making Castleton students eligible for student assistance. In 1967, NLN deferred action on initial accreditation and asked for a progress report within the next three years. Although there were a number of commendations made concerning the sound leadership, the interest and enthusiasm of faculty, and the strong administrative support, the lack of master's-prepared faculty and questions about proposed curriculum prompted the board to defer accreditation.

In 1968, the program's chairperson, Marjorie Meyer, cited two seemingly insurmountable problems: the difficulty obtaining and retaining qualified faculty, and the nonacceptance of associate degree education by hospital nurses and administration and by the Castleton faculty. If problems with faculty could not be resolved before the end of the school year, it was recommended that admission of students be stopped and the program at Castleton be phased out.

By the end of the 1968 school year, all nursing faculty had resigned. However, the college chose to continue to support the nursing program, and in August hired Fanny Hager as director. She was faced with the formidable task of finding all new faculty and having a curriculum in place for the entering students and returning sophomores in September. Incredibly, she did it! All faculty were not master's-prepared, but were experienced in nursing education and strongly supported associate degree education. The strongest factor was that they were residents of Rutland County and had potential to provide a stable faculty for the coming years. Shortly afterward, the nursing department moved to Black Science Building, occupying all of the top floor. There were ample faculty offices, telephones, and a secretary, as well as a large lecture hall and an adequately equipped college laboratory. In 1969, the Board of Nursing gave full approval to the Castleton nursing program, citing the improvement in support, plans, facilities, and personnel.

In 1970, Fanny Hager wrote to NLN asking for an extension of time

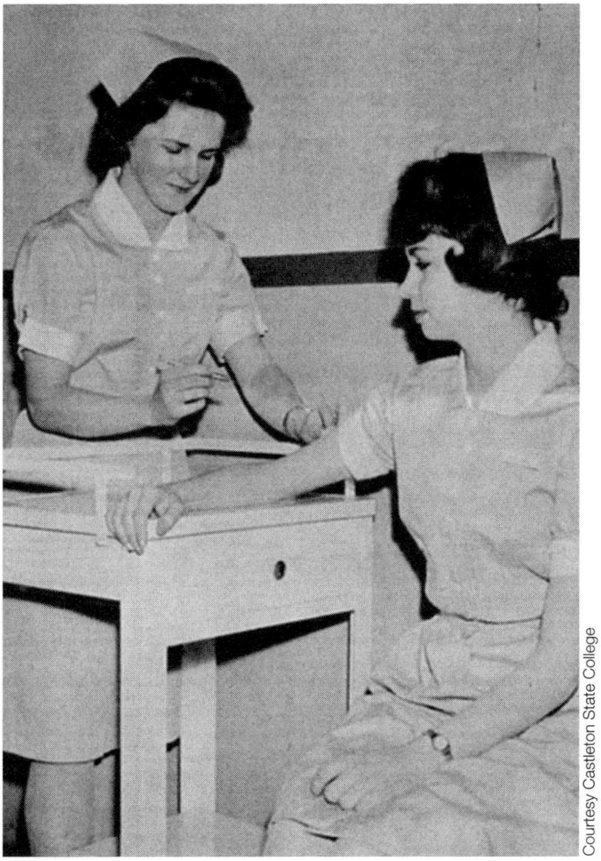

Students practicing nursing skills at the college infirmary, George Adams Ellis Hall, Castleton State College, 1963.

to prepare a report of the school's status. Although there had been revisions of curriculum, improvement in faculty preparation, consultant visits by NLN, and meetings with the associate degree faculty at The University of Vermont (headed by Virginia Allen), Hager felt that the program was not ready for the NLN visit.

In 1971, Chancellor Robert Babcock, faced with a financial crisis, recommended closing the Castleton State College nursing program, citing its high per student cost and student enrollment of only thirty-five. He suggested that all nursing education might be centered at The University of Vermont, with clinical training centers throughout the state. The proposed closure of the nursing program came at a time when there was a national and state-wide shortage of nurses. A whirlwind of opposition resulted—letters were written, petitions presented, and a delegation of local community members, faculty, graduates, and students attended the meetings of the Vermont State Colleges Board of Trustees to protest closure.

The Rutland community felt the program was needed because of recent expansion of Rutland Hospital and additions to several area nursing homes. There was also fear that a large number of nursing students who were commuters would not attend a program away from Castleton. Strong statements of support were made by Representative John Mulligan of Castleton; John Richwagen, Administrator of Rutland Hospital; Richard Young, Executive Director of Vermont Hospital Association; as well as Mary Thompson, President of Vermont State Board of Nursing. Dr. Edward Reiman, a Rutland dentist and avid supporter of the Castleton nursing program, was now on the Board of Trustees of Vermont State Colleges, and argued for continuance.

In February, a resolution asking for continuance of the nursing program was brought to the floor of the House by the Health and Welfare Committee. It won strong support! The *Rutland Herald* headline of February 12, 1971, stated "Castleton Nursing Program Dead!" but the next day read, "Nursing Program Alive." So it went—back and forth until March 1, when the college trustees agreed to continue the nursing program at Castleton.

Ironically, the number of applicants for admission was higher than it had ever been. The college admitted sixty-one freshman nursing students in the fall of 1971.

In spite of all the conflicts and problems, the faculty, working diligently, had made the Castleton nursing program into one that was strong in curriculum and clinical instruction. During the years 1964 to 1971, 90% of Castleton's 105 graduates passed state boards!

Elaine Armstrong became the department chairperson in September, 1972, and preparation began immediately to meet NLN accreditation standards. The department had received two grants from the Department of Health, Education, and Welfare. The first was to be used to identify the needs of the program, to establish priorities, and to effect change. The second was for general support of the program. The grants allowed for extensive curriculum revision, NLN consultant visits, the development of auto-tutorial instruction, increased library holdings, and two additional faculty. A full-time instructor was hired for the college laboratory, and Minerva Potter was hired to help with integration of mental health concepts throughout the curriculum. Clinical experiences outside of the hospital were developed. Students rotated to Brattleboro Retreat, local nursing homes, Brandon Training School, and Vermont Achievement Center.

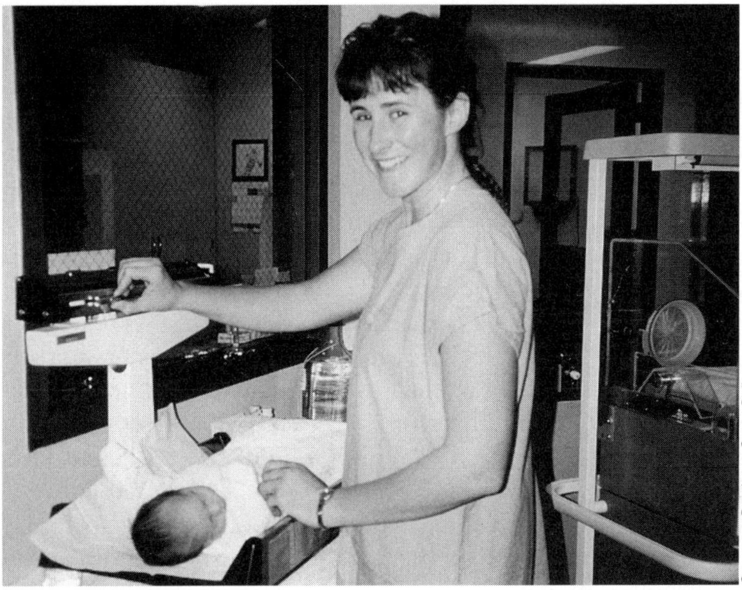

Castleton State College student during maternity rotation

The program grew into a well-respected program (both on and off campus) that attracted many students. NLN accreditation was scheduled for the fall of 1975. However, due to several faculty changes and a fiscal crisis, the program was not accredited until 1977.

Under Shirley Belock's leadership, innovative changes occurred. They included licensed practical nurse (LPN) challenge exams for articulation into the second or third semesters (1974), establishment of a re-entry program (1976), and a baccalaureate two-plus-two program for registered nurses (RNs) (1976).

A baccalaureate nursing program was approved in September 1975 by the Castleton Curriculum Committee with hopes it would begin in January of 1976. It was to be self-supporting from tuition and fees, and the first such program in the state. There was a need within the state for advanced education of RNs, as agencies were encouraging staff to return to school and obtain Bachelors in Science in Nursing degrees. The baccalaureate program was unanimously approved by the Castleton State College board in March 1976. The program was to be two years in length but since the program was designed for working RNs, the courses were not sequential to allow students to begin during any semester. The program was very popular, enrolling large numbers of RNs on campus as well as off campus at outreach programs in North Country Hospital and Veterans

Hospital in White River Junction. Eventually, part-time faculty were replaced by full-time faculty. In 1982–83 the program was completely revised with the assistance of grant funding.

The baccalaureate program continued for twelve years. Student numbers started to decrease as the pool of nurses in the area was depleted. Costs increased and progress toward accreditation was slow. In 1990, the faculty recommended to President Lyle Gray that the program be phased out. He suggested placing the program on hold for two years and then reviewing it. It was reviewed in 1992, and the faculty voted to close the program.

In 1976, the first of the Helene Fuld Health Trust grants was received. It was for the purchase of audiovisual equipment and library books. In addition, videotapes and film strips were received. A later grant allowed the college to purchase a van to transport students to Rutland Hospital (1979).

In September 1979, Dennis Ross was appointed assistant professor. He was one of the first—if not the first—male nurse educator in Vermont schools. This was a time when the number of men entering nursing was rapidly increasing. As the woman-dominated profession began to accept male nurses, the job mobility, and improved salaries and benefits of nursing made it more attractive to men. Over the years, Dr. Ross has served as an excellent role model for male students and has had positive influence in promoting the role of men in nursing.

The associate degree program celebrated the twentieth anniversary of its first graduating class in May, 1984. One of the highlights was the implementation of another Helene Fuld grant for computer-assisted video instruction. This grant was written by Chairperson Louise Esiason in collaboration with Dr. Robert Gershon, media program director.

The nursing program applied for and received NLN re-accreditation in 1985. In 1987, Castleton hosted a state-wide forum on Utilization and Credentialing of Associate Degree Nurses in celebration of the thirtieth anniversary of associate degree nursing education. Keynote speaker was the noted nurse educator, Dr. Mildred Montag, professor emerita at Columbia University.

By the late 1980s, faculty who had worked together since the late 1960s and early 1970s started to retire. Shirley Belock, Louise Esiason, Barbara FitzGerald, Elizabeth Wolcott, and Jean Lertola all left within five years. They had seen many changes in the program, survived a number of crises, and lived through three NLN accreditation visits.

The following years were quiet ones. Now all faculty have Master of Science in Nursing degrees, and one faculty member has a PhD. The Department is housed in a new building that includes a large multi-

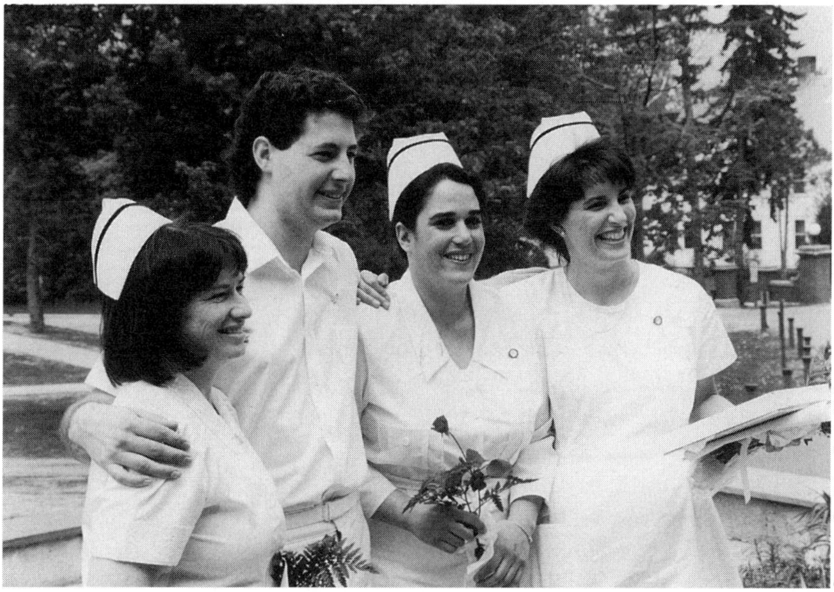

Castleton State College graduates, May 1989

purpose audiovisual room, a computer center, and a large, well-equipped college laboratory. The program continues to be one of quality, with high passage of state boards. The program was reaccredited in 1993. It enjoys excellent support from the administration and continued strong support from the community. The student population is one mainly of nontraditional students who live off campus. A high percentage of graduates remain in Vermont with a concentration in Rutland County. Nursing alumni, now numbering over 900, are in every U.S. state and several foreign countries. Many have advanced degrees and work in diverse fields as midwives, nurse anesthetists, nurse educators, nursing administrators, and health field entrepreneurs.

Much has changed in the thirty-five years since the program was started. A *Rutland Herald* article of July 2, 1962, carried the headline, "Castleton Still Taking Girls in Nursing Course." The article referred to "training" and described the chairperson as "a young, attractive brunette." We have come a long way. . . .

—JEAN F. LERTOLA, RN, BSN, MA

Memories of an Associate Degree Student

A Personal Account

IT SEEMS SO LONG AGO, but memories quickly return whenever I help our own daughters make college decisions. The year was 1967. I knew for sure that I wanted to be a nurse, but I was confused as to the route to take.

Touring hospitals, I observed three-year diploma students in action. Of course I was impressed with their efficiency. But a new kind of nursing program had made the scene and my mother and aunt encouraged me to look into an associate degree program for nursing. They argued that I could attend Castleton's program, live at home and save money, and eventually complete my bachelor's degree. These women were wise, almost prophetic, for their time. As a daughter in a working-class family, it made perfect sense to take advantage of a program so close to home. My father paid only a few hundred dollars for me to attend Castleton. What the lab lacked in luster, the faculty made up for in dedication. Those teachers became my mentors and friends, not only as a student, but as a graduate, and eventually as a new faculty member at Castleton.

We all remember the ugly and uncomfortable student nurse uniforms, the psychiatric nursing experience at institutions, and the crowded hospital wards. Though perhaps not as sophisticated as nursing education today, the nursing programs of old are to be credited with providing a solid foundation from which many of us blossomed in our nursing careers.

—SUSAN FARRELL, RN, MAED, MS

Southern Vermont College Nursing Programs

SOUTHERN VERMONT COLLEGE (SVC) has its roots in Saint Joseph College, a business school established by the Sisters of Saint Joseph in 1926. In 1974, the college, which no longer has a religious affiliation, was moved to its current location on the 371-acre Everett Estate in Bennington and re-named Southern Vermont College.

The only other nursing program in Bennington County is the Putnam Memorial School of Practical Nursing. In the early 1980s, the Putnam Health Corporation, which was the parent organization of both the Practical Nursing School and Southwestern Vermont Medical Center, determined that there was a significant need for registered nurses in the county. With a small seed grant, the Associate Degree Program for LPNs was established at Southern Vermont College as a three-semester, advanced placement program admitting only licensed practical nurses. The Associate Degree Nursing Program was initially accredited by the National League for Nursing (NLN) in the fall of 1990. Shortly thereafter, it was recognized that given the rural nature of the area, the geographic obstacles to travel, and primarily the pressing need for professionally prepared baccalaureate nurses, a BSN program was needed. However, the nearest baccalaureate program in Vermont, one of only two at the time, was a three-hour commute, with the alternative being out-of-state travel to New York or Massachusetts.

Using grant monies from the Putnam Health Corporation, the original BSN program was established as an accelerated program for registered nurses (RNs). Requiring many courses both in nursing management and in general education, the curriculum prepared a generalist practitioner. Lower-level nursing course credits were transferred into the program and the nursing component built student competencies in areas such as health assessment, case management, and moving patients across the continuum of care. The first class of baccalaureate-prepared RNs graduated in 1994.

In 1993, the curricula of both programs were evaluated for relevance in the rapidly changing health care environment, taking into account demands for professional nurses prepared as generalists practicing in non-traditional areas. There followed an extensive period of curricular refinement in both the associate and baccalaureate programs. In the bac-

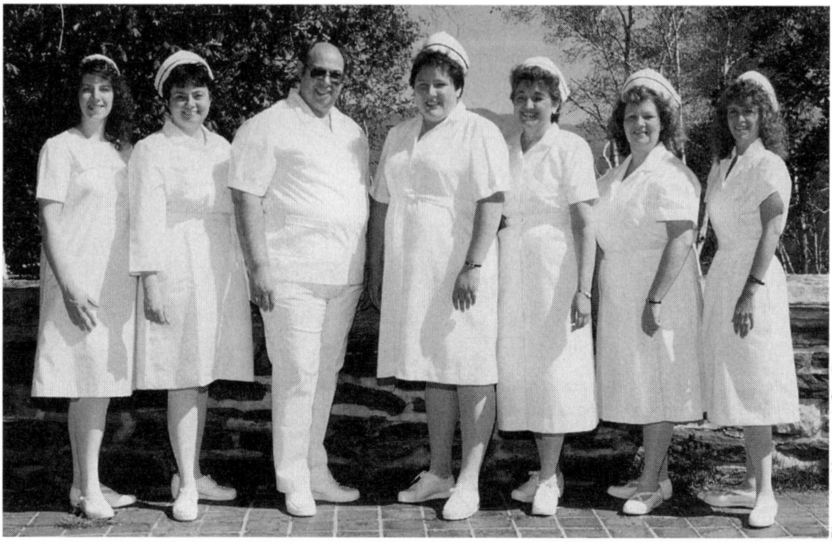

Southern Vermont College Class of 1988.

calaureate program these reviews addressed specifically the characteristics of higher education in nursing identified by NLN, the health care needs of a larger population, and the increased technology of nursing, especially in the nontraditional setting. This review of the RN/BSN program resulted in a strengthening of the philosophy, conceptual framework, and curriculum content in relation to the role of the RN prepared at the baccalaureate level in the present and future health care system.

During the summer of 1995, meetings were held by the director with the administration and the Admissions Office to investigate the need for a "generic" associate degree program for individuals with no prior experience in the health care field. It was determined that such a program was needed, as the college received numerous inquiries, only to respond that SVC had programs only for those already licensed as LPNs. A curriculum was developed, approved as a "two-plus-two" model requiring National Council Licensure Examination (NCLEX) after the first two years, and was implemented for the first time in the fall of 1996. Program enrollments continue to be kept very low, in keeping with the college mission and program philosophy of individual attention and availability of faculty. Current enrollment in the first semester of the new ADN program is limited to only twenty students, with twenty-seven LPNs joining them in the spring and graduating a year later. Current enrollment in the upper division baccalaureate nursing classes is thirteen.

Southern Vermont College meets the educational needs of individuals with licensure as RNs and LPNs, as well as those with no prior health care experience. The effect is a program design that reflects a career ladder from generic associate degree to baccalaureate degree. Receiving praise and encouragement from the Vermont State Board of Nursing and the National League for Nursing for a model curriculum and conceptual framework, the director, faculty, and college administration work together to maintain quality programs.

—Wendy L. LaFage, RN, MS, MA

Vermont College/Norwich University Nursing Programs

VERMONT COLLEGE (VC), a private junior college for women in Montpelier, Vermont, initiated a two-year nursing program in September 1961. It was the first such program in the state, and VC became the only private school in New England offering two-year nursing education.

President Dr. Ralph Noble stressed that the College was inaugurating nursing education as a public service in response to the documented need for more nurses in Vermont. He acknowledged Eleanor Diack, Director of Nurses at Barre City Hospital, and M. Ferry Chastney, Administrator of Heaton Hospital in Montpelier, for their invaluable support of the program.

In January 1961, Ruby Carr was hired to head the program. She wrote, "It was a real challenge to find faculty to assist in developing the program. However, we finally found two willing nurses who found the associate degree concept a challenging adventure: Marion Gorham, RN MSN, and Anita (Fregosi) Ristau, RN, BSN."[1]

These instructors and Mrs. Carr were responsible for developing the philosophy, objectives, and curriculum, and for teaching the first-semester Fundamentals of Nursing and Maternal Child Health courses. In the second year, Doris Macdonald and Erna Goodrich were hired to develop and teach courses in physical illness. Psychiatric Nursing was offered in a short summer program by Alice Robinson until Louise Davis assumed that responsibility in 1963. In the early years students received their clinical experience at Heaton Hospital (Montpelier), Barre City Hospital, and the Vermont State Hospital (Waterbury).

Twenty-nine students were admitted to the first class. They wore distinctive navy blue uniforms designed by Carr, and a cap emblazoned with a blue stripe designed by the college's art department. Twenty-two would graduate.

Mrs. Carr wrote: "The headquarters for the nursing program began with its offices and laboratory in the basement of Heaton Hospital Nursing Residence. It also served as a dormitory for the nursing students. It was not too convenient since the students were compelled to walk from

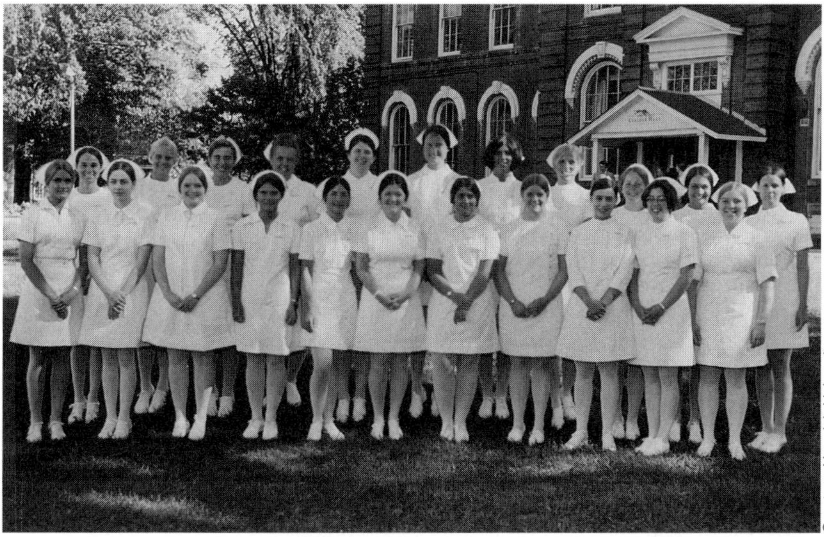

Courtesy Norwich University

Vermont College, Class of 1971

Heaton Hospital to the VC campus for their liberal arts classes. However, by 1962 Stone Science Hall was built and ready and the nursing department became truly a part of the VC family by setting up headquarters there in September 1962."

The program was approved by the Vermont State Board of Nursing in 1963. It went on to receive National League for Nursing (NLN) accreditation in 1964—one of less than ten two-year programs in the country to obtain this distinction at that time.

Dr. Mildred Montag, founder of associate degree nursing education, visited the program in 1962. She was so impressed with the curriculum that she urged Gorham and Fregosi (Ristau) to write an article for publication on the unique way maternal child health (MCH) was taught. In July 1964, *Nursing Outlook* published the article, "Our MCH Course Begins with Adolescence."

Ruby Carr resigned from her position in 1963. Marion Gorham succeeded her and served as chair until 1967. Carr returned to her former position, directing the program until her tragic death in 1973 from an automobile accident.

In 1972, Vermont College underwent a major change when it merged with Norwich University. The intent was to continue to offer a residential civilian campus in Montpelier called the Vermont College Division of Norwich University.

The nursing program continued to grow and attract a diverse group of individuals. Louise Davis, who succeeded Carr as chair, wrote in her report for the academic year 1971–72: "The first two men were admitted to the program, along with a married couple, a nun with a master's degree and 20 years of teaching experience, several students with bachelor's degrees, a licensed beautician, and three transfer students, two from diploma schools and one from a BSN program."[2]

In 1977, the nursing program received a three-year Health, Education, and Welfare (HEW) grant. This grant application was spearheaded by faculty member Sister Saint Thomas to establish a Learning Resource Center for the nursing students. The basement of Stone Science Hall was renovated for a media and video room and clinical simulation laboratory. Selected modules were developed for individualized learning which supplanted the traditional lecture format. That year saw freshman enrollment reach seventy-two students, a peak that was never exceeded.

In 1978, Norwich University responded to the aspirations of nurses wishing to further their education when it established the first upper division baccalaureate program in Vermont specifically geared toward RN students. Ristau, now chair of the associate degree program, introduced the new offering as a two-plus-two concept designed to mutually reinforce and build upon the associate degree program. Jane Hayward was hired to implement and design the program.

Suzanne Kusserow was hired in 1979, followed by Linda Ellis and Barbara Boise in 1980, to serve as the first baccalaureate faculty. The program was accredited by the NLN in 1981.

The college continued to be innovative and committed to meeting the varying needs of students, particularly adult learners. Through federal grant funding, the first satellite programs were established in 1982 in St. Johnsbury and Springfield. Videotapes of campus lectures were provided to the sites, and clinical instructors from the area offered clinical instruction at the local hospitals. The upper division program was presented by faculty traveling to the sites. St. Johnsbury and White River Junction were the first BSN sites selected, but through the years the faculty would travel for late afternoon and weekend classes to Brattleboro and Burlington, as well. This effort reenforced the faculty's commitment to adult learning needs.

A summer associate degree nursing (ADN) program was established in 1983 primarily for licensed practical nurse (LPN) students. It allowed LPNs to complete the AD curriculum in one calendar year by challenging the first semester and taking the second semester in the summer.

In 1983, the organizational structure was again revised. Nursing became one of eight divisions at Norwich University. Ristau was appointed head of the Division of Nursing and Ellis chair of the BSN program.

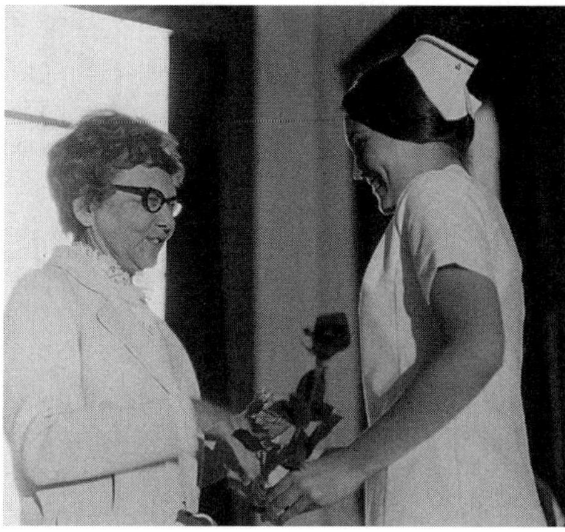

Courtesy Norwich University

Ruby Carr, first chairman of the Vermont College Associate Degree Program, at pinning ceremony, 1973.

When enrollments started to plummet in the mid-eighties, the Division began once more to experiment and diversify its academic options. An on-campus weekend ADN program was first presented in 1987. Students were able to obtain an associate degree in nursing in three years by attending classes every other weekend, allowing them to work while attending school.

The weekend baccalaureate program began one year later in 1988 and was located in Putney. This was also created as a three-year sequence with faculty traveling to the site to teach the courses.

The most innovative program, however, was the contract initiated by Joe Caldwell, Chief Nurse at the Veteran's Administration Hospital (VA) and the Nursing Division and negotiated with the VA hospital in White River Junction in 1988. This initiative was the first in the nation to provide an entire nursing degree program on-site at a health care facility. The VA contracted for a specific sum directly to Norwich University. Under this contract, the hospital staff was able to matriculate into the program free of charge, and in five years obtain an associate or baccalaureate degree, depending on the student's prior academic status. The *New York Times*, all the local papers and Vermont television, as well as *RN Magazine* and *Nursing '88* ran stories touting this unique way to stave off the nursing shortage and increase enrollments.

The VA contract was later expanded to include staff members at Dartmouth Hitchcock Medical Center in Hanover, New Hampshire. In 1990, Rutland Hospital contracted with Norwich University to offer the Upper Division Program at their site.

In 1993, after thirty years in Montpelier, all traditional programs moved to Norwich's military campus in Northfield. Ristau resigned from her administrative position at that time, and was succeeded by Ellis. In 1995, Norwich instituted a generic baccalaureate program, largely in response to the students enrolled in the corps of cadets.

Carr quoted an unknown source in the preface of her ten-year history of VC: "A program to survive must be sufficiently stable to sustain the ideal which gave it birth, and sufficiently responsive to remain relevant to the society which supports it."

Norwich has met this challenge and is proud of its rich history in providing innovative nursing education to both traditional and adult learners since 1961.

—Anita F. Ristau, RN, MS

NOTES

1. Ruby Carr, "Ten Years of Transition," unpublished manuscript on the history of Vermont College at the Norwich University Archives, Northfield, Vermont. Subsequent quotes from Carr are also from this work.
2. Louise Davis, Vermont College Nursing Faculty Minutes, June 1972. Norwich University Archives.

Continuing Education for Nurses at The University of Vermont

REFLECTING the land grant philosophy of The University of Vermont (UVM), one of the missions of the School of Nursing, since its beginning in September 1943, has been to provide lifelong learning for nurses in the State of Vermont. During the first seventeen years of the program, the majority of the offerings were formal classes for diploma graduates who practiced in community hospitals. In addition to conducting the basic nursing program and the program for graduate nurses, Faye Crabbe, first director of the baccalaureate program, traveled throughout the state to conduct continuing education offerings on ward management, trends and developments in nursing, and pharmacological aspects of care. The Department of Nursing cooperated with professional nursing organizations (Vermont State Nurses' Association, Vermont League of Nursing) and various voluntary health agencies (such as Vermont Heart Association, Vermont Diabetes Association) to offer continuing education programs. From 1943 to the 1960s, continuing education offerings were provided by the School of Nursing only sporadically.

The 1960s: Development of a Formal Continuing Education Program

During the 1960s, nurses in general were not receptive to the nurse whose basic preparation was at the associate or baccalaureate level. Nurses were less supportive of continuing education offered by nurses than by physicians. In the local communities of Vermont, as well as on the state level, there was competition between and within professional groups, between and within state service and educational agencies, between regions of the state, between voluntary and official health agencies, between Burlington and the rest of the state, between neighboring towns, and between certain groups within some towns.[1]

In the early 1960s, the Board of Directors of the American Nurses' Association approved the first statement that defined continuing education for nurses. It set forth that *continuing education* 1) can assist the individual to develop one's potential either personally or professionally, 2) can minimize the gap between knowledge and practice, and 3) can provide a forum by which one's ideas and practices can stay current, with the ultimate goal to elevate the standards of patient/client care. The introduction of the statement included the following, "No nurse today, regardless of the type of program in which she was prepared, can continue to provide skilled care if her education stops with the conclusion of the basic program."[2]

In the 1960s and again in the late 1970s, nurses and employers of nurses, through surveys, requested that the School of Nursing establish a coordinated plan for providing continuing education for nurses. They asked that the program serve nurses with different levels of education; serve nurses with roles in different types of nursing (education, administration, research, or service); serve nurses requiring different levels of expertise in different types of clinical practice; and offer programs to enhance knowledge and skills, as well as attitudes. Surveys indicated that the provision of continuing education for nurses should be the responsibility of a higher education institution.

From 1962 through 1964, Winifred Griffin, Associate Director, Regional Nursing Programs of the New England Board of Higher Education, and nurse consultant to the New England Council on Higher Education for Nursing, in conjunction with the School of Nursing at UVM, held work conferences for nurse managers at hospitals, city, and state health departments and visiting nurse associations; for persons interested in establishing associate degree programs for nursing within schools in the New England states; for nurse educators interested in teaching in associate degree programs; and for faculty conferences dealing with curriculum issues. At the same time, Norma Woodruff, chairman of the UVM nursing program, held lengthy discussions with the Extension Service about a possible joint endeavor in offering continuing education for nurses. This joint endeavor did not materialize at that time.

In 1962 and 1967–68, the New England Board of Higher Education held short-term regional nursing programs in conjunction with UVM, entitled "Training in Leadership." The program's goal was to assist supervisors or head nurses in hospitals to prepare nurses in assuming a management and teaching role with ancillary staff members (orderlies, practical nurses, nursing aides) on their nursing units. In addition, this project assisted nurses in teaching beginning nurses and inactive nurses who were returning to an active role in the profession. Aline Demers, a faculty member of the School of Nursing, was the conference director of the program in 1967–68.

During 1963–66, a demonstration project in the provision of continuing education for nurses in a rural state was based in Vermont through the auspices of the School of Nursing. The project was funded and managed by The American Nurses Foundation. It was titled "Development of a Continuing Education Program for Nurse Practitioners* in Upper New England on the Utilization of Research Findings in the Improvement of Patient Care." Lois C. Meier directed the project (1963–64) and was succeeded by Mary E. Beam (1964–66). Two hundred and thirty-nine participating nurses were assisted in utilizing research findings within nursing practice. The project involved three areas of the state: Barre-Montpelier, Rutland-Castleton, and Southeastern Vermont (from South Windsor to the Massachusetts border). The project was a community-centered continuing education program,† that focused on problems of direct patient care. The continuing education offerings had been identified by the local nurses and were delivered in various regions of the state. Preceptor assistance within the nurses' specific practices was made available in order to assist the nurse in utilizing the additional knowledge when administering patient care. Some of the programs for nurses were coordinated with those provided physicians in local or regional areas, so that the local nurses could discuss newer trends in the nursing care of patients with specific problems at the same time physicians were studying the newer trends concerning medical care of the specific problems. Seminars conducted included "Pain and Its Alleviation," "Care of an Individual with a Cerebral Vascular Accident," and "Rehabilitation Nursing." A few of the nursing faculty involved in the project were Mary Thompson, Lee Oakley, Rose Forgione, Mary Ellen Palmer, Sister Evaline Barrett, and Aline Demers.

From 1966 to 1972, with the support of faculties of the School of Nursing and Northern New England Regional Medical Program, a full-time Continuing Education Program for Nurses was offered under the direction of Mary Beam; a position assumed later by Ruth Adams and Judith G. Whittaker who previously had been Executive Director of the American Nurses' Association. Libraries with audiovisual capabilities (tape cassettes, film loops, slides, and movies) were established in local hospitals (e.g., St. Johnsbury and St. Albans). In 1969, two-way radio conferences for nurses in conjunction with Albany Regional Program were offered on nursing care in emergency situations, and reached forty-two hospitals in New York State and Vermont. In 1970, Dartmouth Medical School and the University Hospital in Hanover, New Hampshire, and The University of Vermont College of Medicine in Burlington became centers for a closed circuit television network called The New Hampshire-Vermont Medical Interactive Communication Network.

---

* The definition of "practitioners" at that time: all nurses who were registered nurses.

† The definition of "community-centered program": a program developed in a geographically circumscribed community center, easily accessible to all participants, that provides for the educational needs of nurses regardless of the setting in which they practice.

Links with approximately thirty small community hospitals, a vocational training school, and a state prison were established, as well as links between distant coronary care units, radiology departments, psychiatry, medical offices, and classrooms. During the 1970s and early 1980s, the School of Nursing used this network extensively for continuing education offerings.

The first year of the full-time Continuing Education Program (1966–67) focused primarily on nursing care problems related to the chronically ill and was financially supported by the Division of Chronic Disease Control of the Vermont Department of Health. Workshops for newly employed school nurses, and school nurses in general, were offered in conjunction with the State Health Department Division of Public Health Nursing. Between 1966 and 1972, various continuing education offerings were co-sponsored with Health Associations (Vermont Tuberculosis and Health Association, Vermont Division of the American Cancer Society, Vermont School Nurses' Association, Vermont Inservice Directors Organization, and Nursing Home Association), and Health Agencies (Albany Regional Medical Program and Vermont Assembly of Home Health Agencies). The American College of Obstetrics and Gynecology and the School of Nursing provided sessions in both New Hampshire and Vermont which focused on issues in obstetrics and gynecology. The Vermont Heart Association held one-day programs for three years (1964–66) for nurses in conjunction with the Vermont State Nurses' Association and the School of Nursing. These sessions were again offered in the 1970s. In 1972, the School of Nursing had to discontinue the program due to budget constraints.

With the development of specialization in nursing practice and the need for highly specialized nursing knowledge in various clinical areas (intensive care, coronary care, oncology), there was a clear need for continuing education for nurses. There was need for self-development, but the nurses also needed the support of others to obtain the knowledge that was required. There was under-utilization of nurses' skills due to lack of educational opportunities. Inservice education was nonexistent in some institutions and inconsistent in others. Thus many nurses with less than master's preparation improved their competencies for work in a specialty area through various programs financially supported by the Northeastern Regional Medical Program. An example of this was a four-week course that the Regional Medical Program conducted at UVM for nurses who worked as coronary care nurses in Vermont and New Hampshire intensive coronary care units. Sister Evaline Barrett stated that ". . . emphasis was placed on the nurse's role in intensive surveillance assisted with electronic monitoring, and on the application of immediate corrective and resuscitative measures."[3]

The 1970s: Preparing Nurses for the Expanded Role

In 1974, financial support was received by the School of Nursing from the New England Council on Higher Education for Nursing to establish a State Coordinated Plan for Continuing Education for Nurses. The project (1974–79) involved nurses, employers, representatives of health agencies, in-service directors, schools of nursing, and the Vermont Assembly of Home Health Agencies to plan, propose, and implement action related to continuing education of nurses throughout the state. Janet P. Brown, representing the School of Nursing, provided co-leadership in this endeavor with Kathryn Lambert, Medical Center Hospital of Vermont; Elizabeth Davis, Visiting Nurse Association of Burlington; Lois Smith, In-Service Director; and Marion McKeon, Vermont Heart Association. The coordinating committee was enlarged to represent special nursing organizations (e.g., American Association of Critical Care Nurses, Emergency Department Nurses Association), Vermont College of Norwich University, Vermont State Nurses' Association, and the Public Health Nursing Division of the Vermont Health Department. The principal focus for the project was communication networking in regards to the availability of continuing education offerings for nurses. A telephone clearinghouse was established through the auspices of the Vermont Heart Association where dates and topics could be cleared while in the early planning stage. A calendar of offerings, listing location, date, time, cost, and sponsorship was made available on a six-month basis. The listing was distributed through newsletters, radio spots, telephone talk shows, and mailings. Some members of the committee collaborated in the delivery of continuing education as well as developing various consortium arrangements. The committee defined the gaps of knowledge, attitudes, and psychomotor skills that needed to be addressed in order to allow the individual nurse to grow professionally, and attempted to utilize various instructional modalities for the delivery of continuing education. The committee developed and disseminated "Guidelines for Financing Continuing Education from an Employee/Employer Prospective." Again, as in the 1960s, discussions were entered into by the School of Nursing and the Extension Service to share resources and jointly service the continuing education needs of nurses. A few programs in the St. Johnsbury area as well as in the southwestern area of Vermont were developed and offered to the nurses of those regions.

In 1973, the Visiting Nurse Association of Burlington identified a need for a nurse practitioner program, and received funding from the Northeastern Regional Medical Program to offer such a program in cooperation with The University of Vermont School of Nursing and College of Medicine. Janet P. Brown, who had been teaching at Boston College, was appointed to the nursing faculty and co-directed this program with George W. Welsh, MD, director of continuing medical education at UVM. In the fall of 1973, the Adult Nurse Clinician Certificate Program was offered to twelve graduate nurses with baccalaureate or master's degrees, who worked with a physician who was willing to serve as a preceptor for one year. This program prepared nurses to function in an expanded role for the care of adults in an ambulatory care setting. In that year monies were obtained through the Professional Nurse Traineeship Program to offer conferences and short courses for practicing nurses.

In 1974, the School of Nursing received a Federal Contract Grant from the Division of Nursing, Bureau of Health Manpower, Department of Health, Education, and Welfare to support a twelve-month on-the-job continuing education family nurse practitioner program that awarded a certificate of completion. This program was offered in cooperation with the College of Medicine and the Medical Center Hospital of Vermont from 1974–77 and 1978–81. The objectives of this program were to:

> Provide a continuing education program for registered nurses who are interested in becoming primary care providers working in collaboration with other members of the ambulatory health team and who are committed to the generalist approach.
>
> Promote the development of health care delivery systems which can be objectively audited.
>
> Assess the impact of extending the role of the nurse, as a primary care provider on improving the quality and quantity of health care afforded to the public, particularly in rural settings."[4]

Some nurses with baccalaureate and master's degrees were eager to enlarge their competencies for work in specialty areas through certificate programs (pediatric practitioner, adult clinician, family nurse practitioner). The need was documented that Vermont, being a rural state, had health manpower distribution problems. The rural areas had few physicians and there were a limited number of ambulatory settings that provided comprehensive services, such as health education, preventative services, early case finding, and maintenance. It was determined that better prepared nurses could meet over 80% of these health care needs. This type of education made it possible for nurse-run clinics to be established, and federal financing was achieved through legislation supported by Senator Patrick Leahy.

The rapid advancement of research, the lack of easy accessibility of continuing education, and the inefficient dissemination of knowledge were factors contributing to the gap between scientific and technological advances and the practice of nursing. The technological advances placed increasing demands on nurses for keeping practice current. Directly and indirectly, changes in nursing practice resulted from alterations in the society. For example, better care was being demanded, population mobility resulted in a high turnover of nursing personnel, and there were shifts in age composition of the clients being served.

As the objectives of the Family Nurse Practitioner Program indicate, the nurse was the principal student, but the entire health team of any particular setting was also involved. As the knowledge and skill bases of the nurse were enhanced, the role of the nurse changed, which meant that the roles of the other health team members had to change also. Experience showed that the receptionist who did the scheduling of patients was key in allowing the roles to change. Janet Brown and George Welsh provided on-going consultation to the nurse student, physician, and health team members for one year, and a post-visit to the practice site six months after the course. Consultation took place by telephone, written letters, closed circuit television, and/or site visits.

Reestablishment of the Continuing Education Program

Recognizing the need for the School of Nursing to redevelop a continuing education program, Director Jean Milligan appointed a continuing education committee in 1974. The committee, chaired by faculty member JoAnn Scranton, planned an offering that year. The committee developed a long-term plan for presenting several short-term programs annually. Some of these were co-sponsored by voluntary health agencies and professional associations. This program served as a foundation for the later grant application.

The American Nurses' Association had not drawn up guidelines for the state associations to use in establishing the process by which the quality of the continuing education offering for nurses could be evaluated. Thus the Vermont State Nurses' Association, with the assistance of the School of Nursing, used the criteria as set forth by the Task Force of Colleges and Universities in granting Continuing Education Units (CEUs). In the late 1970s and into the 1980s, until the Vermont State Nurses' Association was accredited as an approver of continuing education for nurses, the Division of Continuing Education of Education at UVM asked the School of Nursing to review all continuing education offerings for nurses that were being given by organizations or groups on campus. This review was to determine if the objectives and delivery of the offering would be recognized by various Boards of Nursing and official nursing organizations as being pertinent for nurses.

In 1978–79, with the support of the University and a three-year special projects grant from the Division of Nursing, Department of Health and Human Services, full-time status for the Continuing Education Program in the School of Nursing was resumed. With the ever-increasing complexity of nursing care, nurses functioning in various capacities needed opportunities to update their knowledge, skill, and attitudes. The goal of the Continuing Education Program at the School of Nursing was to provide an organized plan of offerings for nurses at all levels in all areas of the state. Programs that could be presented in collaboration with other health and nursing groups in the state were given high priority. Most of the offerings were one-day sessions, and the subject matter was intended to have immediate application by the learner. Some of the offerings required a defined level of knowledge and were restricted to specific groups of nurses. Selected offerings were open to senior nursing students (e.g., Pharmacology and Pharmacokinetics, Physical Assessment Skills). At least one session each year was planned for other disciplines (physicians, physical therapists, social workers, and dieticians). In order to offer improved communication and service to the entire state, the state was divided into four geographic regions. A master's-prepared part-time coordinator, who lived and worked in the area, was employed for each region (e.g., Nedra Willard of Peacham, Georgeana Hunton of Norwich, and Pat Allen of Middlesex) and an advisory committee of representatives of providers of continuing education, employers of nurses, and a variety of groups with an interest in continuing education for nurses was organized in each region. A continuing education needs assessment of each region was done by the advisory committee each year. Using the results of the needs assessment, an annual program was developed for each region and the state as a whole. Primarily the program served nurses in Vermont, New Hampshire, and northern New York, with some attending from Maine and northwestern Massachusetts.

The Philosophy of Continuing Education for the School of Nursing was the following:

> The faculty in the School of Nursing of the University of Vermont believe that education is a continuous process of developing each individual's potentials. We believe that opportunities for life-long learning should be afforded all individuals and that the School of Nursing has a responsibility to provide continuing education for nurses.
>
> We believe that continuing education consists of planned learning experiences beyond basic nursing education and that these experiences should emphasize emerging nursing concepts and the progressive development of competencies required to enhance changes in the health care delivery system. It is our belief that continuing education should develop each individual's potentials within his/her professional role. We believe that the School of Nursing should work within the continuing education structure of the University and cooperate with institutions of higher education and agencies in providing leadership to upgrade nursing practice."[5]

The 1980s: Maintaining the Continuing Education Program

In 1980, to improve accessibility, offerings were delivered via nontraditional teaching techniques (video, computer-assisted instructional modules), as well as more traditional methods (e.g., closed-circuit television, teleconferencing, and self-learning packages). These teaching techniques made offerings more easily accessible to nurses, helping them to recognize that there were multiple ways of receiving continuing education, such as "self education" through reading, listening to tapes, use of self-learning packages, correspondence courses, as well as educational television.

After the termination of federal funding for the continuing education program in July 1981, the School of Nursing continued the program throughout the state with financing from UVM, registration fees, cosponsorships, and grants. It continued as a full-time program until 1985, and then as a part-time program from 1985 to 1987.

The School of Nursing Continuing Education Program was well known both on and off campus. Administration and faculty of the University have commented positively on the "outreach" efforts of the program. As the program's staff traveled in Vermont, they received positive comments about the quality and "outreach" efforts of the School of Nursing. Evaluation of the offerings and the program by participants have been ongoing since 1976 and have been consistently positive. From 1979 to 1981, the Center for Evaluation and Policy Research was asked to evaluate the Continuing Education Program for Nurses. The formal evaluations of both the offerings and the program were favorable. The participants in the offerings indicated that the instructors were of good quality; that the knowledge, skills, and attitudes taught were put to some use; and the project staff was responsive to their needs. The drawbacks identified in the evaluative study were the cost of the programs, the distance participants must travel to attend some of the offerings, and the limited support—either financially or "time off"—provided by employers.

The evolution of continuing education programs within the School of Nursing indicates that the commitment to make lifelong learning available to nurses has been ongoing since the beginning of the school. Unlike formal educational programs, where there is always some percentage of financing available, financing of continuing education programs has not been consistent. Without the availability of consistent funding and without nurses and/or their employers willing to pay their share of the cost of programming, consistent continuing education programming was and is hard to maintain.

Over the years, the School of Nursing has explored various ways of financing the continuing education offerings so that fees could be maintained at a level that was attractive to Vermont nurses. Co-sponsorship of offerings with other agencies, the receipt of grants, and contracts with state and federal agencies helped to keep fees at an acceptable level. There was a concerted effort to educate nurses to the need to budget each year for their continuing education. With employers, there were discussions of the principles of cost sharing and the possibility of financial support for continuing education as a fringe benefit for their employees. Persons were encouraged to buy gift certificates for their nurse friends. The Office of Development talked about the possibility of friends of the school leaving money in their wills for use by the School of Nursing for continuing education activities.

Employers' involvement in providing their own form of continuing education offerings is very crucial to the continuous development of nurses. Bigger institutions may afford having their own in-service departments, but consortiums of smaller agencies are another way of being certain that in-service and continuing education needs can be met. Not only are employers critical in supporting such efforts financially, but equally important is making it possible for employees to have "time off" to attend offerings. Employers are in an excellent position to observe nurses in practice, and to determine educational needs. Also, they have knowledge of the emerging new trends, technologies, and/or equipment. The "downside" of employer involvement in providing continuing education is the diminished number of potential attendees at offerings sponsored by the School of Nursing or other agencies offering continuing education.

—Janet P. Brown-Wolff, RN, EdD

NOTES

1. Mary E. Beam, "Report of a Project for Development of a Continuing Education Program for Nurse Practitioners in Upper New England on the Utilization of Research Findings in the Improvement of Patient Care" (New York: The American Nurses Foundation, Inc., June 1966), 10–13.
2. American Nurses' Association, "First Position Paper on Education for Nursing," *American Journal of Nursing* 65 (1965): 106–11.
3. Beam, "Report of a Project," 264.
4. School of Nursing, "Objectives of the Family Nurse Practitioner Program" (Burlington, Vt.: The University of Vermont, 1978).
5. School of Nursing, "Philosophy of Continuing Education" (Burlington, Vt.: The University of Vermont, 1 April 1985).

An RN with a New BS Reflects

A Personal Account

TODAY when a person decides to become a nurse, (s)he is more likely to enter a degree program than a diploma program. When I entered nursing school in 1967, the reverse was true. The diploma program was more prevalent and well known. By the time I graduated, three years later, I had become more aware of the benefits of a college degree. These benefits included enhanced professional standing, additional professional opportunities, and personal satisfaction and growth.

I started college [the University of Connecticut–West Hartford] almost immediately after graduation, working toward my degree in nursing. I found out that many colleges with nursing programs were willing to give credit for experience and prior education provided that the student demonstrate that (s)he had the equivalent knowledge by taking and passing challenge examinations. Up to 50% of the required credits could be accumulated in this way, depending on the college chosen. Later on I also discovered that many nonnursing courses could also be challenged through the College Level Examination Program (CLEP) administered by the Educational Testing Service in Princeton, New Jersey, and available in Vermont. Credits in history, English, microbiology, and other subjects can be earned by passing tests which are similar to SAT and College Board Examinations. As a result of my nursing and some independent study, I was able to accumulate a large percentage of the 125 credits required for graduation in this manner. While this method gave me an advantage over beginning college students, the remaining credits (about 80 in my case) had to be acquired by taking college courses in the "normal" manner by attending classes.

One of the reasons I persevered in working toward my degree was that I found through my hospital work that a college degree enhanced a nurse's professional standing. Hospital administrations seemed to value BSN graduates more—as reflected in salary as well as consideration for promotions. I also observed that there were branches of the nursing profession,

---

Reprinted from *Vermont Registered Nurse*, August, 1984.

such as school nursing, occupational health nursing, and public health nursing, that give hiring preference to BSN graduates. In these fields the nurse must assume a major teaching role. The academic program of a BSN graduate is particularly designed to develop the ability and skills for the role of teaching.

Although it took me over ten years of part-time study (because of my commitments to raising a family and part-time work), I enjoyed the challenge and the work. In the nonnursing courses I found that I enjoyed learning about music, literature, history, mathematics, philosophy, and other subjects which were not a part of my nursing background. Taking these courses rounded out my education—which is, of course, one of the goals of a college education. As a part-time student in these general education courses, I also had the opportunity to interact with students in other majors with other points of view. This type of experience helped me put my career as a nurse into perspective with respect to other fields and career possibilities. It helped me see the advantages as well as disadvantages of a nursing career. Needless to say, from my personal point of view, the advantages have outweighed the disadvantages. I found my senior year—the only two semesters I went full time—to be especially exciting. While the nonnursing courses helped me expand my personal horizons, the nursing courses I took in my senior year expanded my professional horizons.

The University of Vermont requires at least one semester of full-time study at the university before graduation, with the option of taking the fall semester part-time. I decided to complete my degree work in one year by taking my entire senior year as a full-time student. This decision gave me a firm completion date and, as a bonus, I thoroughly enjoyed the two semesters. Part of the excitement of my senior year was the community nursing program. This program allowed me to gain experience in two nursing fields which were entirely new to me. During the first semester I functioned as a school nurse in a nearby locality. I enjoyed working with the children in the classroom and administering to their health needs. I also learned a lot about community funding of school health programs in the process.

During my second semester I worked as an occupational health nurse in a local industry. My responsibilities included doing physical and health assessments, providing first aid care for industrial injuries, and teaching preventive and promotional health care measures. The other course work during my senior year was not as exciting, but again included much new material such as our research.

I found that the faculty was very supportive and gave me and the other RNs in the program more freedom of choice than the generic students. The faculty tailored their supervision to fit our needs. I felt that this was an expression of the confidence they had in our prior education and experience. I also found that interacting with the generic students was revitalizing and inspired in me an enthusiasm which I hadn't had since I graduated from nursing school.

Now that the excitement of the graduation ceremonies is past and I've had a chance to relax and to resume my family life, I am looking back at the past year and feel a sense of accomplishment and great personal satisfaction. I also am grateful to my husband and children for all of their support. I am looking forward now to going back to the nursing work I enjoy.

—Janet Yantachka, RN, BSN

Practical Nursing Programs

Practical nursing education in Vermont began as early as 1907 in Brattleboro, when one student enrolled in a training program initiated by the Brattleboro Mutual Aid Association, an outgrowth of the Thomas Thompson trust fund. The money from the fund was "for the relief and support of poor seamstresses, needlewomen and shop girls, who may be in temporary need for want of employment, sickness or misfortunes in the town of Brattleboro, Vt. and Rhinebeck, NY." Students were called Mutual Aid Nursing Attendants and they cared for the sick in their home and "the mother and baby in childbirth."[1] This was the beginning of the Thompson School for Practical Nurses.

Thirty-eight years later, in 1945, the second school of practical nursing was established—the Putnam Memorial School of Practical Nursing in Bennington. The graduates of these programs, however, were not licensed or approved by the Vermont State Board of Nursing until 1951. Minimum standards for licensed practical nurse (LPN) programs were adopted by the board on September 18, 1951. On October 16, 1951, both the Thompson and Putnam schools were fully approved by the Vermont State Board of Nursing.[2]

In July 1951, the graduates of the practical nursing programs were given an option to be licensed by waiver or examination. A licensure examination was given for the first time in November 1951 to eighteen practical nurse candidates. The passing grade was 70%. Fourteen of the candidates passed the exam, four failed, and one repeated the exam on May 9, 1952, and passed.[3]

In June 1957, Legislative Act 273 enabled the Vermont State Board of Education to approve practical nurse education after a statewide search identified the need for nurses. The opening of the Fanny Allen School for Practical Nursing in Colchester in November 1957 was in direct response to this need. The school was approved by the Board of Nursing in the same year. The cost of the programs at this time was approximately $300–$400 during the first sixteen weeks. There were three-and-a-half hours of classroom theory per week, and the rest of the hours were at the bedside. Generally students were provided meals and given a $60 per month stipend. If the school was affiliated with a hospital, as all three schools were, the state contributed 75% of the instructor's salary and the affiliating hospital contributed $100 directly to the school. In 1970, Bennington County legislators petitioned the state for additional financial assistance to operate the Putnam School.

Under the provision of federal vocational education legislation, funds were available to support the training of practical nurses. The money was granted in 1971 and the practical nursing schools' parent organization became the Vermont State Department of Education–Vocational Division. The schools changed over time from offering three classes a year to two per year and eventually, in 1986, one class was admitted in August and graduated students after forty-five weeks of training.

In 1992–93, the Vermont Department of Employment and Training (DET) secured a grant through the Job Training Partnership Act to assist underemployed individuals to gain employment via an educational program. The Fanny Allen program partnered with DET to sponsor practical nursing education, utilizing Vermont Interactive Television to deliver theory-based courses. This program was offered in the most rural area of Vermont's Northeast Kingdom. The one-year program graduated thirty-four practical nurses who became part of Vermont's health-care workforce.

Legislative bill H.781, 16 VSA §2651, was enacted in July 1994 "to assist existing schools for practical nursing and to assist in the establishment of a School for Practical Nursing under the direction of the Board of Trustees of the Vermont State College System." This act delineated provisions for the transfer of Fanny Allen, Putnam, and Thompson schools, and one full-time director, three full-time site directors, 7.4 full-time equivalent instructors, and 2.7 full-time secretaries to the state college system. Vermont Technical College was designated as the controlling institution, and personnel were granted all the rights and privileges of this system.[4]

In 1994–95, Vermont Technical College and DET partnered with one another to offer another grant-funded practical nursing program to under-employed residents of the Northeast Kingdom. Twenty-seven students were admitted in the fall of 1994. Twenty students graduated in the spring of 1995. Distance learning technology was utilized to efficiently deliver this educational program.

Under the college system, the LPN programs merged into one program but maintained their identity at each site. The courses became credit-bearing in 1996 and part of a one-plus-one concept linking the practical nurse programs with associate degree programs in Vermont.

—Anita F. Ristau, RN, MS

NOTES

1. Florence Wells, "The First School," *Journal of Practical Nursing* (September 1958).
2. Vermont State Board of Nursing, Minutes of 16 October 1951, 4. Vermont State Archives, Office of the Secretary of State, Montpelier, Vermont.
3. Ibid., 9 May 1952, 7.
4. State of Vermont, "No. 145, An Act Relating to Transfer of the State Nursing Education Program," Public Acts, 1994 Session, 114.

Thompson School for Practical Nurses

THE OLDEST CONTINUING SCHOOL for practical nurse education in the United States, the Thompson School in Brattleboro, began with one pupil in 1907. It was founded for the purpose of caring for birthing mothers and to give home care to children of mothers who were in the work force.

Brattleboro Memorial Hospital did not have a resident trained nurse when it opened in 1904. A group of fifteen local church women were called together in 1907 by Richard Bradley, one of the three first trustees of the Thomas Thompson Trust Fund. This group, the Brattleboro Mutual Aid Association, had as its purpose "to supply those needs in sickness that are not now properly covered by hospital service, the visiting nurses, or by unorganized private nursing."[1]

A training course, operating out of a house on Harris Place in Brattleboro, was instituted to ensure the standards of selected women—to be called Mutual Aid Nursing Attendants—who would care for the sick in their homes. From this humble beginning, Thompson School for Practical Nurses began.

Charlotte MacLeod was employed as the first director of the school in 1909. Prior to her appointment she had established the Victorian Order of Nurses in Canada. Seven women enrolled in the first class which extended over twelve months. The first class graduated in 1911.

The Alumni Association was founded in 1926 and was instrumental in improving the hourly pay schedule. In 1934, the graduates were paid $25 a week after the first year with four hours of free time a day. By 1945, they were receiving $35 a week for a twenty-hour day, $30 for a twelve-hour day.

In 1956, the Thompson School found it could not provide room for an extra class of students at its Brattleboro site. Barre City Hospital volunteered to cooperate with the training of LPN students by having the students affiliate at that hospital for a 32-week clinical session. "Any girls and men who have had at least two years of high school or older persons up to 50 years of age" could apply.[2]

The curriculum in the 1950s and 1960s was twenty weeks of medical-surgical nursing, four weeks caring for children, three weeks caring for mothers, three weeks caring for newborns, and two weeks in the diet kitchen. Male students studied urology in place of maternity care. During the clinical period, students received four hours of classroom theory a week. The Vocational Education Division of the Vermont Department of Education paid part of the instructor's salary and students were given a $7 per week stipend.[3]

In 1994, the Thompson School of nursing joined the other Practical Nursing programs and came under the organizational structure of Vermont Technical College.

—Rose-Marie Tarbell, RN, MEd
Faculty and Site Director
Anita Fregosi Ristau, RN, MS

NOTES

1. Florence Wells, "The First School," *Journal of Practical Nursing* (September 1958).
2. "Barre City Hospital to Cooperate in Training of Practical Nurses," *Barre (Vermont) Daily Times*, 19 July 1956.
3. Ibid.

Putnam Memorial School of Practical Nursing

THE PUTNAM MEMORIAL School of Practical Nursing was established in 1945 by the Board of Corporators of the Putnam Memorial Hospital, Bennington, Vermont, and functioned as an integral part of the hospital. In 1949 it became the eighth school of practical nursing in the country to be nationally accredited by the National Association for Practical Nurse Education and Service, Inc.

In the early years, the students were involved in an apprentice-type, service-oriented program. Licensure was permissive rather than mandatory. When the school was established, it was a two-year school and the program accepted two classes per year. There were eight graduates in the first school graduation.

In 1951, the Putnam Memorial Hospital School of Practical Nursing was approved by the Vermont State Board of Registration of Nurses, and in 1967 the school was accredited by the National League for Nursing. In the 1950s, there were approximately thirty-two graduates for both classes. The spring classes were smaller than the fall.

In 1970, the Board of Corporators of the hospital, through Bennington County legislators, petitioned the state Legislature for additional financial assistance to operate the school. This was granted to the hospital under a Congressional Act which provided for aid to education in the health occupations, in cooperation with the state. The next year, however, the school's parent organization became the Vermont State Department of Education.

Room and board was provided at the school until 1976. After that time, students were responsible for their own room and board. In the 1960s to the 1980s, graduating classes contained thirteen to thirty students, again with the larger classes being in the fall. There was a part-time program for two years which started in 1983.

In 1984 a career ladder program was organized with Southern Vermont College to enable the students to continue their education. At this time the courses were not credit-bearing and it was difficult to transfer the program's courses to college credits.

In July 1994, Putnam Memorial School of Practical Nursing became a program of Vermont Technical College. In August 1996, a credit-bearing curriculum was implemented in an effort to assure that graduates could easily continue their education. Presently the program is a ten-and-a-half month program and accepts one class of approximately thirty students per year.

—Mary McMahon, MS, BSN, RN
Faculty and Site Director

Fanny Allen Memorial School for Practical Nursing

THE FANNY ALLEN Memorial School for Practical Nursing was founded on June 28, 1957, and the first class entered on November 18, 1957. The school was housed in the Fanny Allen Hospital.

Legislative Act 273 was enacted in June 1957 in response to a statewide search to identify a need for nurses. This survey was conducted by Harold Graeme, supervisor of Trade and Industrial Education in conjunction with Dr. Louis Thabault, Dr. Jeremiah K. Durick, and Sister Marion Chaloux.

The Fanny Allen School of Nursing was established under the leadership of Sister Marion Chaloux as a result of this legislation. The mandate was that "candidates will be trained in the care of medicine and surgery patients, in diet kitchens, with the aged, with mothers, with newborn infants, and with children."*

The curriculum for the program was based on that proposed by the National Association for Practical Nursing Education Services and the cost of the program was $300–$400 during the first sixteen weeks. Three-and-a-half hours per week were devoted to the classroom, and the rest of the hours the students were at the bedside, for a total of thirty-two weeks.

Affiliating hospitals such as Fanny Allen Hospital in Winooski, Brightlook Hospital in St. Johnsbury, and Kerbs Memorial Hospital in Newport, were expected to recruit ten students and secure an instructor for the clinical experience. The state contributed 75% of the instructors' salaries. The affiliating hospitals contributed $100 to the Fanny Allen School for each session in which it had students. The money was used for teaching, supplies, and reference books. The affiliating hospitals also provided a classroom and classroom equipment, and a schedule of work to give the student a well-rounded experience in nursing. Students spent the first four months at Fanny Allen, then upon completion of clinical experience at affiliating hospitals, came back to Fanny Allen for graduation from the program.

---

* *Burlington (Vermont) Free Press,* 7 November 1957.

The school admitted three classes a year from 1957, and added affiliations in the 1960s to include DeGoesbriand Memorial Hospital and Fletcher Allen Hospital in Burlington, and Orleans County Memorial Hospital in Newport.

In 1978, the school moved its central offices from Fanny Allen Hospital into a building provided by the hospital. It was on the grounds of the hospital and was an excellent facility for staff and students. During 1984 and 1985, only two classes were admitted. Since 1986, one class a year has been admitted in August, with graduation at the end of forty-five weeks.

In 1993, the school moved from the Fanny Allen complex to the Dupont Building at Fort Ethan Allen, owned by Saint Michael's College, and is currently at that location.

The directors for the school were as follows:

Sr. Marion Chaloux, RHSJ	1957–1964
Jane Mullen	1964–1965 (Interim)
Rollande Irvine, BSN, RN	1965–1981
Shirley Stockwell, BSN, RN	1981–1984
Patricia Nolin, BS, RN	1984–1986
Jeanne Howrigan, RN, BS	1986–1990
Phyllis Iorlano, BS, RN	1990–1993

The parent organization changed from the Vermont State Department of Education to Vermont Technical College in 1994, with a state director for Vermont's three practical nursing schools (Putnam Memorial, the Thompson School, and Fanny Allen) and a site director at each school. Mary Wright, RN, BA, was named site director at Fanny Allen in 1993.

The Fanny Allen Memorial School for Practical Nursing has had Vermont State Board of Nursing approval from its beginning in 1957. Accreditation was given by the National Association of Practical Nurse Education and Service, Inc. until 1986. From 1986 until the present, the National League for Nursing has been the accrediting body.

The total number of graduates from this program from 1957 to 1999 is 1,909. In 1999, the 100th class was graduated.

—Mary Wright, RN, BA
Faculty and Site Director

TWO

Nursing Practice

Nursing Practice: Introduction

In 1941, *We Who Serve: A Story of Nursing in Vermont*, was published.[1] That year found the United States preparing for war. The Lend Lease Bill, which had formalized this country's support of the Allied War effort, had brought an end to the Great Depression of the 1930s as the economy geared to produce the materiel of war. The all-volunteer army disappeared with the passage of the Selective Service Act in September 1940. By early 1941, Vermont draftees were on their way to basic training. In the spring of 1941, the Vermont National Guard was called to active duty. Following the attack on Pearl Harbor on December 7, 1941, war was declared against the Axis powers (Germany, Japan, and Italy). The energies of all Americans became directed toward supporting the war effort to a victorious outcome. It is interesting to note that the state of Vermont had already declared war on Germany and Italy in September 1941.

In Vermont, as throughout the country, the challenge faced by the nursing profession was to meet the needs of the armed forces as well as those of the civilian population. It proved a tough task. The Vermont Council on Defense, later called the Vermont State Nursing Council for War Service, was organized in 1942. Its objectives centered on attracting graduate nurses to Vermont as well as recruiting student nurses. To this end, in November 1942, the Vermont State Board of Registration of Nurses lowered the applicant age to 17½ years, waived chemistry as a high school requirement, accelerated training courses, and accepted New York registrants without examination.

In 1942, the Federal Cadet Nurse Corps was established as a means of recruitment. Many young women were attracted to the profession by the offer of a subsidized nursing education, a monthly stipend, and—I speak for myself—a snappy gray uniform with regimental insignia that I thought made an impression on all who saw it. The Cadet Nurse Corps proved an excellent recruiting program.

The nursing crisis persisted. An article about Heaton Hospital that appeared in the *Montpelier Argus* of August 6, 1946, related that in World War II, two doctors entered the service from the hospital staff and 35 Heaton Hospital nurse graduates served in the armed forces. The article continued: "Last year and the year before Red Cross Nurses' Aides rallied

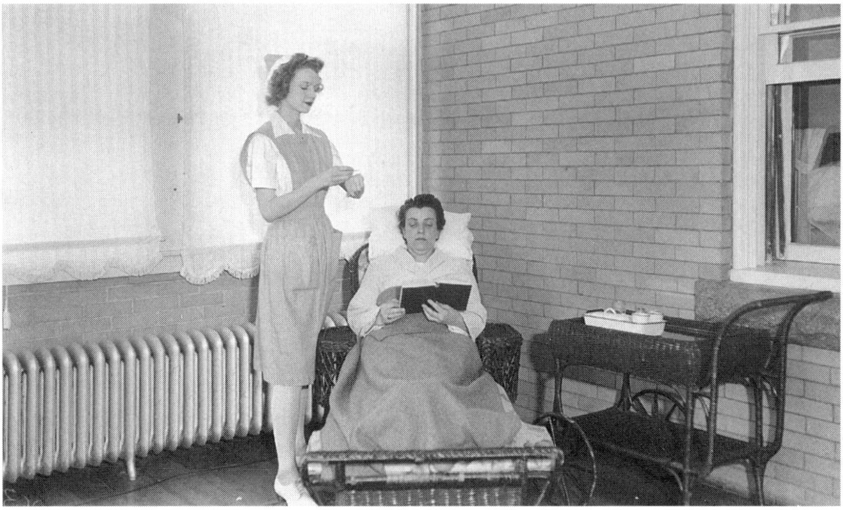

Courtesy Houston Photograph Collection, Vermont State Archives

Red Cross volunteer, Heaton Hospital, and patient, Montpelier, Vermont, 1943.

to the assistance of the hospital in maintaining adequate and efficient services to the community."[2] Norma Raymond of Montpelier was one of these Red Cross volunteers. She relates that in 1943 a notice appeared in the local paper requesting volunteers to participate in a Red Cross training course to help out at the hospital. Katherine Blakely, RN, taught a group of 15 Montpelier area women. Following completion of the training course, these volunteers worked at the hospital on twelve-hour shifts, including holidays and weekends. Norma reports that she gave "hands on patient care" and also worked in the "sterilization room" (cleaned and sterilized supplies for use in patient care).[3]

In December, 1944, at the request of Hortense Harwood, chairman of the Vermont State Nursing Council for War Service, a meeting of the Committee on Personnel Policies and Practices was held at Rutland Hospital. In attendance were Abbie Starkey, Executive Secretary of the Vermont State Nurses' Association; Sister Bisson, Vermont State Board of Registration of Nurses; N. Gertrude Sharpe, Superintendent, Springfield Hospital; Dr. B. F. Cook, State Medical Society; Laurence C. Campbell, State Hospital Association; and Timothy Dale, Commissioner of Public Welfare. As a result of the meeting, it was recommended that a survey of working conditions—including salaries and hours worked—be conducted by hospitals throughout the state. Twenty-five hospitals agreed to be surveyed. In May 1945 the results were published: Salaries for staff nurses ranged from $85 to $125 per month, salaries for per diem nurses ranged from $3 to $6. The working day ranged from eight to twelve hours. There is no evidence that the survey changed the economic status quo for staff nurses.

During the war years, the shortage of graduate nursing staff meant that student nurses became responsible for much of the nursing care in Vermont hospitals. It was truly a baptism by fire—a learning by doing. Periods of hospitalization were often lengthy and nurses came to know their patients well. Cleanliness was obviously considered next to godliness, from the early AM care in the dawn hours, to the morning bedbath, to the late afternoon PM care, to the evening care at bedtime, patients and their environment were scrubbed, cleaned, and comforted. Mealtimes often called for an exercise in patience by the nurse when feeding patients needing assistance, pacing the forkfuls of food to the capacity of the patient to chew and swallow. And yet these acts of intimate bedside care gave the nurse the ability to better identify the patient's physical, emotional, and spiritual needs, while providing a special measure of comfort. Moreover, the nurse developed an acute ability to assess even minor changes in the patient's status and call for early intervention.

Unfortunately, for more than seventy-five years the role of family support in the healing process was not well understood. In hospitals, visiting hours were strictly enforced. Initially this was to control transmission of infection. In discussing parental visitation with hospitalized children, Barbara Brodie, RN, PhD, FAAN, in the seventy-fifth anniversary commemorative edition of *Reflections*, writes,

> Nurses understood that ill children required extra kindness and consolation but they believed their womanly natural capabilities for healing and compassion effectively substituted for mother's attentiveness. Moreover, the behavior of the child—often fretful, tearful and uncooperative—diminished many mother's ability to maintain physician's prescribed regimens. It was considered prudent to limit visits to twice a week. However, studies by Anna Freud and Dorothy Burlingham on English children during World War II, and by Renee Spitz on hospitalized children, concluded that separating children from their mothers often left children emotionally traumatized."[4]

Within a few years it became the norm for parents to spend extended periods of time with their hospitalized children.

The administration of treatments and medications was a complex affair. Equipment used daily (e.g., catheters, intravenous (IV) bottles and tubing, and hypodermics) required cleaning and sterilization—by nurses. The words "throw away" were not yet part of the hospital lexicon. Every golden anniversary nursing graduate recalls the emery used to sharpen and resharpen—and sharpen again—the hypodermic needles used in the frustrating chore of drawing up and then administering to some poor patient the milky, viscous dosages of penicillin; and the spoon and alcohol lamp and sterile water which made preparing a dose of morphine a time-consuming procedure. In rural Vermont hospitals, nurses were often called upon to perform tasks and procedures that were not normally a part of nursing practice. Nurses often assumed the responsibility of "dropping" ether for obstetrical anesthesia, or for administration of IV medications. There were needs and no one else to meet them. In today's litigious society things are different.

Nurses laugh a lot and draw strength from camaraderie. A gathering of older grads always initiates hilarious stories. One of my favorites, told to me years ago by a graduate of Jeanne Mance School of Nursing, relates the tale of the young student who was assigned the task of cleaning her three patients' false teeth. A short time later, she approached the charge nurse with a worried smile and three sets of immaculate false teeth sitting in a basin. Imagine the rest of the story. Nurses exposed to pain and sadness as part of their daily work have always found that a sense of fun and humor have made the hard times easier to endure.

And so the war ended. Joan E. Lynaugh has written, ". . . the watershed event we called World War II did permanently alter American society, and in particular, it shook the world of that long-ago 'woman in white.' "[5]

It could be said that the private duty nurse became a casualty of the post-war era. Prior to that time, private duty nurses made up the largest group of practicing nurses in Vermont. Many used nurse registries, located in various areas of the state, as job referral resources. The registry rules were stringent. The registry run by the Graduate Nurses' Association on Colchester Avenue in Burlington provides an example. To list a few of the registry rules, published in June 1943:

> Any nurse registering and whose name is first or second on the list shall keep the registry informed of her whereabouts.
>
> Nurses registering at 16 Colchester Avenue must have a telephone and reside within a fifteen mile radius of Burlington. Such nurses must be able to answer any call within an hour's time of call.[6]

Compensation for cases is as follows:

> Regular cases, 12 hours, $6.00, 20 hours, $8.00.
>
> Mental Cases and obstetrics with care of baby, 12 hours, $7.00, 20 hours, $8.00.
>
> An additional fee of $1.00 per day may be charged for each extra patient in the same house. For fractions of days, 6 hours or less, $3.00. More than 6 hours, $6.00-hourly nursing, first hour, $1.50.[7]

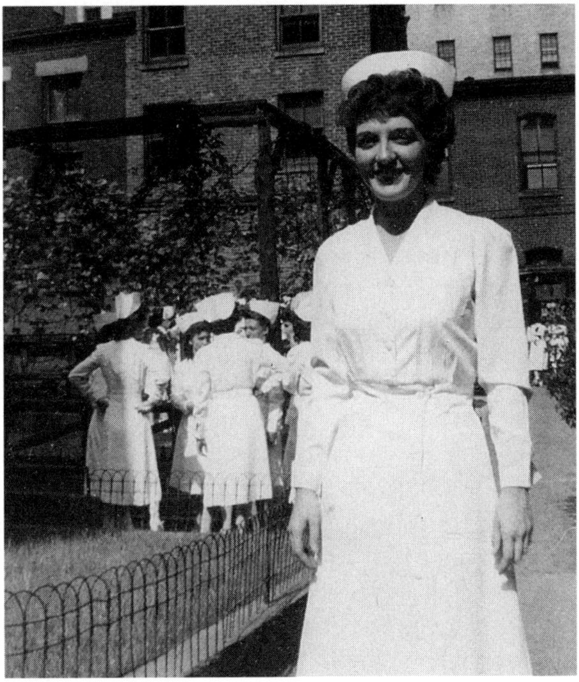

A "woman in white" circa 1947.

The private duty nurse was essentially self-employed. Many nurses cared for patients of a particular physician—elective surgery might even be postponed by the physician until that nurse was available. Sally Sample, RN, reports that her father, a surgeon in St. Albans, would plan elective surgery around the availability of Ruth White, RN, to care for his patients following surgery.[8] These relationships might be said to have formed the first collaborative practices.

In 1949, there were 2,262 RNs in Vermont, 415 of whom were private duty nurses, comprising the largest group of practitioners. However, by 1954 an article in the *Vermont Registered Nurse* by Frances B. Courville, chairman of the private duty section of the Vermont State Nurses' Association, reported that few new graduate nurses were attracted to private duty.[9] The acute nursing shortage following the war, the increased number of patients covered by health insurance, and the increasing complexity of patient care, all contributed to the decrease in the number of self-employed private duty nurses.

Another change precipitated by the postwar nursing shortage was the introduction of differentiated levels of nursing education and practice, and the use of ancillary personnel. The increasing complexity of health care called for an expanded knowledge base and skill level. Added responsibilities often shifted the nurse from primary care giver to primary care overseer. Currently, the delegation of nursing tasks is an integral part of nursing practice.

Out of the tragedy of World War II came tremendous advances in medical treatment and surgical techniques. The discovery of penicillin and other antibiotics meant that former lethal infections were treatable. Penicillin was used for every conceivable ailment—in the 1940s it was even available as a throat lozenge! But by the mid 1950s, the emergence of resistant organisms began. *Staphylococcus aureus*, "the golden killer," made its appearance. Hospital nurseries were at particular risk. Vermont was not spared.

In 1952, there were 250,000 cases of tuberculosis in the United States. In Vermont, there were 352 cases. Two sanatoria—in Barre and Pittsford—provided care for patients with active disease. Nurses provided inpatient care. In the public health area, they were active in case finding and follow-up. Introduced in 1952, antibiotics swiftly decreased tuberculosis morbidity and mortality. Exuberant patients celebrated their new lease on life. By 1967, Vermont had only six reported cases of tuberculosis.

Until 1955, poliomyelitis was the most dreaded epidemic in the United States. A discussion of the ways Vermont nurses met the challenges of the disease is reported in a separate article.* Let it be said that by the late 1950s both poliomyelitis and rubeola had become preventable diseases. Nurses were able to transfer their role from one of bedside care of these diseases to community education regarding their prevention.

The second half of the twentieth century witnessed tremendous societal and cultural changes in American life. The role of women in the culture changed dramatically. In 1941, a woman's choice of a profession was usually limited to nursing or teaching. Moreover, a woman's career was considered as a waystation on the road to matrimony and life as a homemaker. World War II became the initial catalyst, as women in large numbers worked outside the home to further the war effort.

Following the war, the economic good times, along with the GI bill for returning veterans, provided educational opportunities never before available. In Vermont the academic preparation of nurses gradually moved from the hospital school to the college campus. Equal employment opportunity and passage of civil rights laws opened new doors.

The advent of the oral contraceptive pill, *Roe vs. Wade*, and the flower-

* See "Vermont Nurses and the Polio Epidemic," pp. 99–102.

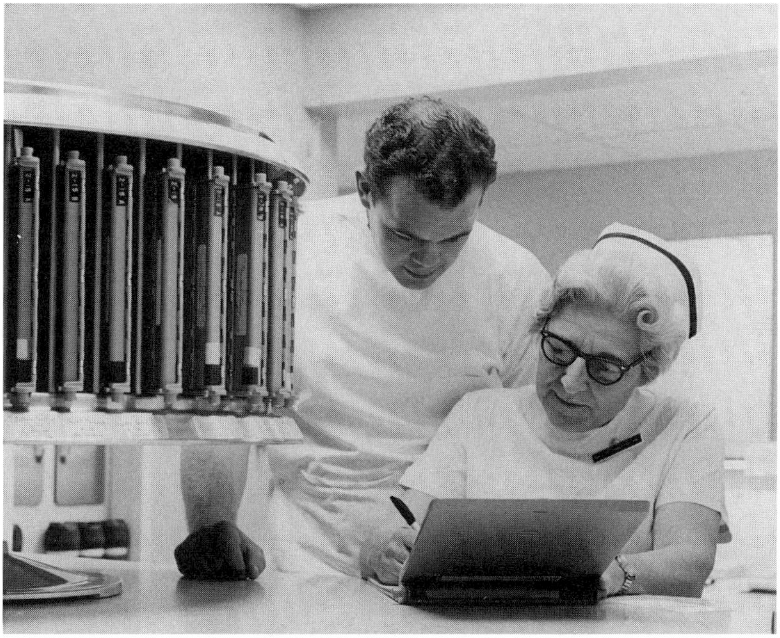

Caeserina Zanleoni, RN, reviews patient's chart with assisting staff member at the recently opened Central Vermont Hospital, 1969.

ing of the feminist movement heralded a change in the traditional role of women. And by popular demand, "women's health" became a specialty area of nursing.

Medicare arrived in Vermont in the mid 1960s, and Medicaid soon followed. These programs revolutionized the delivery of health care. Home health care agencies experienced explosive growth as services became available to poor mothers and children and to frail elderly in the home. The community health nurse quickly moved into the role of case manager and patient care advocate. The political climate of the time was one of "guns and butter," as the Johnson administration's War on Poverty introduced a multitude of new social programs while the country was embroiled in an increasingly unpopular war. By 1983, as health care costs soared, the introduction of Diagnostic Related Groups (DRGs) heralded the advent of managed care.

Changing demographics caused by increased longevity brought new challenges to Vermont nurses. In 1963, Janice Littlejohn wrote an article for the *Vermont Registered Nurse* after attending a workshop on improvement of nursing care of the aged:

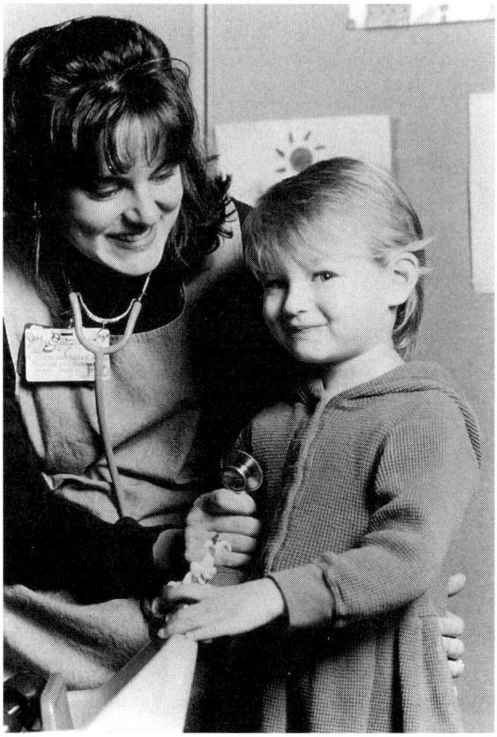

Courtesy Public Relations Office, Fletcher Allen Health Care

A smiling child, a smiling nurse: a happy pediatric experience

> Due to improvements and research in medicine people are living much longer lives. I learned many ways to help care for the elderly patient—the main purpose being to help the elderly to live and maintain as independent lives as possible. This new field of nursing to me is one with a lot of satisfaction. The elderly patient has more emotional problems and is much slower to adapt. It takes a lot of the nurse's time, patience, and understanding, but she will obtain more satisfaction from a long hard job well done.[10]

Geriatrics and long-term care became career choices within the nursing profession.

In 1965, an innovative pilot program to train pediatric nurse practitioners was introduced at the University of Colorado by visionaries Loretta Ford, RN, EdD, and Henry Silver, MD. Twelve nurses were enrolled. In an interview with *Advance for Nurse Practitioners*, Dr. Ford discussed the founding of the program.[11] As a community-based nurse she had become frustrated with not having the clinical skills or established protocols to make needed clinical decisions regarding the women and children she served. She began to create a curriculum for a public health pediatric nurse practitioner. The time was right; there was a physician shortage and a public need for the type of pediatric practitioner Dr. Ford envisioned. Dr. Silver and the University of Colorado Department of Medicine provided collaborative support. Thus the nurse practitioner movement was born. Soon programs to educate adult and family nurse practitioners, as well as pediatric nurse practitioners, were established throughout the country. Despite resistance—much of it from nursing colleagues—the role of the advanced practice nurse remains alive and well. There are now 346 advanced practice nurses endorsed in Vermont.

Integral to nursing practice has been health education and counseling. This has become especially important as a person's life style has increasingly impacted the quality and the length of life. In 1980, G. E. Alan Dever wrote, "Death certificates code diseases, they do not code causes. Traditionally we ask: What is the cause of death? Traditionally we answer: heart attack, lung cancer, automobile accident, suicide and so on. We *should* answer: lack of exercise, inadequate diet, smoking, excessive drinking, drug abuse, depression."[12] The first hospital outreach health education department in Vermont was established at Fanny Allen Hospital in 1978. Marie Clorey, RHSJ, RN, was the director. She and her successor, Amy Raiser, RN, introduced innovative programs which have been emulated throughout the state.

These fifty-five years have not been comfortable for nursing. Many of the problems that plagued the profession in the 1940s—shortages, economic inequity—continue today. In a keynote address before the Vermont State Nurses' Association convention in 1968, Dr. Beverly Dunsten discussed specific questions nursing struggled with at that time:

> How can nurses get back to the bedside?
> How can nurses maintain the nurse/patient relationship?
> How do we work with new health workers below the LPN level?

She identified the origins of these problems:

> Reliance on outmoded systems of care.
> A myopic view of nursing as a dependent occupation.
> False allegiance to technical and managerial skills.
> Narrow perspective of health services.
> Recalcitrant attitude toward change.[13]

Today nursing's response might be: "We're trying!"

And so it has gone. The professional woman in white has become the professional woman in scrubs and Birkenstocks. Patients have become clients, and we are no longer a single gender profession. Along the way we have spread our wings, have met new challenges and discovered new possibilities.

As science and technology have made dramatic inroads into the prevention and treatment of life-threatening diseases, health education and counseling had been directed toward the promotion of wellness, helping individuals to assume greater responsibility for their own well being. This has become especially important as a person's lifestyle increasingly impacts the quality and length of life. Nursing has been in the forefront of this effort. The voices of Vermont nurses attest to the fact.

—Jane P. Campbell, RNC, FNP, MEd

NOTES

1. Vermont State Nurses' Association, *We Who Serve: A Story of Nursing in Vermont* (Winooski, Vt.: Vermont State Nurses' Association, 1941).
2. Mary Perry, "Heaton Hospital Today Celebrates Its Founding Just 50 Years Ago," *Montpelier Argus*, 6 August 1946.
3. Norma Raymond, personal communication to the author, 13 September 2000.
4. Barbara Brodie, "Mothers and Pediatric Nursing, Changing Values 1800–1960," *Reflections* (magazine of Sigma Theta Tau International) 43, no. 3, 34.
5. Joan E. Lynaugh, "Values in Conflict, The 1950s," *Reflections* 43, no. 3, 26.
6. Graduate Nurses' Association, "Registry Rules," revised June 1943. Vermont State Nurses' Association Special Collection, Library Research Annex, The University of Vermont, Burlington, Vermont.
7. Ibid.
8. Sally Sample, personal communication to the author, 1999.
9. Frances B. Courville, "The Private Duty Section of the Biennial," *Vermont Registered Nurse* (April 1954): 3.
10. Janice Littlejohn, "Utilization of Research Findings in the Improvement of Nursing Care of the Aged," *Vermont Registered Nurse* (July 1963): 4.
11. Mary S. Hahn, "A Woman of Substance: Advance Talks to Loretta C. Ford, RN, EdD, FAAN," *Advance for Nurse Practitioners* (July, 1996).
12. Jane Campbell, "Wellness in an Academic Setting," (master's thesis, St. Michaels College, Colchester, Vermont, 1988): 20.
13. Beverly Dunsten, "Collective Unity and Action for Progress" (a keynote address to Vermont State Nurses' Association Convention, 23 September 1968), *Vermont Registered Nurse* (November 1968): 2.

Nursing Changes and Challenges, 1942–1975

A Personal Account

I WAS BORN December 19, 1920 in Wilder, Vermont, a sixth-generation Vermonter. I spent the majority of my elementary and high school years in Claremont, New Hampshire. I received my three-year nursing diploma from Massachusetts General Hospital (MGH) in February 1942. That spring my class had not yet been advised of the outcome of our nursing "boards." We were therefore ineligible for military service in Europe with the MGH unit which left at that time. However, we received positions at MGH upon graduation that normally wouldn't have been available to us with our paucity of experience.

I was assigned as "supervisory float nurse" under the direction of night supervisors Marie Hinkley (medical) and Adele Corkum (surgical). Each night brought new challenges as I was sent "where needed." These fine administrators instilled in me a great appreciation for flexibility, and an ability to adapt to change, which has been a definite asset for me in nursing.

My most memorable experience at MGH was on November 28, 1942, the night of the Coconut Grove fire in which 492 persons lost their lives. (The Coconut Grove was a popular Boston nightclub.) Ambulances poured up to the Emergency Room as I went on duty. Dr. Edward Churchill, chief of services, ordered the war burn protocol that had been established at the start of World War II. All medical students and hospital personnel were called to report for duty as able. From 10:30 PM until 12:45 AM 114 injured presented; 75 were dead on arrival (DOA) and 39 later assigned to White 6, a surgical floor. I was on the triage team administering morphine for pain and marking sites in red with time and amount. The casualties were assigned for debridement as ordered. Those who were DOA were placed in the "Brick Corridor," an area between the White and Bullfinch buildings. Later that night, I was sent to White 6 to help move the surgical patients who usually occupied the floor, because it was to be on reverse precautions—for burn patients only. The surgical patients were transferred to the Bullfinch medical unit, which made it necessary to transport them through the "Brick Corridor." I will never forget the smell of burnt flesh, hair, and clothing permeating the area, and the chaos as family members looked for their loved ones. It was a heart-wrenching experience. Subsequently, I spent many nights on White 6 caring for burn victims. For the first time in the Boston area, penicillin was used.

While my husband was overseas, I returned to Claremont, New Hampshire, and did floor duty at the local hospital. I also taught a Red Cross Home Nursing course at the local high school. Many of these students became nurse's aides and were later "waivered" as licensed practical nurses, both categories quite new at the time.

After World War II, while my husband attended the University of New Hampshire, I worked at the college infirmary, Hood House, and at Portsmouth Hospital on the maternity floor. Upon his graduation we moved to Lyndonville, Vermont. There my good friend and mentor, Dr. Ralph Jardine, encouraged me to do private duty to "keep my hand in nursing" while I raised four children. My mother lived with us during the winter months, so I was able to work occasionally while she or some of my friends took care of my "brood."

At St. Johnsbury Hospital I did night duty, for which I received $8–$10 a shift, from 8:00 PM to 7:00 AM While my patients slept, I really enjoyed working with the Catholic nursing sisters and often helped them fold dressings and make other supplies that they sterilized themselves.

My most memorable private duty case was at Brightlook Hospital in St. Johnsbury in the early 1950s. Three well-known national club women, on their way home to Chicago from a conference in Boston, were in a serious automobile accident in the White Mountains. One of the women died at the scene. The two others were severely injured. One, whom I will call Mrs. B, had several limb fractures; the other, whom I will call Mrs. C, suffered serious head and facial injuries. Because air transportation from this area was limited in the late 1940s, Mrs. C was specialed for two months in St. Johnsbury. Her facial injuries were especially severe. The surgeon who reconstructed her face told us that he had only "imagined" what she had looked like by using a picture of her from the Boston papers. He felt she would require extensive further plastic surgery after the initial healing. While healing she became severely depressed, ate very little and refused to have a mirror in her room.

I specialed Mrs. C on the 3:00 PM to 11:00 PM shift. As Mrs. B recovered, she was able in her wheelchair to visit Mrs. C. Mrs. B and I became friends, as most of Mrs. C's communication was through us. When they finally returned to Chicago, I received regular letters from Mrs. B for several years. These missives from Mrs. B described several additional reconstructive surgeries for Mrs C, with attendant periods of depression. My experience with Mrs. C, as well as my undergraduate affiliation at McLean Psychiatric Hospital in Waverley, Massachusetts, are responsible for the many years I later spent in psychiatric nursing.

From 1960 until 1975 I worked at Brattleboro Retreat. Shortly after moving to Brattleboro, while I was on the staff of the Town of Brattleboro Public Health Nursing Service, I bumped into a former classmate of mine who had worked with me at McLean Hospital during our student affiliation. His name was Joseph Lavoie, RN, MS, and he was director of nursing at Brattleboro Retreat. Dr. J. Butler Tompkins, also from McLean, had been appointed the sixth superintendent of the Retreat in 1949, and he was later joined by Dr. Douglas Sharpe as staff physician, also from McLean. Joe, his wife Shirley (also a classmate), and I renewed our friendship and he asked me, "Why aren't you at the Retreat? There are some real changes taking place in psychiatry." After the birth of my sixth child and when my mother moved to live with me, I joined the Retreat staff.

In order to give a picture of the various areas at the Retreat, I will list them as they were in 1960. Tyler IV, where I was assigned, was the admissions and only locked unit, with approximately 100 patients. Osgood infirmary held over 100 infirm geriatric patients. The Main Building had administrative offices in the front section and two large patient services—West for males and East for females—housing 386 patients. Linden Lodge had just been accredited by the state as a nursing home. It was formerly called the Marsh Building, named for the Retreat founder, Anna Hunt Marsh. This building had formerly held mostly "well to do" ambulatory patients.

I was excited about the new psychiatric drugs of the time, and to hear that electro-convulsive therapy (ECT) had been stopped in the late 1950s at the Retreat to better evaluate the new treatments without its use.

The entire staff was very educationally oriented. In 1958, a course had been given to fourteen selected and experienced attendants, leading to exams and licensure as waivered LPNs. I grew to know this group very well, and found them particularly eager allies as several programs I was involved with were developed. In the Tyler building, regular rounds were held at which cases were presented to medical, nursing psychology, and social service staff. These were great open forums for education and interaction. Nursing care plans were being promoted throughout nursing at this time and though many balked at "all the paper work," I found them a challenge. Hence Mr. Lavoie asked me to move to Main Building East service as supervisor and see what I could effect regarding change there.

As I became acquainted with the patients and staff of East, I learned through reading case histories that there were many incorrect myths about patients who were mostly known only by diagnosis and observed behaviors. Little was known of their background or family history. Daily at report I would give a synopsis of a case history and present a couple of care plans. Lois Pease, an LPN ally, shared my enthusiasm and soon everyone wanted their cases to be reviewed. About this time, Mrs. Barbara McAlister, RN, the Main Building West supervisor, moved to Linden Lodge as director there, and I was asked to supervise West as well as East. The new ideas and nursing care plans were incorporated on West and again effected a positive response from staff.

The two Main Building services were composed primarily of committed state patients. The men who were able to be out, worked at the Retreat farm, which had a renowned registered Holstein herd, a piggery, and gardens covering a very large acreage. They were supervised by farm managers. The women worked in the sewing room making shapeless garments. A few worked in the kitchen and laundry. I loved "snapping" green beans and shucking peas on the back porches with the patients, who loved to chat and thought it was neat when the staff took part.

An alcohol counselor from the state, Mr. Ronald Beck, held occasional Alcoholics Anonymous meetings with a group of court-committed alcoholics. Alcohol as a disease was just beginning to be talked about. It upset me that the alcoholics who had sufficient funds were out and about in the Tyler building, while those needing state funding were given six-month inebriate committals by the courts. Chronic repeaters were given longer committals.

About the time I started working in the Main Building, Mr. Lavoie left to pursue a master's degree. Mrs. Hilda Packard, RN, BS, the supervisor in Tyler, was appointed director of nursing. Under her aegis, the registered nursing staff decided to "give nursing back to the patient." The licensed practical nurses worked with registered nurse supervisors to help design a whole new style of administration. The registered nurses were assigned to work with a specific doctor as psychiatric clinicians, and the licensed practical nurses became ward and unit managers. The National LPN Association had recently written a ward management course individually planned for nursing homes. We were able to use this course to help our LPNs in their new roles. Mrs. Packard also assigned two fine young graduates to work with me on Main East and West.

While working on East and West, the Retreat sent me to Marcy State Hospital, New York, to learn a technique called "remotivation" for working with long-term institutionalized patients. On my return I was able to teach aides, who then started groups with their patients. The course used visual aids and group discussions and was well received. On completion of the course, the aides received a certificate and a pin with the "remotivation" logo.

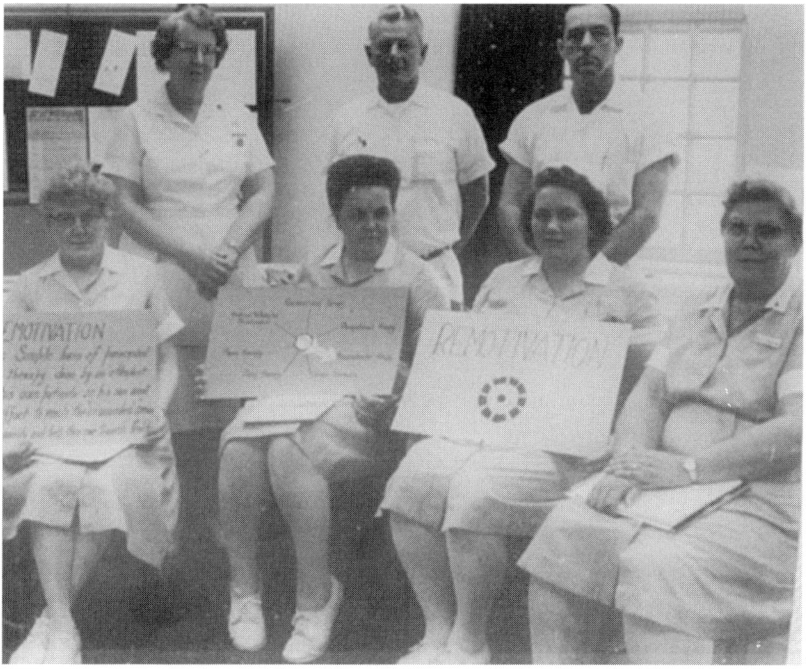

Courtesy Viola McGinn

Viola McGinn, RN (*back row, left*), with graduates of the remotivation program for the long-term mentally ill at Brattleboro Retreat, 1963.

When the Joint Commission for Accreditation of Hospitals (JCAH) mandated in-service education at all hospitals, I was assigned as director of in-service education. The New England Board of Higher Education made available—through the Vermont State Nurses' Association and The University of Vermont—a two-year course to be given in three- and four-day sessions to help prepare the "adult learner" for these in-service positions. I attended this with Mrs. Amy Yearley, RN, BS, from Brattleboro Memorial Hospital, and extended my fellowship with other nurses in Vermont in a most productive venue.

From the principles learned at the education courses at UVM, I set up several courses for employees, along with regular in-service filmed discussions, seminars, etc. The Retreat provided excellent facilities for these seminars, with leaders in the field participating. The most popular course was Psych Nursing III, where members of the medical staff taught the various diagnostic categories of mental illness. Students from Castleton State College, Antioch New England College, University of Massachusetts, and Windham College did work-study programs and were able to receive academic credit from their schools.

In the fifteen years I was at the Retreat, several major changes took place that significantly affected the patients and the hospital administration:

1. Patient census dropped due to use of new drugs and earlier discharge (after World War II admissions had greatly increased).
2. Medicare onset allowed the older patient population to have a monthly allowance, many of whom had previously had no funds available to them. Some were no longer allowed to work within the hospital. The state changed rates paid for care per patient and many financial constraints were felt in the delivery of mental health care.
3. The state decided to assign patients to the geographical areas they were from. On April 12, 1970, twenty-six patients were moved from the Main Building to the Vermont State Hospital in Waterbury. A month later, twenty-eight more were relocated there. To most of the patients, Brattleboro had been home for many years. They were in tears, as were the employees who had cared for them. Their departure is a very unhappy memory of mine.
4. The Kennedy family had long been interested in psychiatric illness and hospitalization. In 1963, the Kennedy Commission found 564,947 persons residing in public mental hospitals, many in deplorable condition. Further, there were scores of communities in America with no psychiatric services available to the people who were able to go home. President John F. Kennedy gave an impassioned speech to Congress, appealing for a "bold new approach" to the problem. Congress responded by enacting public law 88-164 appropriating $950 million to assist states in building community health centers.

   Planning grants were also available for implementing the following (my shortened version):

   A. Inpatient and outpatient services and emergency care
   B. More hospitalization in general hospitals
   C. Many more community services interaction—i.e., police, clergy, welfare departments
   D. Diagnostic, preventive, and rehabilitation services
   E. Research and evaluation

Since the 1960s, I have maintained a keen interest in the evolution of President Kennedy's hopes for these "bold new approaches."

—Viola (Rusty) Chase McGinn, RN, BS

Vermont Nurses and the Polio Epidemic

During the 1940s and into the mid 1950s, poliomyelitis, or infantile paralysis as it was popularly called, was the most dreaded epidemic disease in the United States. For Vermont parents, as with parents across the country, the late summer months when most cases occurred were anxious times. The incidence or severity of the disease within the population could not be predicted. Children and young adults were the usual victims.

In 1938, the National Foundation for Infantile Paralysis (NFIP) was established, supported in great part by public contributions to its "March of Dimes." The fact that President Franklin Roosevelt was a victim of the disease served to heighten public generosity. The NFIP then joined with the American Red Cross (ARC) to aggressively address the problem and to help local communities meet the challenge of an epidemic. Prior to this time, the ability to deal with an epidemic on a local level was compromised by a lack of facilities to care for the patients and a lack of health care personnel educated and experienced in the care of the polio patient.

Throughout the 1940s, the NFIP invested millions to remedy the situation. The Joint Orthopedic Nursing Advisory Service (JONAS), sponsored by the National League of Nursing Education and the National Organization for Public Health Nursing, and supported by the ARC and the NFIP, accepted the task of educating staff and general duty nurses in the care and treatment of polio patients. Institutes and workshops were held throughout the country. Polio courses were offered each year at principal medical centers in the country, financed by the NFIP. Schools of nursing were urged to teach students the basic nursing procedures unique to polio nursing.

Volunteer nurse coordinators were also invaluable to local communities experiencing an epidemic. The job of the nurse coordinator was to aid hospitals in evaluating the need for recruitment of nurses in the case of an emergency situation. The volunteer coordinator acted as a liaison between the hospital and the recruited nurse, and helped orient the recruited nurse to the community.

Recruited nurses were paid $275 a month for general duty and $300 for supervision. They agreed to serve a minimum of two months, but could be released at an earlier date. Much of the financial support for this program came from the local chapters of the NFIP.

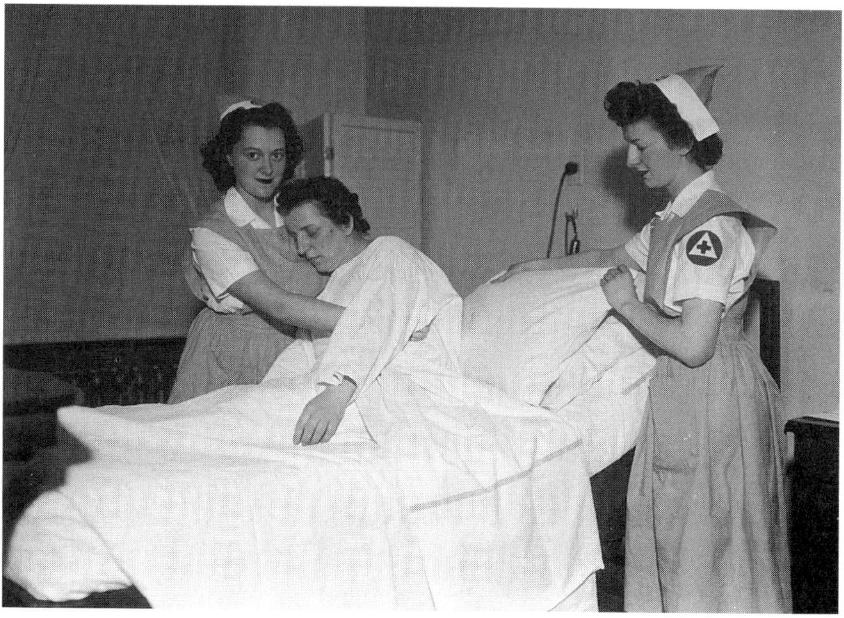

Courtesy Houston Photograph Collection, Vermont State Archives

Red Cross volunteers with patient, Heaton Hospital, Montpelier, 1943.

In 1949, volunteer nurse coordinators listed by district were:

District 1	Miss Veronica Cullinan, RN	Burlington
District 2	Mrs. Katherine Blakely, RN	Montpelier
District 3	Mrs. Mary Lowe, RN	St. Johnsbury
District 4	Mrs. Claire Elaine Stewart	Rutland

In March 1950, the following Vermont nurses were recognized by JONAS as being prepared and/or experienced in the care of the polio patient:

Dorothy A. Montague, RN*	Underhill
Lena Mildred Plaisted, RN, PT*	Burlington
Priscilla Raymond, RN*	Stowe
Pauline Mongeon, RN*	Winooski (Fanny Allen Hospital)
Irene Moyse, RN*	Burlington (Mary Fletcher Hospital)
Sadie M. Tobin, RN*	Burlington
Mrs. Jos. W. Blakely, RN	Montpelier
Mrs. Hildur J. Chadbourne	Burlington

In July 1952, the Vermont Polio Planning Committee was organized to promote better professional education. Bernice Frechette, RN, repre-

* Supervisors

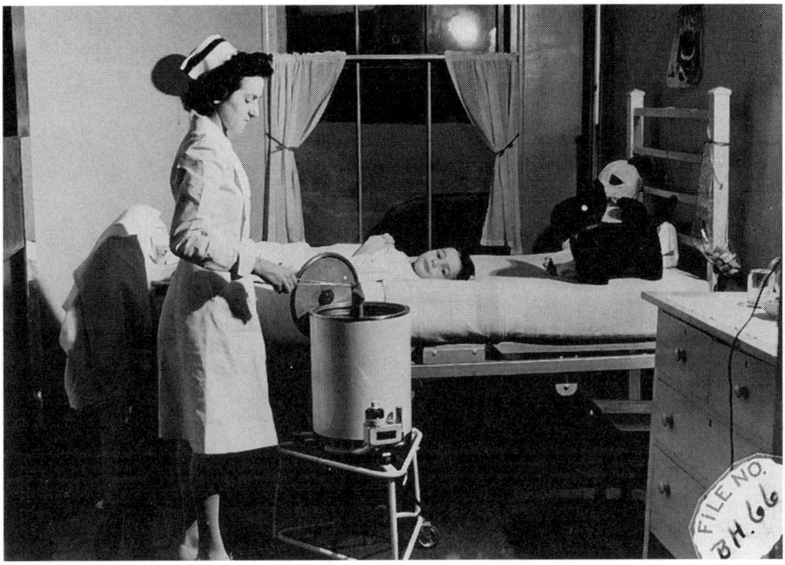

Courtesy Central Vermont Medical Center

Nurse and young patient with Sister Kenney Hot Pack Machine used in treatment of poliomyelitis, 1944.

sented the Vermont State Nurses' Association. John Bell, MD, director of the Crippled Children's Division of the State Health Department, became the first chairperson. Because the polio season was on its way, an educational program, directed by the subcommittee on nursing education, was postponed until June 1953. Nationally, the number of polio cases increased almost eight-fold between 1940 and 1950. In 1940, there were 9,804 reported cases. In 1952, there were 57,879 reported cases. In Vermont the largest number of cases occurred in 1949 (151), 1953 (120), and 1955 (121).

The disease affected the spinal cord, causing paralysis or weakness, usually of the extensor muscles. Bulbar polio, a more severe form, affected the respiratory system.

Nurses who have worked with polio patients remember vividly the late summer heat as they labored in isolation gowns and masks (there was no air conditioning), the Kenney packs (steamed flannel cloths applied to affected limbs to relieve the pain of acute muscle spasm), and the endless bellows sound of the iron lungs that resembled large cylindrical oil drums, with apertures through which care could be delivered. Nurses rejoiced when a youngster was discharged with minimal need of rehabilitation, and knew sorrow when the disease claimed another young victim.

It is not difficult to imagine the joy that was felt when Salk vaccine became available in the mid 1950s. By 1958, the number of polio cases in Vermont had declined to five, and since 1964 there have been no cases of polio in this state.

—Jane Campbell, RNC, FNP, MEd

BIBLIOGRAPHY

American Red Cross and National Foundation for Infantile Paralysis, Joint Orthopedic Nursing Advisory Service, Polio Nursing, "Procedures for Recruitment of Temporary Nurses for Poliomyelitis Care," pamphlet, 1952. Vermont State Nurses' Association Special Collection, Library Research Annex, The University of Vermont, Burlington.

Joint Orthopedic Advisory Committee correspondence to Vermont State Nurses' Association, 31 March 1950. Vermont State Nurses' Association Special Collection, Box 5.

Cohen, Victor, *Sister Kenney, The Woman Who Challenged Doctors.* Signet Books, 1975.

The Nurse Practitioner: A New Trail Blazed

A Personal Account

After graduation from a diploma school of nursing, I married and did a stint of hospital staff nursing, followed by private duty at the hospital, a hitch of camp nursing, and then advanced in my career to being a full-time mother of five. I say advanced because, looking back on it all now, I realize what a broadening wealth of experience it awarded me, as it was during this time that my professional garden was unknowingly tilled and seeds were planted.

In my spare time, I launched into community activities such as Girl Scout leadership, a Parent–Teacher Association (PTA) presidency, teaching (progressing to director of) twelve grades of a church school—among other things. In 1966, I became a single parent. These experiences and my life surrounding them gave a fertility to this aforementioned professional garden that I was to realize in a future bloom of creative and innovative nursing positions. I believe it brought an authenticity and relevance to my nursing practice that no degree could have.

With family economics forcing me, I reentered hospital nursing in 1967. I'd had a hiatus of thirteen years and what a hiatus it was! I was appalled at the degree of technical progress and, what I felt was regress of bedside nursing. I was distressed at how the new procedures (e.g., measuring central venous pressures) were overriding the bedside nursing component, leaving less time for educating or helping patients to understand their illness, emotionally preparing them for surgery, and comforting with backrubs to allay anxiety and apprehension. I was surprised at the presence of ancillary personnel doing hands-on care. It concerned me that they lacked the skills to use their time for valuable one-on-one teaching at the bedside, which I, as a professional nurse, had been educated to give. I was concerned, too, about safety issues, and my conscience brought me to speak with the director of nurses, Sally Sample, who heard me well and wondered if I might find visiting nurse work more satisfying. She was right on, and the Visiting Nurse Association (VNA) proved to be my cup of tea for thirty years.

The VNA caseloads consisted of two categories: morbidity and maternal child. In the morbidity area we did medications, nursing assessment, counseling, and personal care—no health aides there! There were few supplies (even disposable needles were a blessing). Procedures like catheterization started from scratch—including making solutions and boiling improvised homefound equipment.

In the maternal child field we checked postpartum mothers and taught newborn care. We did case finding for multi-problem families and those with inadequate immunizations. We did five well-child clinics each month in various locations, including one at the Moose Club in Burlington where examinations were done on pool tables, necessitating emptying ashtrays and wiping up beer from the night before. Medical students and a pediatric resident did the exams, and the nurses did immunizations and interviews that lent themselves to health and developmental-behavioral counseling. I felt like I was doing important work, possessing relevant personal experience to draw on with my years of single parenting on a strict budget and coping with child-raising challenges.

It was also our domain to motivate parents to bring their child to the Emergency Room when we found serious symptoms. This wasn't easy, there being a lack of knowledge and trust on the part of those who'd had "run ins" with judgmental MDs who had no idea of the multiple day-to-day survival problems these people faced. Many lived in slum housing conditions, as this period preceded urban renewal or any ordinances regarding housing standards. Welfare was in the hands of each town's Overseer of the Poor, and Medicaid, though on the way, was not yet operational. Much of the care had to be free (up to the visiting nurse to arrange); otherwise, fear of a huge bill stood in the way, and pride superceded the need to be seen medically. Communication blocks were a big factor, as the educated medical establishment often couldn't speak poor folks' language and vice versa. Hospital personnel were turned off by the lack of clean clothes worn by these patients, while the visiting nurse knew that they lacked a washing facility or money to pay the water bill. Advocacy was our thrust, but was often met with resistance.

I found myself as frustrated as the families, and felt a new focus was needed to give them a better chance at life and their children a better start. I voiced this to my nursing director, Betsy Davis, always a creative and sensitive listener and innovative pragmatist. I found my concerns were in sympathy with others who were also aware of the glaring need in our community. Betsy sparked an idea with Dr. Joan Babbott, the director of Maternal Child Health at the Vermont Health Department, who had heard of an experimental new way of delivering pediatric primary care by pediatric nurse practitioners.

These two dynamic leaders spawned a plan, and I was the lucky one to implement it. Through an incredible alliance with The University of Vermont (UVM) College of Medicine, the Winooski Model Cities Project (a federal program under the Johnson administration), the Health Department, and the Visiting Nurse Association, a vision was transformed into a new paradigm of primary care delivery in which a nurse and physician collaborated. This was a new way of being for each—replacing the nurse as handmaiden to the doctor with a trusting partnership between them. It took mutual courage and patience. It was also an education for the physician to learn to appreciate the nurse's experience, judgment, and capability.

Dr. James McKay, the chief of pediatrics at the Mary Fletcher Hospital, and also president of the American Academy of Pediatrics, was my sponsor. I was off to Boston's Massachusetts General Hospital and Northeastern University each week for didactic instruction, and back for practicum in Burlington, doing physical exams with UVM medical students, supervised by Dr. Carol Lee Phillips of the UVM College of Medicine pediatric faculty. I graduated in 1970 as the first pediatric nurse practitioner in the state. (I believe Nina Trumper of Brattleboro was in a class before me, but worked in Massachusetts.) Susan Heath of the VNA followed a year or two later, graduating from the Denver program, and she and I were to later work together providing pediatric care to low-income families in Chittenden and Grand Isle counties.

The summer before and the summer after I completed my program (1969 and 1970), I participated with child psychologist David Egner in directing a summer preschool screening camp—first in Burlington and the following year in Winooski—as part of the Model Cities program. To my knowledge, these were the first preschool screening programs of this type in the state. In fact, the Burlington camp was filmed for video demonstration. Using the video, I gave the keynote address at the state PTA convention, citing the preschool camp as a method of identifying children with special needs. The Winooski camp had input from Dr. Arnold Golodetz, and culminated in my publishing a paper in *Nursing Outlook* entitled "A Stitch in Time" (vol. 19, no. 7, 1971).

In the spring of 1971, we (the VNA) opened the Winooski Family Health Center on the second floor of the VFW. It was to be part of the Model Cities medical component. It was also financed by a grant from the U.S. Department of Health, Education, and Welfare (HEW) and the War on Poverty money. Winooski was, at that time, an urban poverty pocket. I had trained a group of local workers as neighborhood aides who would go from door to door spreading the word about this new center where Winooski children could be seen free for well and sick care and immunizations. "If you build it, they will come." Eligible children from newborns through age twenty-one soon filled the waiting room at the VFW building on Maple Street.

The Health Center staff consisted of myself, health aide Bernie Newsom, and secretary-receptionist Shirley Reardon, both Winooski residents. Bernie prepared the patients (height, weight, and temperatures), cleaned and stocked exam rooms, and served as community liaison. Shirley made appointments, filed charts, and transcribed all my notes from dictation. They were invaluable resources with their ties to the community and their wise counsel in this regard.

My medical backup was the Department of Pediatrics' residents, and we were under the supervision of Dr. Phillips. Each week a resident and several observing medical students would spend part of a morning seeing children whom I had identified with abnormal findings on routine physicals, and children whose acute illnesses had not resolved with treatment within the expected time frame. I had protocols with my collaborating physician from which I prescribed appropriate antibiotics for infections such as strep throat. (An incubator was on site and I read the cultures.) I also treated urinary tract, middle ear, and gastrointestinal infections, along with other common childhood illnesses. I became an expert on lice, scabies, chicken pox, mumps, and rubella, as well as rubeola.

The weekly excursions for the medical students and residents were valuable because they were able to see a nurse in action and were exposed to psychosocial problems that affected a child's health or illness. I presented each child from the perspective of the whole child, not just the symptom or disease entity that we were seeing. I would say that each child came from a whole family, no matter how fragmented or dysfunctional. This was a new concept. Each family was a part of the community of which we also were a part. This was in fact the philosophy of the Health Center that made it unique and kept me dedicated to it. It was a real turnaround from the old days, which had so frustrated me and families. Early intervention and strong prevention goals had far-reaching effects.

An illustration that comes to mind is that of two very undernourished boys who exhibited nervousness and darting, apprehensive eyes every time I saw them. Their single mother was very poor but was genuinely loving and conscientious, coming to the nutrition class that I held regularly and keeping all appointments. After weeks of getting to know and trust me, they shared a secret which explained everything. The cockroaches in their apartment were so bad they couldn't eat. They would drop off the exposed hot-water pipes onto their toast as they brought it to their mouths. With information like this, we could get environmental help for the family through the Model Cities network. Subsequently, we saw a gradual weight gain and a calmed demeanor when they returned for followup appointments. A similar case was the "failure to thrive" baby whose bottle nipples were being chewed by rats as she lay in her crib. These made for very good learning situations for residents who otherwise might have remained ignorant of such circumstances in the artificial enclosure of a hospital.

In addition to physicals and sick child exams, I held classes for mothers on good nutrition, obesity, child development, and common childhood problems. I worked closely with the schools, both parochial and public. Many of the children discussed were those that I had in preschool camp the previous summer. All of these activities contributed to greater continuity of care and more thorough data collection.

Another aspect of my position included counseling, supervised by Janet Munt, ACSW, psychiatric social worker at the VNA. There were many psychosocial issues, including alcoholism, domestic violence, and of course, child abuse. Mine was an appropriate role, as the family members felt comfortable with me. In 1975, I became a member of the Child Abuse Team at the Medical Center, composed of chair Theresa Tomasi, ACSW, several pediatricians, Dr. John Tampas, radiologist, and Janet Munt. This later evolved into the Child Protection Team. It encompassed representatives from various agencies such as Howard Mental Health, Agency of Human Services, Family Resource Center, and Spectrum.

Another outgrowth of the nursing position I held was membership on various committees feeding into state policy on daycare rules and regulations. It was prestigious for nursing to be called upon and listened to for input into such important issues. Prior to this time, organized daycare was nonexistent.

The wonderful things about the Health Center as it grew were the sense of community and the sense of trust, which had emerged, in me—a nurse practitioner—as their primary caregiver. This was a new role in health care and the Health Center was new entity. The people used it more and more, feeling that here was a safe place where they could be heard without being judged. They were glad their children felt good about physicals and even shots, and that they had someone to talk with about their problems. I went on 24-hour first call (no answering service) and had a special "hot line" installed in my home. If I was unavailable they called the pediatric resident who might know them through previous consulting. Emergency room visits and hospital admissions declined, although this was difficult to document in those days when we did not have computer access.

All good things must come to an end, and so did the Model Cities Project for Winooski. Because the Health Center was such a success, we were designated as one of the three state locations to receive money from the Vermont State Health Department by way of a Children and Youth

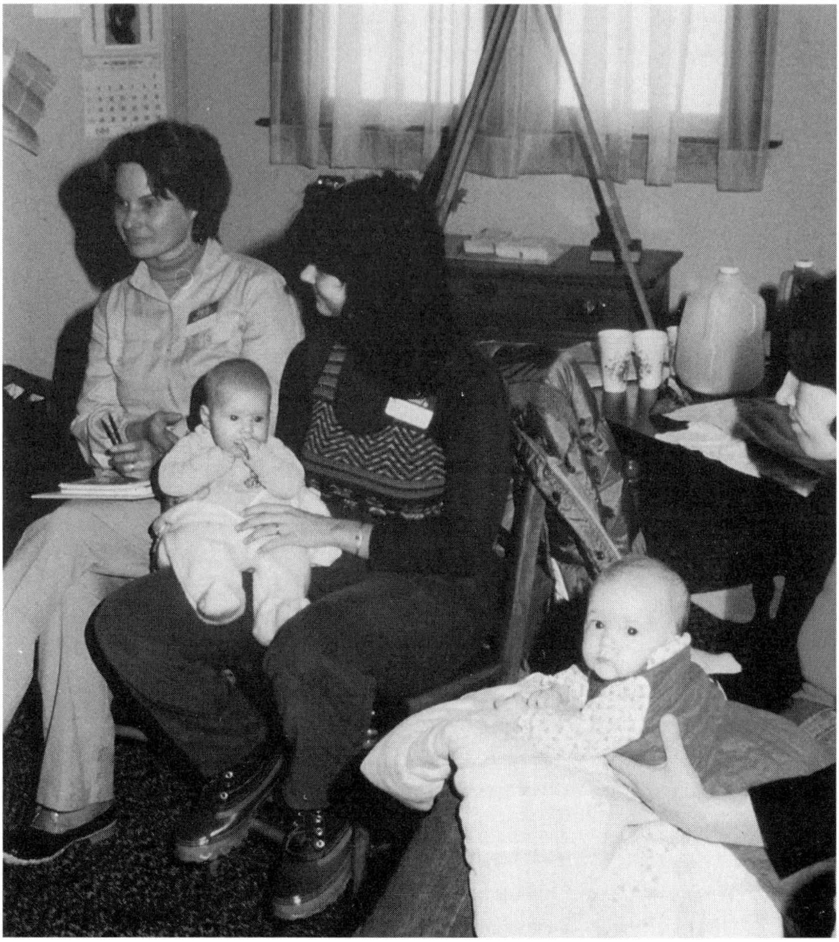

Courtesy Vermont Department of Health

Jan Campbell, RN, leads a parent-child group, Burlington, 1985.

grant (another federal program) out of HEW. There were many guidelines to follow. It was to be a multi-disciplinary interface with the families we served, namely the working poor. We hired another pediatric nurse practitioner, a social worker, a nutritionist, a coordinator, another health aide, and a medical typist. Our pediatrician was Dr. Paul Young, and later Dr. William Hodgkin, who were on site one half-day each week. Our facility was housed on the second floor of a renovated Winooski landmark. On the first floor was a dentist, also part of the project, and a low income daycare, an outgrowth of the Model City project. We collaborated on our mutual children, and were an enriching resource for each other.

A playgroup was supported by the various disciplines. A one-way mirror allowed the parents and me to observe children's interactions and developmental skills. The group was led by Lisa Simon, a woman of considerable capability. She acted as a role model for the observing parents. My membership in the Child Protection Team continued as well as my counseling. Again, the trust that was present due to my nurse practitioner role was pivotal in helping families understand my responsibility to report suspected child abuse. Reporting was always done with the family's knowledge.

The Winooski Valley Family Health Center (we now were also serving Colchester) ran successfully until 1980 when political expediency reared its head in the way of budget cuts under the new administration. Public outcry, meetings, letters to the editor, newspaper articles, television reports, petitions, even the pleas of Chittenden County senators failed to sway the prevailing powers. Federal cutbacks ruled the day and there was no compromise to be had. Funding was eliminated despite the admonition that the decision was penny wise and pound foolish.

Recalling these twelve years of my nursing life raises many thoughts for me. What role should and does nursing have in society? If nursing had spoken with one voice against the closing of the Health Center, might we have influenced public policy? Nurses have the unique privilege of foreseeing the results of poor health care decisions. However, we are pragmatists and so busy doing what we do so well that we often fail to speak out about those matters that impact our patients and our profession. We have important things to say and we need to say them—together.

Our model was outrageously ahead of its time. Unfortunately, politicians trying to save money by failing to fund these clinics short-shrifted children for years to come. Now in the 1990s we are paying the price of neglect. Many of the current crises of domestic violence, abused children, and children with emotional, physical, and spiritual problems might have been averted by the multifaceted interventions modeled by the Health Center.

On another tack—my preparation for pioneering this new nursing role of pediatric nurse practitioner involved all my life experiences. As a diploma graduate of a progressive school of nursing, and as a woman with family-leadership experience, I was able to be admitted to a leading edge program at a time when the philosophy stressed capability and performance rather than academic credentials. Nurse practitioners of that era proved that nurses in advanced practice have a great contribution to make. In so doing, they have blazed the way for others to follow.

—Jane Packard Bryant, RN, PNP, CHTP

Nursing Intervention: Parenting Skills

A Personal Account

Born in 1942, I grew up in West Virginia and later in a suburb of New York City. I was sheltered, protected from the realities of the world. As a teen, it was clear that the acceptable career choice for my peers and me was to become a wife and mother with responsibility for making a comfortable home for a husband and children. However, my grandmother was a stern woman who believed in women learning. She had completed college and worked as a teacher until the birth of her four sons. I was allowed to work summers in high school and to go to college.

The last two years of high school I worked as an "aide" (no training and very little supervision) on the maternity floor of a small hospital near us. Every day I was allowed to bathe and feed newborn infants and to "make them pretty" for their mothers who were "resting for the transition to home." Mother and baby stayed in the hospital at least 10 days. Four times I was allowed to watch deliveries. In every instance, the mother was sedated and the physician managed the delivery with forceps. I was curious, overwhelmed, and awed by the infants who were born tiny, bluish, and crying for life.

Although I was unaware of it at the time, great strides were being made in the understanding of infants, mothering, and the interaction between parent and child. World War II was a time when thousands of infants and young children were separated from parents because they were sent out of cities to "safer" ground, or because they were orphaned in the tragedy of war. Building on the work of Piaget, Ames, Ilg and Gesell, and others were exploring and defining for parents "normal behaviors" of infants and young children. Benjamin Spock wrote his bestseller encouraging parents to follow their common sense in understanding what was needed in caring for their infants. In the mid-to-late 1940s, Anna Freud and Rene Spitz were exploring children's response to trauma and separation. This was the beginning of understanding children as special people who come into this world with a specific need for interactions with parents or other responsible adults; with a need for caring and nurturing without which they literally fade away and die. The focus of research at this time was either on children who were mentally ill, children diagnosed as schizophrenic or autistic, or on exploring the physical and cognitive capacity of children. It was the foundation of understanding developmental ages and stages and the impact of environmental trauma.

As I was progressing through my latency, pre-teen, and teen years, John Bowlby was doing his seminal research on attachment and separation. Margaret Mahler and others were developing the theories of the psychological development and the evolution of emotional object constancy in infants. Mothers were discovered as important and powerful in the lives of their infants. Conversely, they were being blamed for mental illness, poor school performance, and other social ills that evolved in the lives of their children.

In 1960, I went to college: Duke University in Durham, North Carolina. The choice was made because I wanted to be a nurse (stemming from my hospital aide jobs) and I wanted to go to college where I would be exposed to a broader scope of learning: languages, history, sociology, art—whatever I could find. What I learned was not expected. Duke University School of Nursing had a strong focus on interpersonal interactions and psychiatric nursing. From the first week continuing throughout the four years, we did weekly detailed documentation of interactions with clients (what the client said, what we said, what we observed of body language, what we felt during the exchange). This exercise consolidated a talent for careful observation of interpersonal interactions.

In addition, Durham, and Duke itself, was still segregated. I was curious and stunned noticing that gas stations had water fountains labeled "white" and "colored." When my friends and I went into town on the bus we always got a seat; no matter that we were young and the bus was full. Although the Civil Rights movement was beginning, it was not a big part of life in the contained world of Duke. My first two years of work in the hospital was on "white" floors. Patients had either private or semi-private rooms. The floors were well staffed and call bells were answered. Nursing students were assigned to two or three patients for the full shift—adult medicine, surgery, obstetrics, orthopedics. There were no black patients. However, in my junior year, 1963, I was assigned to work on a "colored unit." My world was turned upside down. These floors had four large rooms with sixteen to twenty beds. One or two nurses were responsible for the floor with the help of four students. Opening up dressers or pulling curtains around a bed caused hundreds of cockroaches to scurry. Rarely did the patients ask for help. I did not understand.

Later that same year, I did a public health rotation. As I drove out into the country, I searched dirt roads and farm lanes to find my patients, all of them black, most of them pregnant. Suddenly I was in a world where large families lived in simple cabins, many with dirt floors, and some without running water. Despite the level of poverty, I found the families warm, welcoming, and surprisingly content. Each of them had a private garden plot so no one seemed hungry. There were lots of children who all seemed welcomed and cherished. No one moved very fast and no one wanted to participate in my public health education "lessons." Each mother was willing to tell me about how she cared for her infant, how each helped the child grow to be "strong and sassy." It was a world I knew I did not understand. I knew that I could not go back to work in hospitals where I saw pain, helplessness, and overwhelming disrespect for vulnerable humans. I wanted to work in a world where clients were more in charge.

For three years I worked for the Visiting Nurse Association of New York on the Lower East Side of New York City. Each day was a cacophony of cultures, mundane and exotic diseases, and survival. The Vietnam War started, and I began to visit apartments where young women and young men lived, drifting, using drugs, withdrawing from the world. The questions of how people survive and how they make choices about their lives came up daily.

I was married and started my own family. In New York, Elizabeth Bing was teaching the Lamaze method of childbirth and we were fortunate enough to have our first child in a hospital that supported fathers attending labor and delivery. We moved, and I learned how unprepared one can be for parenting; how lack of support systems and maternal role models interfere with the transition to confident, competent mothering. I was teaching childbirth classes and learning about the stress of other young transient mothers and about the resonant stress of infants. I was learning to understand depression.

In 1969, we moved to Vermont. Expecting my second child within months, I learned that there was no preparation for childbirth as I had experienced it. Fathers were not yet allowed in the delivery room and infants stayed in the nursery. However, by this time women had a voice. There were models for collective action. Research focused on growing concern for parent–child interactions: LeBoyer's gentle birth, Klaus and Kendal, newborn attachment and bonding, Thomas and Chess on infant temperament, Brazelton, and the more ominous writing from Ray Helfer and others on the battered child, and the cycle of abuse. The Visiting Nurse Association in Burlington hired me. Linda Abbott and I started childbirth preparation classes and worked with other members of the community to advocate for fathers' attendance during labor and delivery, and for rooming-in of infants. I began to understand the power of birth as a time of transition and growth, the potential for life change when women learned to define need, make choices, and feel successful during labor and delivery. I learned to support women in knowing their infants before they were born, to enhance the sense of being a mother and of attachment during pregnancy.

By 1974, I had worked with hundreds of families preparing for childbirth, attended births, and provided home visiting support in the immediate postpartum period. During the summer of 1974, my colleagues and I did followup visits to all infants in Chittenden County who were between twelve and eighteen months of age. By this time, it was clear to me that one could, during the pregnancy, identify families who were likely to have difficult adjustments to parenting. With the help of Dr. Herbert Durfee, chair of the Department of Obstetrics and Gynecology, Medical Center Hospital of Vermont, I obtained a contract with the largest community practice of obstetricians. In the early 1970s, Dr. Durfee had hired a nurse midwife from England to join the practice. For three years I was able to work with the midwives and physicians. In the down time of waiting in the examining room, I talked to women about their expectations of labor, of the infant, of their support systems. If they had no support system, if they were ambivalent about the infant, unsure of parenting, or if they revealed issues of concern (domestic violence, substance abuse, mental illness, history of protective services) they were offered home visits for up to two years following the birth of the baby.

During the four years of this project I learned to observe parent–infant interactions, to understand the impact of family dynamics, and to understand the cycle of repeating the parenting of one's own childhood. I learned the power of nursing. People in general perceive nurses as helpful and therefore let them into their lives as agents of change. At the Visiting Nurse Association we developed a team of maternal and child health nurses with the purpose of increasing expertise and focus on young families. In 1978, under the direction of Janet Munt, MSW, we applied for and received a large federal grant to develop a program, based on nursing interventions, for the prevention of neglect and abuse of children. Using principles of health promotion, health education, supportive counseling, and relationship building, we worked with families to support attachment, develop parenting skills, and help parents become careful observers of their infant's development.

In the early 1980s, Selma Fraiberg, Burton White, and Stanley Greenspan were expanding the body of knowledge related to infant emotional development. Tiffany Field, Kathryn Barnard, and Joy Osofsky were part of the explosion of writing related to the impact of depressed mothers on infants, on infant cues, on "the dance between parent and child." Side-by-side with parents, we were learning what works and what

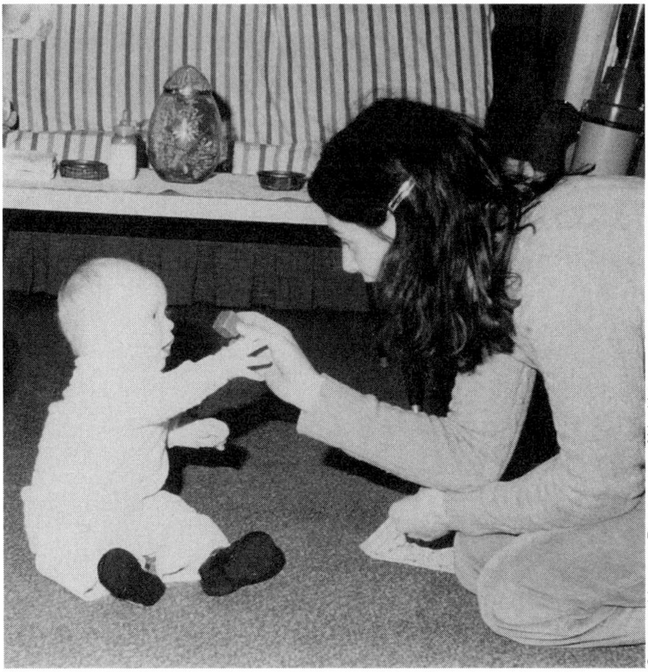

Kathleen Ready, RN, assesses child development during a home visit, circa 1985.

doesn't work, how people grow (both parent and child), and what circumstances interfere to a degree that parents need permission to take care of themselves and to feel good about letting go of their children and their parenting. Research on the impact of alcohol, cigarettes, and poor nutrition forced increasing concern on intervention before and during pregnancy. In 1986, we started the Family Room in the H.O. Wheeler Community School in Burlington. Drawing on the expertise of early childhood education, we built a place where isolated parents could find community, with an opportunity to learn to play, and to learn to observe and support their children learning. The focus on children in families in the school setting allowed an opportunity for primary prevention information on environmental safety, good nutrition, exercise, and skills training for adults as well as for children.

The 1990s have brought an increased awareness and focus on the role of fathers and other important adults in the lives of children. We are learning to support and strengthen this extended network for children. The National Institute for Clinical Infant Studies has brought us the HeartStart work, so we can now assess and support development of curiosity, feelings of competency, impulse control, capacity to communicate, and capacity to empathize. Current brain research leads us toward an increasingly complex understanding of timing and the long-term impact of missed opportunity. Social and medical research continues to reinforce the impact of violence and neglect in destroying the health and the potential of our children. We have moved from simple understanding of physical and cognitive development of the child to curiosity about the interaction between mother and child, to understanding more about the power and impact of the child on the interaction. Now we are moving toward an increasingly complex understanding of the role and the work of the broader systems of family and community in the lives of our children. With an interest in maternal child health, community health nurses have a unique opportunity to utilize skills of assessment, the role as educator, and basic characteristics of nurturing to improve family health and, by extension, community well-being.

—Elizabeth Allen, RN, BSN

Pediatric Rehabilitation Nursing at the Vermont Achievement Center, 1987–1995

THE VERMONT ACHIEVEMENT CENTER was established in Rutland in 1937 as the Vermont Association for the Crippled. Founded by an organization begun by seven women's groups—including the Vermont State Nurses' Association—it became best known by its acronym, VAC. In the 1970s, the name was changed to the Vermont Achievement Center to better reflect the broadening scope of children being served. From 1972 to 1995, there was a pediatric inpatient unit at VAC in Rutland that provided rehabilitation nursing to infants, children, and teenagers.

The founders' 1937 statement of purpose included plans for an inpatient pediatric convalescent service for children from birth to twenty-one years of age. This part of their plan was to be finally realized in 1972. The twenty-bed unit was known as the PCS (Pediatric Convalescent Services) unit, and was built as an addition to the original building at 88 Park Street with funds appropriated by the Vermont Legislature. Children were admitted to the inpatient unit by medical referral if they had a nursing, medical, or rehabilitation need. Many children were there for long-term care, for short-term postconvalescence requiring skilled nursing care, or for intensive rehabilitation. The Center had its own staff of speech/language pathologists, occupational and physical therapists, as well as teachers. Other children came for progressive casts, wheelchair education, bowel/bladder programming, medication adjustment, and program evaluations. In *The Vermont Achievement Center: 40 Years of Service* (Rutland, Vt.: Academy Books), author George Bellerose reported that the late 1970s found the twenty-bed unit often with empty beds. This was also true into the late 1980s, when I arrived. Some of the diagnoses of the children served by the PCS unit at that time included cerebral palsy, shaken baby syndrome, autism, seizure disorders, failure to thrive, neuromuscular disorders, prematurity, and bowel/bladder incontinence.

In 1989, the unit expanded its services and changed its philosophy to encourage more family participation. In July 1989, The Medical Center Hospital of Vermont in Burlington began a new surgery for some children with spastic cerebral palsy. It was known as selective posterior rhizotomy. The surgery was long and intensive. It utilized electromyelography in the operating room to identify which particular nerves were causing the spasticity. These nerves would then be cut by the surgeon to reduce the spasticity. Each child would then spend a few days in the Medical Center before being transferred to the PCS unit for a six-week intensive therapy program. Parents and siblings would come to the Center and stay in the parent apartment so that the parents could be involved and reassured of the progress of their child. It was very stressful for parents—more than they anticipated. Previously, their child walked with a spastic gait. The surgery removed the spastic gait, and the child was therefore temporarily unable to walk immediately after surgery and on arrival on the PCS unit. The rehabilitation team—consisting of parents, nurses, therapists, and social workers—provided an intensive six-week rehabilitation program concentrating on helping the child learn to walk anew. The child was then discharged with a therapy program for home and intermittent outpatient visits.

This was the beginning of moving our practice toward family-centered care. We had always been patient-centered, but the family is the center of a child's life. We needed to professionally support these families in caring for their child. We were the professionals in our disciplines, but the families were the professionals in the care of their child. The families helped open our eyes in ways we had not even considered. Family-centered care—frequently challenging, but always rewarding and dynamic!

Next, we began to take medically challenged children. Infants with bronchopulmonary dysplasia needing oxygen, apnea monitors, and pulse oximeters were admitted. Adolescents with neurological challenges from head injury, brain tumors, and cerebral vascular accidents were another new group we served. Both groups required nurses to update their clinical skills to manage our changing population and to meet the child's individual needs. Many of the children we had served were school-aged. Babies and teens were expanding our expertise in addressing the developmental needs of a broader range of ages.

Just when we thought we had all bases covered, something would develop that would indicate a need for additional resources. One toddler who had a tracheotomy tube most of her life would pull out the trach tube and throw it across the room when angry or bored! Med-Surg 201 and Pediatrics never prepared us for this! This highlighted for us that a child might benefit from a behavioral program in order for the rehabilitation goals to be met. It was a boon to parents to have the professional support to help them follow through the program during the nonprogram hours when they would be in the parent apartment with their child.

Activities were an important part of the PCS unit. Each year, children from the VAC school program and our PCS children went to the Vermont State Fair in Rutland. In the winter, they enjoyed the snowmobile rides from VAST (Vermont Association of Snow Travelers). Dairy Day in Montpelier was always a big attraction. And, close at home, swimming in VAC's therapeutic pool was always fun. Dances with real DJs were a favorite with the teens.

Since our actual license was that of a skilled nursing home, we fell under federal and state regulations for nursing homes. Needless to say, we were a bit of an anomaly as a pediatric nursing home. In 1987, new federal regulations promulgated under Public Law 100-203 required all nursing assistants working in nursing homes to have specific core education and be tested on these in order to work in any nursing home. To study for the test, our nursing assistants had to learn all about dentures, at the same time our unit orientation required learning about the tooth fairy and orthodontia!

The census rose on the PCS unit as we added our new services. But times were changing. More services became available to medically fragile children in their homes. The Vermont Achievement Center closed the doors of the PCS unit in 1995. There would now be a greater need for pediatric rehabilitation nurses in home care.

—Faith Brothers, MS, RN, CRRN

Maternal Child Health: The Hospital Experience

THE BABY BOOM began in the late 1940s as men returned from the war and families were reunited. The hospital had become the location of choice for labor and delivery. The popular thinking was that hospitals provided a safer environment than the home. Physicians encouraged it—it helped to ease their heavy workload when all their patients were in the hospital; and the increased number of families with hospitalization insurance supported it. For hospitals, space became a significant problem. At times, delivery rooms resembled assembly lines. The Hill Burton Act of 1948 helped hospitals to build and expand to meet the need for more beds. Between 1948 and 1953, a total of 102,000 hospital beds were added throughout the country.*

Early prenatal care was encouraged, and for women who could afford it (there was no Medicaid), the first visit to the doctor was after they were "sure" they were pregnant—which meant a few missed periods and confirming symptoms. Test strips were a long way off.

Labor and delivery units were sterile, alien places, certainly not "user friendly." Anesthesia was usually administered during delivery. In rural hospitals, the nurse often "dropped" ether onto a gauze mask which covered the patient's nose and mouth. Forcep deliveries were common.

Obstetrics was a male specialty. In 1955, Sister Gallant, RHSJ, was assigned to DeGoesbriand Hospital in Burlington. She was a nurse midwife who had received her midwifery education at the highly valued Santa Fe, New Mexico, program. However, Vermont was not yet ready to accept a nurse-midwife—a loss for her professionally, a loss for residents and students who could have learned from her, and a loss to those women who might have been her patients.

Postpartum hospitalization averaged five days. For mothers with large families—and there were many of them—a hospital stay often meant respite time. Babies were only brought to the mother for daytime feed-

---

*Susie Berg Waldman, "What Good Nursing Means To You," U.S. Public Affairs Pamphlet No. 60A, 1955, 6. Vermont State Nurses' Association Special Collection, Library Research Annex, The University of Vermont, Burlington.

ings. Few women breastfed and it was not encouraged. In between times, Mom and Dad could peek through the nursery window to observe their beautiful babe. Fathers had a passive role in the birthing process. Most men, after delivering their wife to the labor unit door—to enter was verboten—went to a waiting room or hospital cafeteria until the doctor came to say, "You have a beautiful baby (sex added)!" So the cigars were handed around and Dad would go back to work—and hold and cuddle his newborn several days later when the baby left the hospital for home.

Many nurses found obstetrical floors happy places to work. Nurses taught the basics of infant care and spent much of their time reassuring new moms that they would do well. As is always the case, nurses had the responsibility of observing and identifying early changes in the status of mother and infant. There were sad times—erythroblastosis was a dreaded outcome of an Rh incompatible birth; low-birth-weight infants might fail to survive; babies with serious birth defects were felt to have little chance to lead productive lives; and the young mother with signs of postpartum depression would need psychiatric care before being able to assume her new role. But for the majority of infants and mothers, the postpartum hospital stay was one of joy and fulfillment.

Since the 1950s, the technical and scientific progress that has taken place has dramatically impacted the way infants and children are cared for in hospitals. To name but a few: The whiskey nipples used for infants requiring sedation for procedures are no longer kept in the medicine cupboard; state of the art anesthesia and pain control is utilized pre- and postoperatively. Croup tents—and the ice that went with them—have melted from sight. Croup is no longer an indication for hospital admission; it can be treated with medication and nebulizers. Kinetic beds, apnea monitors, pulse oximetry, vaccine for formerly life-threatening diseases, phototherapy, rhogam, Apgar scores—all have made a difference in the care and treatment of infants and children and in the nursing skills required to provide that care. Advances in pediatric surgery, including the miniaturization of needles and instruments, has allowed a meningocele to be operated on within twenty-four hours of birth, and cleft palate repair to be done on infants. And lest we forget, we rejoiced at the advent of antibiotics that proved to be the blessing of pediatric acute care—and all too often the bane, as drug-resistant organisms have proliferated.

In the early years, in most hospitals, low-birth-weight newborns and those needing closer observation were kept in a separate area of the newborn nursery. Seriously ill newborns were "specialed" on the pediatric unit by acute care pediatric nurses. In the late 1960s, the Medical Center Hospital of Vermont (MCHV) in Burlington established an intensive care nursery in proximity to the newborn nursery. Staff were recruited from

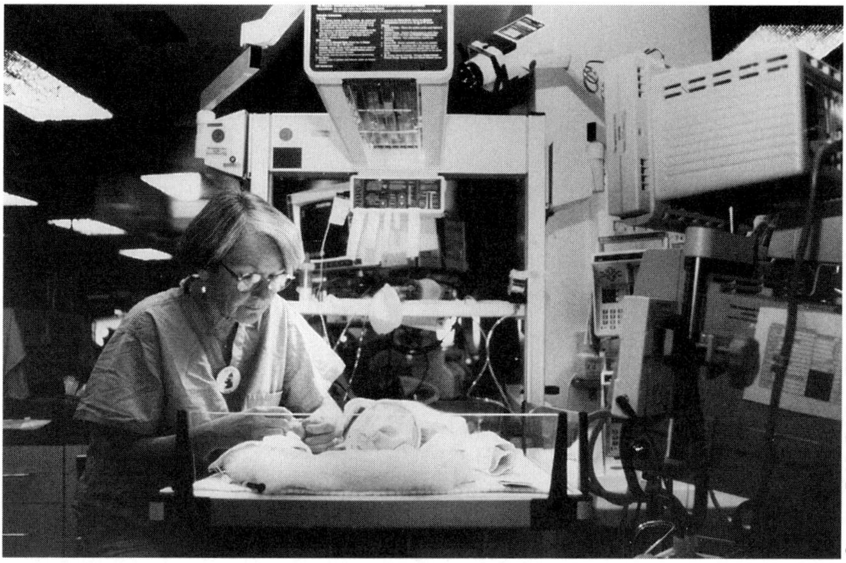

Courtesy Public Relations Office, Fletcher Allen Health Care

Nursing in neonatal intensive care nursery

pediatrics and the newborn nursery to receive further education in neonatal intensive care. Rose Anderson, RN, was the first nurse coordinator of the intensive care nursery, which in 1973 became a regional neonatal intensive care nursery (NICU).

At that time, Dr. Jerrold Lucey and Dr. Alastair Philip of MCHV, and Dr. George Little of Dartmouth-Hitchcock Medical Center, Hanover, New Hampshire, established the Vermont/New Hampshire Regional Neonatal Intensive Care Program. Early research (Stanley Graven) had promoted regional centers, where skilled staff and special equipment situated in a specific locale could better serve the critical newborn. If indicated, prenatal patients were admitted for delivery at the regional centers, or if delivered at a local hospital, the newborn was transported to the center by specially trained teams, consisting of a nurse and pediatric resident. St. Michael's College Rescue provided ambulance coverage for transport. This protocol is still in effect. In 1979, the Vermont Regional Perinatal Program became a separate entity. Martha Grady, RN, became the nurse coordinator, and served in that capacity from 1979 until her retirement in 1998. The current coordinator in Vermont is Mary Ingvoldstad, RN, BS.

Despite advanced technology, there has always been significant morbidity attached to the NICU. Babies with early gestational ages and low birthweights who never would have made it in past years now survive. Nursing research helped to initiate change that has transformed the

NICU from the usual noisy environment of a critical care unit to one that is darkened and quiet. It has been demonstrated that this has reduced neonatal stress and has decreased oxygen consumption.

Parents are partners in care with the staff of the NICU. Parent education is an integral part of the total care of these infants. As a baby shows consistent improvement, he or she may be assigned to a special room on the pediatric unit or transferred back to the local hospital. Complicated special equipment is now rarely needed for the infant at discharge; if it is indicated, the nursing staff is responsible for instructing the parents in its use.

Nursing has effected positive changes in the environment of the pediatric unit. White uniforms have been replaced or covered by brightly printed aprons or colorful tops, more appealing to young children. As an undergraduate at The University of Vermont, Katie Geran's senior project ("Child Life") proposed the development of a play program in pediatrics. In 1980, when she came back to MCHV as administrator of the Women and Children's Program, she brought her project to fruition. Sylvia Wilson was head nurse and Peggy Mahoney Sharpe was assistant head nurse. They were enthusiastic. With the support of Rosemary Dale, director of nursing, and Dr. James McKay, director of pediatric medicine "Child Life" became a reality. To implement the program, Ellen Good became the first "play lady" who acted as a tutor and addressed developmental issues. The program has become an integral part of the pediatric unit and continues to grow. Nursing has fostered efforts to make pediatric care child- and family-friendly. From the days of the 1940s when parents were allowed to visit a few hours weekly and discouraged from holding the child for fear of cross-contamination, has come the 24-hour stay and partnership with nurses in the care of their child. In the maternity unit, babies now stay in the room with their moms prior to discharge, usually twenty-four to forty-eight hours after delivery.

The 1980s and the advent of managed care witnessed significant changes in pediatric care. Hospital stays shortened and pediatric high tech home care became the norm. In-hospital patients were sicker and required more nursing skill and knowledge. Specialty practices including oncology and neonatal nurse practitioners began to evolve. Pediatric critical care units came into being.

Meanwhile, the hospital nurse forms one link in the chain of pediatric nursing care. Pediatric nurse practitioners provide primary care in many settings. Pediatric oncology has become a nursing specialty. Community health nurses work toward early intervention and maternal/child education and counseling. Breast feeding support has brought the credentialing of the lactation consultant. School nurses are asked to provide advanced care for children with special needs, along with participating in health

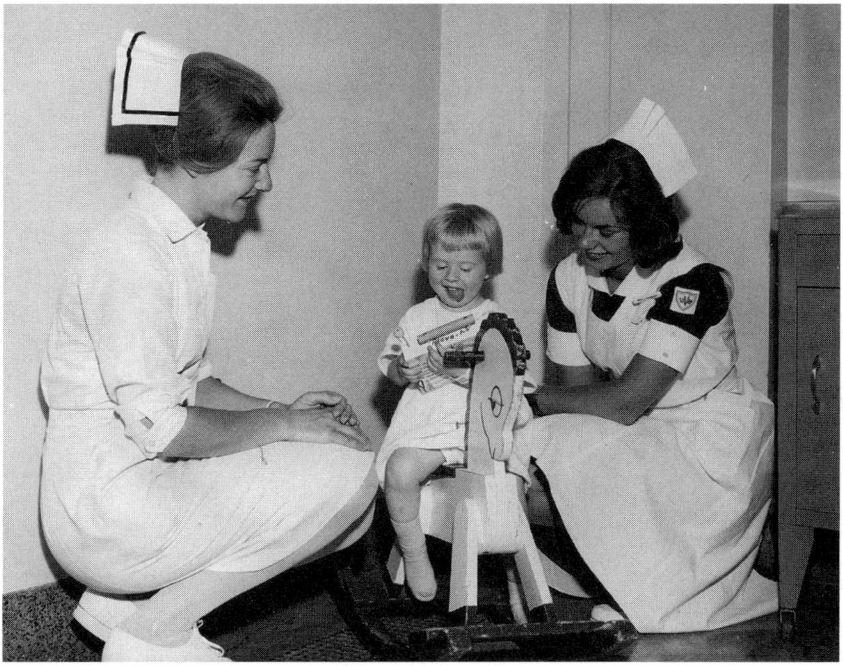

Courtesy The University of Vermont School of Nursing

University of Vermont faculty member and student with pediatric patient, 1965

education in the classroom. Collaborative practice has allowed physicians and nurses to learn from one another. Other disciplines have contributed to the breadth of care that can now be delivered.

The problems and frustrations that affect the nurse in maternal/child health are the same that affect the greater nursing community: the lack of respect and value given to the work of the nurse; the continuing struggle with nursing practice models, including the supervision of ancillary personnel; and an increasing work load where the bottom line and not quality of care becomes the primary consideration.

But the 1990s have reaped rewards also: the variety of opportunities and different avenues within the profession that a nurse can choose to follow, an increasing collaborative relationship among nurses and other members of the health care community, continuous improvement in the way care is delivered, and a heightened awareness of the power of nursing's collective voice to effect positive change for the good of their patients.

—Jane Campbell, RNC, FNP, MEd
with contributions from
Kathleen Geran, RN, MS
Martha Grady, RN, MSN
Margaret Mahoney Sharpe, RN, BSN

Nurse-Midwifery in Vermont

THE GROWTH of nurse-midwifery in Vermont during the 1960s was directly related to the growing women's health movement and consumer demand for family-centered care, decreased technology in birth, and increased use of birthing rooms. Consumers were demanding a choice of providers, choice of location for birth, and alternative options in how their births would occur. Childbirth education classes and availability of nurse-midwives went hand-in-hand with the similar goal of educating women and couples about pregnancy and options for natural childbirth.

In 1968, Vermont was one of the first states in the nation to initiate nurse-midwifery into the care of pregnant women. The pioneer in this early success was John Maeck, MD, then-chair of the Department of Obstetrics and Gynecology at Medical Center Hospital of Vermont. Dr. Maeck clearly recognized the importance and value of incorporating midwifery care into the traditional obstetrical approach, and he understood that through this professional collaboration, women and their families would be better served. The partnership of nurse-midwives with obstetricians combined the supportive woman-focused approach of midwifery with the medical-technological approach of specialty physicians. Dr. Maeck saw this as a necessary synergy in providing the best care possible. He also provided the leadership and vision necessary to gain support from the entire medical faculty and other physicians in the state.

As Dr. Maeck brought nurse-midwives into Vermont, he gained the enthusiasm and support of Mrs. Claire M. Lintilhac of Stowe, Vermont. Mrs. Lintilhac was a British-trained nurse and midwife who was raised and educated in China before coming to the United States in the 1950s. This partnership provided a solid supportive foundation on which nurse-midwifery in Vermont has been able to thrive.

Dr. Maeck hired the first nurse-midwife to practice in Vermont in 1968. Her name was Josephine Morgan, a British-trained midwife. This expansion of the obstetric team was a direct result of the growing realization by the medical staff that as obstetric care shifted from general practice to obstetric practice, medical staff were becoming increasingly involved in normal routine obstetric care. To serve the needs of low-risk pregnant women, and to ensure that women at higher risk for obstetric problems received adequate attention, the Department of Obstetrics and

Gynecology decided that certified nurse-midwives (CNMs) could help provide the full range of comprehensive, efficient, and cost-effective services to all obstetric patients. The added skills of the CNMs in childbirth education, counseling, and labor support were recognized as assets for comprehensive obstetric care. Miss Morgan spent most of her approximately three years at The University of Vermont introducing the professional and lay community to the concept and potential of nurse-midwifery. Although Miss Morgan practiced in office clinical practice, the majority of her efforts were directed toward exploring the possibility of developing a nurse-midwifery educational program. The latter never materialized, but with the addition of Virginia Rudick (also from England) in 1970, and the growing receptivity toward nurse-midwifery care by patients and physicians, the antepartal clinical practice grew and Miss Rudick began labor and delivery care as well. When Miss Morgan left and Betty Bradbury, CNM, arrived, efforts were directed toward further development of the clinical aspect and teaching of medical and nursing students. Marylee Mantz, CNM, was hired in 1973 to expand the program.

Between 1968 and 1979, the nurse-midwifery staff at the Medical Center Hospital of Vermont (MCHV) evolved from one that provided only prenatal care and limited labor and delivery care to one in which four, full-time CNMs followed a specific group of women throughout the reproductive cycle.

In 1977, the Lintilhac Foundation granted funding to expand the midwifery program. From 1977 to 1979, the four CNMs on staff were Deborah Spurlock, Audrey Linn, Mary Hatton, and Kathleen Keleher. These four CNMs provided greater availability of nurse-midwifery care for the full scope of practice—prenatal, postpartum, and coverage of labor and delivery. The percentage of CNM deliveries at MCHV grew from 1.8% to 16%.

In 1979, CNMs were also hired at Northwestern Medical Center, St. Albans (Ruth Johnson) and Gifford Hospital, Randolph (Karen Odato). These practices broke new ground in establishing midwifery care into Vermont hospitals and responding to consumer demand for more responsive family-centered care. These early efforts have grown, so that currently eight of fourteen Vermont hospitals (Fletcher Allen Health Care, Burlington; Northeastern Vermont Medical Center, St. Johnsbury; Porter Hospital, Middlebury; North Country Hospital, Newport; Southwestern Medical Center, Bennington; Copley Hospital, Morrisville; Gifford Hospital; and Brattleboro Memorial Hospital) employ nurse-midwives and CNMs who attend 12% of the births in Vermont—one of the highest rates in the country.

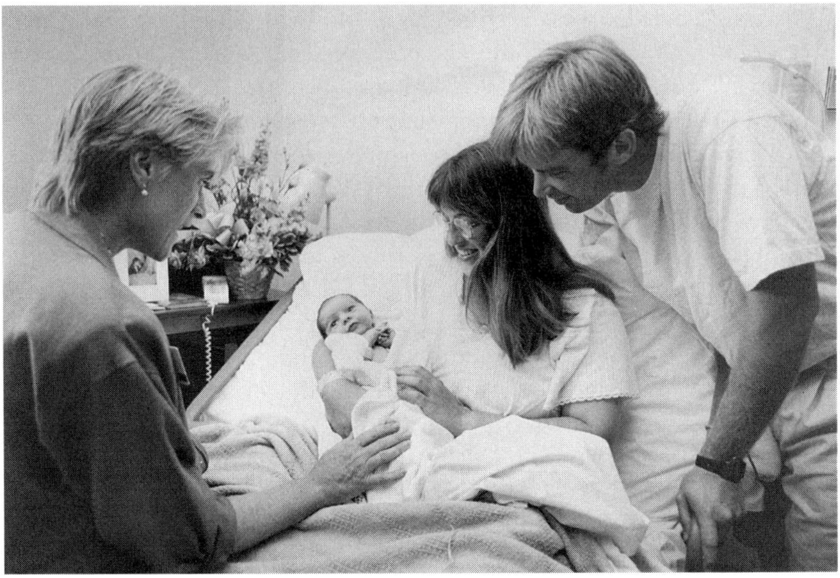

Courtesy Fletcher Allen Health Care

Kathleen Keleher, CNM, with Elizabeth and Edward Coleman and infant daughter, Kaylie, 1995.

As nurse-midwives began attending births in hospitals, there also came the transformation of hospital labor rooms into labor-delivery-recovery/postpartum rooms—one room care—which provided for continuity of care for the laboring mother and avoided the unnecessary routine of moving the woman to the traditional delivery room. Delivery in upright, squatting, or side-lying positions became commonplace. Episiotomy rates and caesarian section rates began to drop, and use of anesthesia during labor declined, in part due to the labor support provided by the CNM.

As Vermont hospitals began hiring CNMs, CNMs started to attend home births. Catherine Gates, CNM, was an early pioneer in CNM-attended home births, leading the way in setting the standard for safely triaged home births. Laura Mann, CNM, started her home birth service in 1993.

Nurse-midwives in Vermont are now active in office practice, hospitals, home birth practices, public health, education, and nursing administration.

In 1981, the Vermont Chapter of the American College of Nurse-Midwives was officially established, which strengthened the professional relationship with the national professional organization.

—Kathleen C. Keleher, CNM, MPH, FACNM

The Role of Nurses in the Evolution of Critical Care Units in Burlington, Vermont

In the early 1950s, Dr. Donald Miller performed the first open-heart surgery on a patient with a ventricular septal defect at the Mary Fletcher Hospital in Burlington. The patient survived the surgery, and operating room nurses monitored the patient, in the operating room, for twenty-four hours. Only then was the patient sent to the medical-surgical unit for recovery.

Since that time, critical care medicine and nursing have evolved to improve the way physicians and nurses serve their critically ill patients in the Burlington area and throughout Vermont. Advancement in critical care practice has dramatically increased the role and responsibilities of nurses, who continue to play a crucial role in these developments.

The Evolution of Critical Care

Modern intensive care units originated as postoperative recovery rooms. As early as 1923, the Johns Hopkins Hospital in Baltimore, Maryland, had a three-bed facility for postoperative neurosurgical patients. World War II, the Korean War, and the Vietnam War all led to significant advances in resuscitation and triage of critically ill patients, as well as advances in anesthesia, postoperative care, and the use of intravenous (IV) fluids and blood products for shock. At the same time, the concept of placing critically ill patients in suitable facilities gained support. Ventilating patients outside the operating room and using other life-sustaining technologies, such as dialysis, external defibrillation, pacemakers, cardioversion, and cardiopulmonary resuscitation (CPR) techniques, brought vital support to the critically ill. Further advancements in healthcare technology offered invasive monitoring devices, pulmonary artery catheters, and other techniques. Together, these improvements led to the formation of a designated space in hospitals—the intensive care unit (ICU)—for continuous physiologic monitoring and life-saving interventions (Calvin, 1997).

The author thanks the nursing and medical staff at Fletcher Allen Health Care for their support and guidance in preparing this article.

Medicare and Medicaid gave more people access to the healthcare system, and their payments allowed hospitals to invest in the most modern technology. As the patient population and their medical treatments grew increasingly complex, the demand for nurses rose. Private duty nurses were responsible for intensive observation and supervision of unstable or critically ill patients. Their presence also fostered increased research. Gone were the days of open wards where many patients could be watched by a few nurses and by other patients who would informally report potential problems.

Economically, it made sense to combine nurses, critically ill patients, and special equipment in a distinct location. Not every ICU had a full-time physician with twenty-four hour coverage. It was the responsibility of the nurse to deal with emergencies until the physician arrived.

During the 1950s, recovery rooms for postoperative patients were burgeoning across the United States. A nurse could pick up subtle changes in a patient's condition early enough to improve outcomes and prevent complications. Iron lungs and rocking beds were advanced technology during the polio epidemic in the early 1950s. All vital signs were closely monitored with the technology of the time and the doctor told the nurse what to do.

Nurses were using "old" technology (sphygmomanometers, chest tubes, metal tracheostomy tubes, catheters) to monitor a patient's condition and provide the necessary physical care. All information passed through the physicians, and then the nurse initiated a therapy based on a doctor's order. Physicians gave a list to the nurses of the things they could do; however, emergent CPR could not be done without a doctor. Nurses saw their limitations and the impact of these limits on patient care and called for more opportunities to learn advanced skills.

Families and other nurses had the highest esteem for these early ICU nurses who controlled the operation of the ICU by virtue of their increasing knowledge and skills. Care was reorganized around physiologic stability rather than medical diagnosis, and doctors and nurses learned together. Doctors and nurses discussed patients in detail, learned cardiac rhythms, and shared their increasing expertise. As these nurses gained more knowledge and skill, their status in the ICU rose (Calvin, 1997).

By the end of 1960, some 95% of hospitals had one or more ICUs; and the Emergency Medical system, funded by the federal government, was refined (Calvin, 1997). Technology advances included EKG monitors, ventilators, and defibrillators. With patients grouped for better observation and convenience, ICU nurses experienced "on-the-job-training." New RN graduates were hired for the ICUs. Physician-nurse collaboration grew as each taught the other. The experiences of physicians and nurses were the basis for developing protocols for managing life-threatening situations in these specialized intensive care units.

In the early-to-mid 1960s, doctors realized that they could monitor the patient's cardiac rhythms and give Lidocaine early in a suitable arrhythmia, thereby changing the mortality rate of myocardial infarctions from 30% to 15%. The only way to do this was to allow nurses to respond to the arrhythmia with the appropriate medication and equipment. This step, of course, was controversial, but it wasn't feasible to have physicians around at all times. New York Hospital (Dr. Killup), St. Vincent's in New York (Dr. Grace), and the Peter Bent Brigham Hospital in Boston (Dr. Lown) were the leaders in developing critical care units (CCU's) staffed and run by nurses and physicians.

The cardiac defibrillator also created an opportunity for nurses to care for critically ill patients. Prior to that, scalpels were outside patient rooms to open the chest for resuscitation. Modern CPR was developed and taught around that time. Nurses had the authority to use independent judgment within protocols.

Critical Care in Vermont

Until 1962, ventilated patients at Burlington's Mary Fletcher Hospital (MFH) were managed on the general nursing units. There was an increased demand for consolidating all patients needing special care in one place, the new ICU, located next to the operating room in the Patrick 3 hub. Such an arrangement saved time for the doctors and respiratory nurses who delivered care to the ventilated patients wherever they were. Joan Blondin, Sally Greenwood, and Ernie Mills worked closely with Respiratory Care and Nursing Departments to coordinate care and educate staff nurses.

Doctors instrumental in supporting the development of the intensive care unit and in educating nurses to care for more acutely ill patients were Dr. John Morgan and Dr. Robert Deane. Later in the 1960s, Dr. Tom Shinozaki joined the ICU medical staff. The Anesthesia Department oversaw the ICU, and respiratory therapy nurses cared for patients on a ventilator. (Bird and Emerson ventilators were used.) Patients with burn injuries, pediatric problems, chronic obstructive pulmonary disease, trauma, and neurological, renal, cardiac, and other disorders were cared for in the ICU.

In 1967, the ICU moved to larger quarters on Patrick Two, continuing under the direction of the Anesthesia Department. Bobbi Lambert was the head nurse in 1969. The unit consisted of eight beds, and many of the nurses were new graduates. The technology included central venous pressure monitors (CVPs) and ventilators that were the new intermittent positive pressure breathing (IPPB) machines. Nurses monitored drug drips, while doctors pushed IV drugs.

At the same time in the mid 1960s, when ICUs were burgeoning, the U.S. government gave money to states to develop CCUs in more hospitals. In Vermont, the goal was to have a CCU in each of the eleven hospitals in the state. Federal grant monies were spent to develop courses for nurses to learn lethal arrhythmia recognition, drug therapy, and defibrillation. The courses were given in Burlington at the Mary Fletcher Hospital; other hospitals in the state sent nurses there to learn. Aline Demers from The University of Vermont (UVM) School of Nursing was one of the instructors. The hospital and the state each paid for half of the six-week course. The Mary Fletcher CCU nurses monitored patients on telemetry in the Bennington Hospital during the year that the nursing staff received CCU training.

Marketing CCU courses to other hospitals became a staff development technique, and basic life support and advanced cardiac life support courses multiplied in the mid 1970s (Arthur Levy, MD, personal communication, 1998).

In 1965, the first CCU beds were opened on Arnold Three at the DeGoesbriand Hospital with four beds on a medical unit. Dr. Bouchard and Dr. Gibson were the directors, and staff was trained on-the-job to recognize lethal arrhythmia and FLBs (funny-looking beats). In 1966 or 1967, a four-bed CCU was also in existence on Shepardson Four at the Mary Fletcher Unit. Colleen Carlson was the head nurse and Dr. Anderson and Dr. Raabe were the medical directors. Nurses had classes on arrhythmia recognition. In January 1968, a UVM grant helped to establish a larger CCU on Shepardson Four South. Dr. Levy and Dr. Bouchard were instrumental in this development. In 1971, the DeGoesbriand Unit and Mary Fletcher Unit merged at the Mary Fletcher Unit, and Suzie Jerger was the head nurse. It was an eight-bed CCU on one end of Shepardson Four with a twenty-two bed step-down unit on the other end, directed by Jackie LaBounty.

At the same time, the DeGoesbriand Hospital was developing a four-bed surgical intensive care unit on the sixth floor in the new Arnold Pavilion. It was merged with the Mary Fletcher Unit in 1968 when the two hospitals merged to form the Medical Center Hospital of Vermont. Attending physicians would make rounds at the DeGoesbriand unit twice every day, and nurses rotated between the two units of the merged facility.

In 1967, Dr. Don Miller and Dr. Larry Coffin were pioneers in thoracic and cardiac surgery, and with Dr. John Davis' support the open-heart surgery program grew. Later, Dr. James Desmueles and Dr. Emil

Blair joined the open-heart team. These patients were cared for in the ICU at MFU, and nursing's responsibilities grew.

In 1974, a new coronary unit was constructed on Shepardson Four South, consisting of eight beds. Shepardson Four North was still the step-down unit which, at the time, was under the nursing direction of Sally Gagnon with Stephanie Feloney as her assistant.

In 1975, financed by a grant from the Vermont Lung Association, the Respiratory Care Unit (RCU) opened on Smith Three with four beds and plans to house nonventilated patients. Patients were to be sent to Smith Three after procedures such as thoracotomy or bronchoscopy; however, on the first day there were six patients and a ventilator. Dr. Robert Deane gave a crash course to nurses on ventilator management and respiratory care, all at the bedside. Nurses from Smith Three received on-the-job training, and new nursing graduates were hired. Prior to working in the RCU, some nurses went to the surgical intensive care unit (SICU) for monitor and ventilator training.

Nursing orientation and education for these new intensive care units was done mainly on-the-job with a preceptor. Some units assigned a nursing instructor or a staff nurse to educate new employees. Technology came gradually, so there was time to learn one thing well before moving on to the next.* Ellen Storer was the first unit instructor in the SICU, when Phyllis Raine was head nurse. Joan Webber-Jones was the unit instructor for the RCU.

Prior to 1978, doctors or nurses taught a variety of skills on the unit. The skills included IV push drugs, cardiac monitors, respiratory treatments, and changes in ventilator settings, taught in informal conferences. The need for more formalized learning was recognized, and in the late 1970s the first CORE curriculum for new ICU nurses was formally developed and presented in a classroom.

Later, an individualized program of critical care learning was developed with objectives, checklists, and a preceptor. The experienced nursing staff was offered formal all-day advanced workshops in advanced cardiac care, intraaortic balloon pumping, advanced respiratory care, CCU reviews, and advanced arrhythmia recognition. Suzette Cardin, Nursing Leader for Critical Care Services in the 1970s, and Susan Urrows, Critical Care Staff Development Coordinator, were instrumental in organizing and delivering these conferences, and teaching much of the content. Rosemary Dale, the director of nursing at the time, developed nursing divisions (Critical Care, Med-Surg, OB, Peds, and others), and each divi-

* Current technology is developing so rapidly it becomes an overwhelming task to orient a new nurse to the myriad of pumps, monitors, and machines.

sion developed protocols, guidelines, staffing regimens, and educational programs for the staff.

Nurses helped teach other nurses, and certification in critical care nursing was offered both institutionally and nationally. Nurses were gaining increasing independence and autonomy. In the early 1970s, Swan-Ganz catheters were introduced for monitoring intracardiac and pulmonary artery pressures, with physicians responsible for the catheters and the machines. Rita Barden, a new CCU head nurse, Pat Drown, head nurse in the ICU, and Suzette Cardin were instrumental in moving the responsibility of monitoring and trouble-shooting this sophisticated equipment to the practice of nursing. Protocols and procedures were developed which increased the nurse's autonomy. Nurses selected for work in ICUs were well-educated, and most physicians respected the nurses' growing knowledge and skills. During this time, a local chapter of the American Association of Critical Care Nurses was started. Its purpose was education and networking.

A minor change in collaborative practice occurred when a few physicians developed reservations about the role of the nurse in the units. The reason for this attitude, as perceived by nurses, was the result of the developing trend toward nursing's increasing responsibility for the delivery of care and influence on patient outcomes. Nurses were not deterred by these tensions, and educational programs for nurses continued. Nurses wanted to know why they were doing what they were doing: "I wouldn't do it without knowing why!" said Charlotte Bova Barewicz, an early ICU nurse (personal communication). By 1982–83, the State of Vermont brought the CCU personnel together to form the Vermont Cardiac Network, to discuss practices around the state, and to supply continuing education for nurses.

In the 1980s the Mary Fletcher Unit of the Medical Center Hospital of Vermont housed a fourteen-bed surgical ICU, a six-bed respiratory ICU, and an eight-bed coronary ICU. Neonates were cared for in the intensive care nursery established in the 1970s. All other seriously ill children were cared for in the SICU.

In 1985, the new McClure wing was added to the Mary Fletcher Unit, which created a sixteen-bed SICU and a sixteen-bed medical intensive care unit (MICU, RCU and CCU combined). The new units had private rooms resulting in a change of nursing care delivery. Patients and nurses were visually isolated and camaraderie and opportunities for collaboration decreased. Nurses had one to two patient assignments and had difficulty keeping up with the status of the other patients. "Covering" for another nurse meant learning about his/her patients and often going from room to room to check on them.

Cross training between the SICU and the MICU began with the idea that nurses could cover shift-by-shift vacancies in either unit. A generic CORE course was offered to new employees. A unit instructor was employed for each unit to facilitate CORE and ongoing in-service offerings. Educational programs, as well as formal preceptor workshops, were marketed. Advanced cardiac life support courses were offered on an ongoing basis, and nurses were sent away to national educational conferences. Physician–nurse collaboration again was growing, and nurses respected themselves. Advanced practice RNs were employed as clinical nurse specialists or nurse practitioners.

In the 1990s, acute care nurse practitioners worked in the catheterization laboratory, in cardiology education programs, and on the acute care floors of Fletcher Allen Health Care (FAHC). Staff turnover, which peaked in the mid 1990s when MCHV became FAHC, is still an issue. Shared governance is in its infancy in critical care services, and is growing. Labor union activity has arisen, and we are in a time of unrest. Changes and challenges will continue in the years ahead.

Nurses, in partnership with other healthcare providers, will continue to play a vital role in crafting and implementing improvements in critical care. Critical care nursing has made great strides in the past thirty years, and critical care nurses will continue to be a visionary part of the nursing community in Burlington and throughout the state of Vermont.

BIBLIOGRAPHY

Ball, C. "Education and Staffing in the ICU: Past, Present, and Future." *British Journal of Nursing* 1, no. 8 (1992): 399–401.

Calvin, J. E. et al. "Critical Care in the United States. Who Are We and How Did We Get Here?" *Critical Care Clinics* 13, no. 2 (April 1997): 363–76.

Cutugno, C. L. "Historical Development of Intensive Care Nursing in the United States." Doctoral dissertation, New York University, 1992.

Fairman, J. "Watchful Vigilance of Nursing Care, Technology, and the Development of Intensive Care Units." *Nursing Research* 41, no. 1 (January–February 1992): 56–60.

Fairman, J. A. "New Hospitals, New Nurses, New Spaces: The Development of Intensive Care Units, 1950–65." Doctoral dissertation, University of Pennsylvania, 1992.

Lynaugh, J. "Four Hundred Postcards. The History of Critical Care Nursing." *Nursing Research* 39, no. 4 (July–August 1990): 254–55.

Lynaugh, J. E., and Fairman, J. "New Nurses, New Spaces: A Review of the AACN History Study." *American Journal of Critical Care* 1, no. 1.

Marvin, A. "Burn Nursing History: The History of Burn Care." *Journal of Burn Care and Rehabilitation* 14 (1993): 252–57.

Development of ICU Nursing at Rutland Regional Medical Center

The first intensive care unit (ICU) at Rutland Hospital was established in 1964 to provide for acutely ill patients requiring continuous comprehensive and detailed care. The early general intensive care unit was initiated with a monitor and a ventricular defibrillator to give care to cardiac and surgical patients requiring close observation and/or more complex technological procedures.

When the ICU first opened, Kathleen Leadford was director of nurses; she was succeeded by Ronald Jacobus. Dea Rotella was the first ICU head nurse; Mary Waite was ICU charge nurse on the 3–11 shift; Elaine Hanlon was charge nurse on the 11–7 shift. Staffing usually consisted of one RN and one LPN. Occasionally, a second RN would be sent to the unit when it was busy. During one high-census period with patients in the hallways, there were thirteen people in the ten-bed capacity unit. Two RNs and one LPN were considered good staffing. In the early days of the ICU, many staff worked in the ICU before taking specialized training; until able to participate in more formal courses, many procedures were learned on-the-job. Education evolved from coronary care courses of the 1960s to critical care courses, advanced cardiac life support, and critical care certification. The advent of the American Association of Critical Care Nurses changed both continuing education and academic education for ICU nurses.

By today's standards, nursing practice in the early ICUs was limited. Intravenous (IV) insertions were usually started by physicians. The evening supervisor could start IVs but usually physicians in the hospital at the time would start IVs, on patients other than their own. The ICU nurses did intermittent positive pressure breathing treatments, attended codes (cardiac arrest) throughout the hospital, interpreted cardiac dysrhythmias, defibrillated patients, and cared for ventilated patients. Nurses also gave IV medications, especially cardiac drugs, and cared for patients

---

This article is a summary of responses to a December 1998 survey of nurses employed in ICUs in southern Vermont hospitals.

who had a temporary or permanent pacemaker, as well as critically ill neurological patients.

Nurses worked closely with physicians during the early years of ICU development. Now, however, there seems to be a more "common ground" for working as a team; the collaborative relationship between nurses and physicians has grown and expanded over time. The ICU nurse of the '90s does hemodynamic monitoring, electrocardiogram interpretation, and physical assessments once done only by the physician. The physicians role has expanded as well.

In 1973, the ICU became two units, one medical and one surgical; all ICU beds became monitored in 1973. As a result of "down-sizing" at Rutland Regional Medical Center, the ICU became one unit again in 1988.

Coping with the daily stress of the job was not difficult because there were good people to work with: Fern Fillioe, RN, Joyce Champine, RN, and Bonny Candon, LPN. Patients appreciated the care and support of Dr. Edward Layden, Dr. William Pratt, and Dr. David Cross. We were all very patient-oriented, and worked well together in new and increasingly challenging roles.

A specific patient situation is still clearly recalled today. The first Hewlett Packard defibrillator arrived with a box and paddles but no monitor. The day staff left their shift advising that it had just arrived and had not been "tested." They also reported that a 36-year-old female patient might need it. We were informed that Dr. Pratt would be in later; but, if the patient appeared to be in ventricular fibrillation, we should not hesitate to use it. We defibrillated her twice that evening. The only physician in the hospital watched and said, "I don't know what you did but it worked!" The patient was later transferred to Burlington for care; but she left Rutland Hospital conscious, alert, and relatively stable.

Another ICU patient, a 31-year-old female, was admitted in 1992 with tetanus infection. The patient had severe pain and spasm but never required ventilator support. She endured great pain, but had a strong desire to go home, and she refused many interventions. Maximizing comfort while maintaining a quiet environment required frequent assessment and communication with her husband and family.

Joan Cota, RN, remembers many ambulance trips with cardiac patients to Burlington, Vermont and Hanover, New Hampshire. One Labor Day weekend she travelled three times with patients with temporary pacemakers in place—ambulanced to Burlington for permanent pacemaker implants. This was before the arrival of Dr. Robert Andrews, the first surgeon in Rutland to implant permanent pacemakers. Another time, in 1994, she remembers defibrillating a patient multiple times en route to Fletcher Allen Health Care in Burlington; the patient survived.

We believe that critical care nursing is a special "calling" within the profession of nursing. There is the ability to use evolving technology and ongoing holistic assessment; and it requires a conscientious commitment to the total well-being of the patient and family, as well as lots of empathy and patience.

—Kathleen M. Ledo, MS, RN, CCRN
Joan Cota, RN, BA, BS, CCRN
Dea Rotella, RN
Mary Waite, RN, BSN, CSN

Nurse Anesthetists

On October 16, 1846, something happened that transformed surgical practice. Ether anesthesia was demonstrated during a surgical procedure at the Massachusetts General Hospital in Boston. The surgical theater was located under the grand dome of the building designed by Charles Bullfinch. That operating theater is still there, and has since that fateful day in 1846, been called "The Ether Dome."

It is interesting to note that in the year preceding 1846 there had been fewer than fifty surgical procedures at Massachusetts General and that all of those operations had been accompanied by intense fear and suffering; they were only consented to as an alternative to death. Yet hardly a year later, many hundreds of surgical operations were being performed around the world peacefully and in freedom from pain.

Of course, surgeons recognized the value of anesthesia immediately. Ether was an easily obtainable volatile agent; the method of administration was quite simple, and in terms of dosage, there was a wide margin of safety. And yet the early days of anesthesia were chaotic and there were many casualties.

Nurses were the first professional group to provide anesthesia services in the United States. Established in the 1880s as the first clinical nursing specialty, nurse anesthesia developed in response to the growing need of surgeons for specially-trained anesthetists.

St. Mary's Hospital in Rochester, Minnesota, was established by Dr. William Worrell Mayo in 1889, and later became known as the Mayo Clinic. Dr. Mayo, along with nurse Alice Magaw—whom Mayo identified as "the mother of anesthesia"—were instrumental in setting up a showcase of excellence in surgery and anesthesia. Both physicians and nurses came to observe and to learn their anesthesia techniques. Alice Magaw documented the anesthesia practice outcomes at St. Mary's Hospital and reported them in various medical journals between 1889 and 1906. During this time, the idea of formalizing the education of nurses for anesthesia practice became popular.

In 1931, practicing nurse anesthetists gathered to form the American Association of Nurse Anesthetists (AANA) to promote increased knowledge and standards in anesthesia practice. Toward that end, the AANA developed and implemented a certification process for nurse anesthetists in 1945 and an accreditation process for educational programs in 1952.

One notable nurse anesthetist in Vermont was Elizabeth (Betty) A. Wells. She graduated from the Mary Fletcher School of Nursing in Burlington in the 1930s, studied with Dr. John Abajian, Jr., and was actively engaged in anesthesia practice at the Mary Fletcher Hospital (now called Fletcher Allen Health Care) from 1941 to 1980. For the next eight years, she worked part-time for the Anesthesia Associates of Burlington. She was a member of the board of directors of the AANA and was a founding member of the Vermont Association of Nurse Anesthetists in November of 1956; she held many offices in that association over the years.

There are approximately sixty certified nurse anesthetists working in almost every hospital in Vermont. Nurse anesthetists were involved in the development of the Vermont State Board of Nursing Rules and Regulations for Nurse Practitioners in 1983.

There have been at least two programs for the education of nurse anesthetists in Vermont, although there are not any at the present time. One program was at Mary Fletcher Hospital in Burlington during the fifties and the other at Putnam Memorial Hospital in Bennington in the sixties and seventies. Beginning in 1998, the minimum requirement for nurse anesthetists will be a master's degree.

—Joe Reilly, BSN, CRNA

Hospital Nursing

A Personal Account

THE YEAR WAS 1977, and the room was small and dimly lit. Too dimly lit to ever be uplifting or calming. The lack of light was probably a very good thing, considering the furniture. The rug was a floral print—big burgundy roses on dark green vines. On the rug was a pair of shoes that I couldn't stop staring at, even though I knew I should stop. The shoes were old, yet well cared for, black oxfords laced up neatly, polished and shined. They were being worn by a man in his early eighties, a man sitting next to me. A man overwhelmed with grief. The old man struggled to control his emotions and did not cry.

I knew I should be able to say or do something therapeutic. After all, I was a sophomore nursing student, working weekends at Graduate Hospital in Philadelphia as a Nurse Extern—even then administrators could come up with titles for untrained personnel to make them sound like they were qualified. I had taken sociology and "Psychology Across the Life Span." I had read Kubler Ross' *On Death and Dying.* I still couldn't think of a thing to say. The nursing supervisor had called me to sit with this man, whose brother had just died. He was alone and a neighbor was coming to pick him up. It was hard not to stare at his shoes, but that was the only thing I felt qualified to do at the moment. It was even harder to figure out a way to help. It was the first of many moments in nursing when I desperately wanted to help and felt ill-equipped to do so. In that moment my education had failed me.

I don't recall the ending of that particular exchange, but I do remember the lesson. There have been many times since that waiting room in 1977 when I have wanted to alleviate a patient's pain or a family's suffering. No matter how much I may want to, there are many sorrows that can't be erased. It is a nursing privilege to be there for a stranger in a desperate moment. Wanting to help and showing concern often times has to be enough.

I was fortunate to grow up in a family that insisted on education. There was never any question that the children in our family would go to college. The only considerations were what we would study, where we would go to school, and how the tuition would possibly get paid.

As I was trying to make my decision, my sister enthusiastically injected, "You want to be a nurse, you've always wanted to be a nurse." I did?

"Yes," she said, "Isn't that why you were a candy striper?"

Well, I had been a candy striper, but I never got out of the coffee shop, and spent my whole candy striper career making ice cream sodas and pouring coffee. I never even saw a patient.

My parents embraced the idea of a career in nursing. It sounded as good as anything else did to me. Also, I knew some nurses. It seemed real and tangible, and I went for it. In retrospect, it's clear there was a total lack of career planning. However, I have no regrets. I do consider changing careers occasionally. Even if I do, I'm glad for the years I've been a nurse. It is a humbling job, one that triggers personal growth.

I graduated from Villanova University with a BSN in 1980. It was an excellent program. I certainly understand our profession's push to define the education entry level. However, without a doubt, some of the finest nurses I have worked with are diploma grads. The difference in clinical practice between a fantastic nurse and a mediocre one has little to do with where they went to school. Nurses who are compassionate, mature, and accountable for their clinical practice are the excellent ones. The individuals who will still read journals, question patient's treatments, and review anatomy and physiology even though they've practiced for twenty years, are the nurses I want taking care of my family.

It was either 1982 or '83 that I first remember caring for an AIDS patient in Vermont. He was a man in his early fifties who had a history of drug abuse. For several years before being diagnosed, he had lived in a commune in Vermont and had been drug-free. His girlfriend visited him regularly in the ICU. She, too, was in her early fifties. We all learned about AIDS together. Then, the only treatment was supportive. Mechanical ventilation, antibiotics, and other palliative therapy were all we had to offer. *Pneumocystis carinii* pneumonia was often the end.

After this first patient died, as nurse manager I received several calls from other members of his commune. They told me that the commune was a "loving, open environment." Relationships were not monogamous, and that first patient had slept with several of the women in the commune. The best I could do was refer them to the Department of Health. It was a sad introduction to a new disease.

In those early years of the AIDS virus, many of the patients we cared for died of the disease. A few nurses refused to care for AIDS patients, fearing the infection themselves. Some nurses were single mothers. It was hard to deny these nurses their fears. It was even harder scientifically to rationalize why some nurses should be exposed, and not others. I researched the data and felt assured our staff was not at risk if using proper precautions. Fortunately, we were blessed with nurses interested in the disease, sympathetic to these patients, and eager to care for them. We were generally able to respect the wishes of the nurses who chose to avoid the AIDS patients. Assignments were made allowing those nurses with an interest to care for the AIDS patients. This method of assigning nurses probably supported misconceptions of the disease. We recognized it at the time. However, nurses are real people, and so are patients. Nurses are asked to do so much. If there's an opportunity to respect an individual nurse's wish, I feel we should work as a team to do so.

Nurses spend so much time taking care of strangers. We need to be better about taking care of each other.

All nurses have moments in their careers that will never be forgotten. I remember once working with a quiet old Vermonter with end stage COPD (chronic obstructive pulmonary disease). His wife was running the farm, but would drive in every day to visit him, even though she didn't like driving into the big city of Burlington. He was mechanically ventilated, and had multiple emphysematous blebs. As his disease progressed and he required increased PEEP (positive end expiratory pressure), the ventilator caused the blebs to blow yielding a pneumothorax. He would get a chest tube each time this happened. His death seemed only a matter of time. In morning rounds, with four chest tubes already in place, he decompensated with yet another pneumothorax. The attending pulmonologist wanted to put in another chest tube.

I was young at the time, and my voice cracked with emotion as I asked this doctor to what ends he intended to treat this man. Sensing my emotions, the doctor asked me if our ICU (intensive care unit) nursing staff had any kind of program set up to help us cope with the endless tragedy we saw. I remember being proud that I still was able to appreciate this patient's suffering. It's so easy to become numb. We are our patient's finest advocate when we can analyze both the benefit and futility that our sophisticated health care has to offer. In the years since, I have learned how to speak on my patient's behalf without being a mush. But I will never regret being able to appreciate a patient's suffering.

The gentleman with COPD died later that day with five chest tubes.

When I graduated from college in 1980, there was a huge demand for RNs. When I interviewed at the Medical Center in Burlington, applying student nurses were interviewed in groups of five. Almost everyone who applied was hired.

Many nurses in practice today entered health care when the floodgates were wide open at hospitals supporting primary nurses and RN-only staff. The problem when I began my career, in the early eighties, was for hospitals to find nurses to hire. There was an intense shortage. Many big-city hospitals instituted the "Weekend Plan" as a staff recruitment/retention program. The weekend plan paid nurses full-time salaries if they would work two twelve-hour shifts every weekend. The rest of the nursing staff would then be able to work Monday through Friday only, no weekends. Talk about retention and recruitment! The weekend plan was a dream come true for nurses in school. The Monday through Friday plan—well, for anyone who has ever been a staff nurse, wow!

With the advent of HMOs and for-profit hospitals, this plan was eventually seen as too expensive, and I'm unaware of any hospitals following this staffing plan today.

Now the pendulum has swung to the opposite extreme, and there has been a dilution of nurses in the workplace. One dilemma I see is that the bulk of nurses are from the same generation I am, and have spent a lot of their careers working with primarily RN staffs. We are now faced with supervising unlicensed personnel, and struggle to do so effectively and safely. I would much prefer to see the former level of RN-to-patient ratios.

The recurring concern for me when I view myself and other hospital nurses is that too often we do not use the brainpower and education we have worked so hard to achieve. All professions have their mundane tasks, but I believe nurses hold on to too many of theirs. Perhaps we can use this dark time in hospital downsizing to come away with the best in assessment skills and accountability to our patients.

Some will think this idea ludicrous, but how about having two call bells for each patient? A bell for an aide, and a bell for a nurse. Too often nurses are pulled away from tasks only they can perform to answer patient requests that any caring individual could satisfy. The argument could be made that patients couldn't differentiate to know which staff member they needed. Yet, perhaps they could. We've all been called to the bedside for pens, changing TV channels, and blankets. Now, I thoroughly believe the patients who need these items are entitled to them, and entitled to ask for them. After all, many are on bedrest, and they're all sick. However, I frown at the system that we have devised in hospitals that lumps all needs together.

The advent of disposable, prepackaged kits has given nurses another dilemma. Many items are less expensive to buy as a disposable one-time item than to reuse and resterilize. Everything from blood gas syringes to hemodynamic pressure transducers, resuscitation bags to bedpans, are disposable. Perhaps disposables save facilities money, but at what cost to our environment? Many nurses feel that we can't waste time putting disposables into various recycle bins. I see recycling as a responsibility to the health of our planet and our children.

Nursing requires compassion to treat patients with the inherent dignity they deserve. Nurses need to be willing to bend the rules. To allow a dying patient to see their dog one last time in the hospital, to treat with fairness the most obnoxious patient ever admitted. Nurses need to empower patients to get the best care they can. Nurses need to enable families to help care for their loved ones in the hospital, to get a drink of water or brush their hair. The average person is intimidated by our huge, sterile hospitals. It is our privilege to deliver the health care they deserve. It is my sincerest wish that nurses have a loud voice in the formulation of how health care is delivered, for we know how to deliver the goods.

—Susan Cucinell Sullivan, RN, BSN

It's the Quality of Care That Counts

A Personal Account

WHILE LOOKING backward for this history, I discovered the driving force of my professional life has been a search for opportunities that will move us all closer to universal, compassionate, quality health care. This is about two opportunities I found in Vermont. Together, they can assure quality in health care.

It was 1948 when I enrolled in the University of Rochester (New York) School of Nursing's three-year diploma course, certain that it would provide quick job training and skills to go out in the world and do good works. After fifty years, good works remain one of those elusive life goals waiting to be reexamined and redefined.

The first examination sent me back to school; post-war health-care technology and information were always just ahead of my skills and knowledge and, in a new understanding of health care, communities needed caretakers as much as hospitals. After another three years to complete a degree in public health nursing in 1954, I followed an academic family from New York to Ohio to Kansas learning valuable lessons about access and quality along the way. I thought I had found an opportunity to move toward my goal when Medicare and Medicaid allowed me to establish home health care in Douglas County, Kansas. And it was an important step, as the Visiting Nurse Agency has just completed its thirtieth busy year. But it was the move to Vermont in 1970 that brought me to an innovative health care system and to pioneering nurse practitioner colleagues—just the opportunities I'd been looking for.

No history of Vermont health care is complete without endorsing the contributions of Dr. Lawrence L. Weed, The University of Vermont Emeritus Professor of the College of Medicine and brilliant visionary, who gave us the problem oriented medical record (POMR) and system to improve the quality of care by organizing medical information. Including his work in a history of nursing in Vermont is especially appropriate because his system expands nursing opportunities in the information component of health care; the other two components are interpersonal skills and manual or technical skills. The interpersonal skills of caring and helping are already nursing skills and there are many examples of expanded technical tasks we can add to our already extensive proficiencies. Putting the information into a computerized tool, as Dr. Weed did in Problem Knowledge Couplers, gives nurse practitioners precisely the help they need to assure quality care.

The Given Health Care Center's (GHCC) mission to establish a general internal medicine practice based on Dr. Weed's POMR and system has captured my attention for the past twenty-seven years. Fortunately, the organizing physicians at GHCC considered advance practice nurses partners of the group and two of us (Louise Bedard preceded me by a year, in 1971) were apprentice-trained as nurse practitioners several years before formal courses for adult care were available. That base—a separate tale of the trial-and-error school of learning—has been expanding ever since, always enhanced by the demands of problem-oriented clinical practice.

Funded by a Kellogg grant, we researched and wrote protocols, designed forms and flow sheets to guarantee that information would be not only available when patients were being seen, but also preserved in the record. Dr. Weed's elegantly simple "subjective, objective, assessment and plan" format kept the record clear to patients, nurses, and physicians alike. Care was an orderly progression from data collection, problem identification, and management to audit. It is a system that anticipated the quality improvement models popping up in industry a decade or more later and the transfer of information from paper to the computer. The patient's own health problems became a table of contents for the medical record, critical information was accessed at the patient problem level instead of the source, and patients received copies of their records. We began designing a system that would keep people well, detect health problems early, and systematically solve and manage health problems.

Meanwhile, nurse practitioners (NPs) began arriving throughout Vermont in the early 1970s. A one-year Certificate Program for Adult Nurse Clinicians commenced in 1973. It was sponsored by the New England Regional Medical Program and the Visiting Nurse Association of Burlington, and was followed by a one-year Certificate Family Nurse Practitioner Program sponsored by The University of Vermont School of Nursing and the U.S. Department of Health, Education, and Welfare (HEW). The co-directors were Janet P. Brown, RN, EdD, and George Welch, MD. Physical assessment skills were taught with the first-year medical students, thereby equalizing assessment skills in both groups. In 1977, some of us—so anxious about missing the very first, one-day opportunity for ANA (American Nurses' Association) certification—spent the pre-exam night in a downtown Boston hotel, fretting over the vastness of our ignorance. With national credentials in place, newly-educated NPs began to care for psychiatric, family planning, gynecology, family practice, pediatric, and general internal medicine patients, joining with already established midwives and nurse anesthetists.

Inevitably, we did what groups of nurses always do—we formed committees for continuing education and creating a Vermont certification that was fair, safe, and secure. Ninety-minute drives to White River Junction for two-hour meetings, then home again, brought us together in a common cause, but it didn't take long to move to blessedly shorter trips. In Montpelier, meetings with legislators and the boards of nursing and medical practice finally produced the rules and regulations for Vermont nurse practitioners in 1986. With great group foresight (I would love to claim credit but a commitment to accuracy prevents me) we had guaranteed collaborative practice and prescriptive authority.

Showing even more good sense, nurse practitioners continued to gather annually for a state-wide conference. For years, little word-processed programs and manila folders with pasted logos designed by Hilary Smith (TAP HEALTH WITH VERMONT NURSE PRACTITIONERS!) were assembled at potluck suppers by a few loyal NPs and midwives. The classy 1998 conference attended by dozens of bright, capable Vermont nurse practitioners and mid-wives proves we are very much alive and well.

I don't know why every American isn't outraged by the current condition of the nation's health care system that has become marketplace medicine, excludes millions, and doesn't give us consistent quality. Just as demystified health information will empower patients to demand quality care, it enhances the power of nurse practitioners as primary care providers. Couplers and practitioners are the powerful forces of change that will help me end my search for universal, compassionate, quality health care.

—MARILYN ROTHWELL, RNC

Independent Nursing Practice: A Path for Healing

A Personal Account

IN 1980, the Visiting Nurse Association received a hospice grant which stipulated twenty-four-hour nursing coverage. I accepted the position of night nurse for both general home care and hospice. It was satisfying to be back in adult medicine, piloting new services. My patients were seriously ill and terminally ill people who were receiving good physical care but whose emotional and spiritual needs were often not addressed.

I became restless with that "is this all there is?" feeling. I wondered about times when I would feel I was just a nurse, and other times when I knew I had been a great nurse. I was attempting to analyze the difference when I attended a workshop in therapeutic touch. I had an immediate "aha!" experience, and it became the experience which launched me into my next nursing life. But not for a while. First I had to become a change agent. The world of Burlington, Vermont, was not ready to embrace this fascinating concept. I was not officially permitted to use my new found treatment on my patients.

As I defined it in a 1996 article in *Home Health Care Nurse*, therapeutic touch is an alternative healing modality based on the premise that all living things are surrounded by a dynamic field of energy. This field is in constant flux and is influenced by factors in our environment and by the energy fields of other living things. This field can be enhanced positively by thought, love, and intent—specifically the intent to heal or make whole. The result is an integration of body, mind, and spirit. The technique utilizes the energy fields of both the patient and the nurse. To implement the process the nurse totally focuses herself and becomes "centered," with the "intent" of helping the patient heal. She proceeds to direct this energizing "intent" through her moving hands, held two to five inches over the patient's body. A peaceful relaxation response is effected that is deeply felt and witnessed. Therapeutic touch is not meant to cure, but to heal through caring.

The concept impressed me and revealed to me the why of those times I had done my best nursing. When the intent was there and I was centered and coming from a place of love and caring, true nursing and healing happened; otherwise, it was just performing a task.

I used the technique with some of my patients, with the provision from our director that I tell each patient I was doing it as a friend and not as an agency nurse. The patients loved it and the peaceful feeling they experienced. I continued to study and use the technique on my family and friends. When the opportunity arose, I asked to present an agency in-service on the topic, and I was ecstatic when I received official go ahead to use therapeutic touch on my patients. By this time, it had become a respected treatment modality in large and prestigious hospital and treatment centers around the country. I initiated and gave courses to interested nurses during weekly brown bag lunches. My article was accepted and published.

Meanwhile, "the times they were a-changin." Managed care was poking through the fabric of our nursing care. There was less and less time available to spend with a patient. The pressure for productivity interfered with the act of centering, which is paramount to the art of therapeutic touch. I felt stifled again, and was also confronted with the chronological fact of being older; I could learn "new tricks," but not ones that seemed to be cutting the caring from nursing.

I had also become attracted to another form of holistic nursing through my membership in the American Holistic Nurses Association. This was healing touch, which incorporates therapeutic touch and other modalities from different cultures and healing systems, always with the intent of reaching harmony of body, mind, and spirit. Frustration with what was happening in home care propelled me to reduce my agency position to parttime and to enter private practice. I found office space and began advertising for patients. As the clientele grew, so did my certainty that I had chosen the right path. It was clear to me that the stresses of organized nursing (or what I felt to be disorganized nursing) were increasing. I retired from my position and aligned myself with other holistic nurses nationwide who had entered private practice. Correspondingly, the medical community began to take notice of "alternative modalities," or to call it by its newest term, "integrative medicine." Some insurance companies have begun reimbursement which makes holistic nursing care an option for many more people.

I believe that nurses in private practice have furthered nursing's image. We demonstrate that ours is an independent profession. Specifically, holistic nursing reaffirms the fact that there is more to healing and caring than our technical and scientific culture generally acknowledges.

—Jane Packard Bryant, RN, PNP, CHTP

Holistic Nursing: The Journey

A Personal Account

As I REFLECT on my experiences of twenty years ago, I remember myself as a young college student majoring in nursing. My first nursing course was structured into the last part of my second year. Before that time, I was taking various liberal arts and science courses that seemed far removed from why I had chosen a career in nursing. Biochemistry and microbiology—even the psychology and human development courses—discussed theoretical rather than interpersonal applications. I was wondering how one took this theory and made a difference with human beings.

My first nursing course was "The History of Nursing," which I enjoyed because it spoke to what had called me to choose a career in nursing. I learned about Florence Nightingale and the difference that one person could make in health care. I learned about providing care that met all the needs of the human. It was care that considered the environment, the belief and family systems of the person, and the many aspects of the individual that made that person unique. I was beginning to see how I could use the seemingly obscure liberal arts courses and make a difference in someone's life. It is the creative side, the art of nursing, that gives the feeling that what was done is important. This is not to negate the science from which we practice.

I began my career as an intensive care nurse. The fast pace appealed to me, as well as the opportunity to gain new skills and the excitement of "saving lives" on a regular basis. The knowledge of the drugs used to minimize side effects of cardiogenic shock or to wean the patient from the intraaortic balloon pump provides the nurse the fulfillment of knowing that one's nursing care has touched a life.

I remember the first time I defibrillated someone. She was a woman in her late 40s, the mother of two young daughters—much too young to sustain a massive myocardial infarction. I remember the feeling of satisfaction as her heart regained a regular rhythm, and I remember thinking about how important it was for this woman to return home.

Days later, it saddened me to realize this woman would never return home. The health care team had saved her physical "life," her heart was beating, and cardiac output was adequate. Yet, frequent efforts at resuscitation and cardiogenic shock had left her brain without the function needed to live as one who is truly alive and present in the world. She would spend the rest of her life in a nursing home, perhaps aware of those around her, perhaps conversing on a higher spiritual level.

At that time, I didn't really consider those options. I saw what was called a "persistent vegetative state"—in other words, a failure. I had no consciousness of the soul's journey and I felt angry that modern medicine couldn't return this woman to her family.

Throughout my experience as an intensive care nurse, I witnessed and was a part of many success stories, people who did return home to a higher quality of life. Like many nurses, I also cared for those who suffered, who passed without family present, who passed being unable to talk to their loved ones at the end of physical life. The biggest frustrations in nursing seemed to stem from being unable to provide care that made a difference.

There were aspects of hospital work that I disliked, but I have always loved caring for patients. I chose a career in nursing education, in part, to share my love for nursing with students. I believed in caring for the whole person, yet I felt restricted in providing holistic care in a hospital environment. While I thought I was reasonably able to provide care that considered mental and emotional factors, I experienced uncertainty about providing care that honored spirituality. I could call the chaplain and respect religious beliefs, but I thought that spirituality was too personal for me to address. With little understanding of the difference between religion and spirituality, I lacked the ability to address what I couldn't grasp.

I resonate with the writings of Margaret Newman,[1] who is influenced by the work of Robert Moss. Margaret Newman considers health and disease on a continuum; it seems that on a soul level neither is better than the other. The purpose of life is to remind us of who we are and why we came. Newman describes a point of tension that frequently precedes growth and change.

In the early 1990s, I began experiencing this tension. I loved my job teaching clinical nursing to university students. Yet, I was struck with feelings of discord, uneasiness, and the quest for something more. As I recall these feelings, I am aware of how my soul was driving my evolution.

In 1994, a colleague and I attended one day of the national conference of the American Holistic Nurses' Association (AHNA) in Burlington, Vermont. What I remember most about that conference was feeling the energy in the meeting room. At that time, I had no knowledge of energy-based healing, yet I felt the joy and excitement of the nurses who gathered there. I was aware that it was like nothing I had ever experienced.

Nurses who gather for the AHNA conferences describe it as a feeling of coming home. In 1995, I attended the AHNA conference in Phoenix. I listened to internationally recognized speakers, staff nurses, nursing students, nurse educators, and physicians who spoke about many aspects of holistic care, including energetic healing.

There were parts of the conference that were outside my belief system at that time, yet there was much that made sense, and I had an inner knowing, an innate wisdom that told me that this was what I had been looking for. I had "come home" to a group of nurses who thought like me and who practiced nursing as I had always envisioned. They practiced holistic nursing that included energetic healing as well as other complementary health care interventions.

What inspired me was that holistic nursing interventions honored and integrated all aspects of humanness, including the spiritual. Holistic interventions also facilitated personal growth (which I have come to recognize as spiritual growth) and they did no harm! Holistic nursing honors the whole person and recognizes that healing occurs on many levels, including standard nursing interventions that reduce physical symptoms. In my heart, I knew I was a holistic nurse; the feelings that created excitement and touched the core of my being were those I experienced during my first nursing class and I was experiencing the same feelings again.

Returning to everyday reality following the conference wasn't easy. I was struggling to integrate the concepts of holism with my past and present jobs. My first passion had been intensive care nursing. As I became more involved with teaching, I was providing less direct patient care; yet my career had begun in a setting that based success on concrete, measurable outcomes: cardiac output, blood pressure, mentation, kidney and liver function.

Working in a specific environment, a person tends to adopt the belief systems of that environment. I had been conditioned to provide care based on scientific research that was grounded in double-blind studies with statistical significance using large patient populations. I had been trained to think "either" this treatment works "or" we try another one. I could usually find answers by taking a course or researching a journal article.

One may not agree with the opinions of an institution, but in order to enjoy one's work, most people follow the principles of the organization and abide with the implied beliefs of the culture. My career choices had helped to define the person I had become and I was doing work that I loved.

My heart and soul were clearly showing me another way to be a nurse, but my brain was telling me that these ideas were unpracticed, unusual, and alternative. I could imagine the looks or comments I would receive from respected professionals when discussing energy field healing. Looking back, I recognize my reaction was based on fear. I didn't want to admit it, but my thoughts at the time were about how holistic nursing would affect my professional credibility.

Mainstream health care tends to divide the human into parts and use techniques to treat the affected part. Holistic health care maintains that we are already complete; we are perfect beings despite our perceived imperfections. Holistic nursing allows the uncertainty, the feelings and thoughts, the joy, sorrow, and learning that is part of the human experience. Holism doesn't divide the person into parts; in each moment we are whole and complete.

Embracing holism meant that I needed to redefine my self-perception, letting go of some of my essential belief patterns in order to integrate the new. In studying holism, I was learning to look inside for answers, to recognize that there were many ways of knowing, and to look past the "either/or" answers that tend to divide humans. Holistic nursing is not about giving up health care treatments that are known to affect disease processes; rather it is about adding to our ways of knowing and being.

At the AHNA conference I heard nurses speaking about "talking the walk" and "walking the talk." These concepts intrigued me! Where were we going? Were we all on the same path? It sounded like a pilgrimage. I came to realize that we are all on the same journey—the journey of life and the manifestation of our soul's deepest desire.

As I become more conscious of myself in each moment of the process of personal growth, I can help others look at their own process. As I forgive myself and accept myself with love, I give others permission to do the same. As I practice nonjudgment, I allow others the same privilege. I have learned that the most important intervention I can use is presence, which is being completely present, loving, and open to the experience of another person. As a nurse, I can offer interventions based on my knowledge base, but I have learned that true healing comes from the inside.

I learned about the difference between thinking and meditating, and about the difference between meditation and prayer. Someone once told me that prayer is when you talk to God; meditation is when God talks to you. I learned that my thoughts are under my control, and about silencing my thoughts so that I could hear the inner wisdom. I learned that our thoughts are forms of energy, and I learned about the importance of intentionality. I learned about letting go of the need to know and accepting the unfolding of the human experience.

At the AHNA conference, I set two intentions: I would become certified in healing touch and I would become certified in holistic nursing. I felt particularly drawn to healing touch, a program of study about energetic healing that in 1995 was taught through the AHNA. When I first learned about the healing touch program, there was never a doubt in my mind that I would learn healing touch. The problem was that it wasn't being offered in the Northeast. I came home from Phoenix exhilarated. "I have got to do this," I told my husband. "I don't know how it's going to happen and I know I'll have to travel but I need to do this." A few months later, I received a flyer that the healing touch program was being offered in Stowe, Vermont—practically my own backyard! I attended the first level of healing touch instruction in December of 1995.

Integrating the physical with the mental, emotional, and spiritual is what drew me to nursing and what drew me to healing touch. The practice of healing touch blends these components of humanness, and treats all components *at the same time*! Perhaps what is most deeply affected by energetic interventions is the part most difficult to describe in words—the spiritual. When I am present with someone for healing touch, the feeling of the work is Divine. There is a sense of time stopping, of the oneness of the Universe, of love. There is also the requirement to let go of attachment to outcomes. While the client and I set an intention for healing, I know that healing occurs on many levels that are all interconnected. Thoughts lead to feelings that may change belief systems, ways of being and impact the physical. Throughout, a sense of love and acceptance is present.

Now I recognize that we are souls going through present life in human bodies. As our soul's longing stirs in our physical bodies, we may ignore it or we may be conscious of our deepest desires. If we are not conscious of that which our soul requires in this lifetime, then the soul will look for other ways to alert us to our longings. The longings of the soul exist individually, but also in community with other beings and with the earth.

As I have begun to integrate the spiritual with the physical, I am learning how to be patient, to trust the Universe, to forgive myself, and how to love myself. I am allowing the not knowing and I am becoming more present in each moment. I am recognizing that I will never have it all figured out; that there are ups and downs on the journey and I still experience anger, fear, sadness, and the everyday annoyances that come with being human. Rather than trying to ignore or explain the feelings, I am letting them be okay, recognizing that they will pass. By acknowledging and allowing all my human experiences, I give others permission to do the same.

Florence Nightingale thought of nursing as God's work. As our culture has become more technologically advanced, many of us forget about why we were called to nursing. At a time when nursing was thought to be women's work, Nightingale cautioned nurses to be wary of prevailing thoughts which she called "jargon." Regarding professional nursing, Nightingale wrote,

> Surely woman should bring the best she has whatever that is, to the work of God's world without attending to [the jargon] . . . [or] . . . listening to the "what will people say", to opinion, to the "voices from without". And as a wise man said, no one has ever done anything great or useful by listening to the voices from without . . . Oh, leave those jargons, and go your way straight to God's work, in simplicity and singleness of heart.[2]

Health care is becoming increasingly technological. Most people believe that this is advancing science. I think we need to pay attention not only to nursing science, but also to the art of nursing, the healing that is done with personal connection such as touch, listening, communicating acceptance.

A person can be a holistic nurse in any setting without taking any course of study. Holistic nursing uses holistic interventions, but it is not about technique or outcomes. Holistic nursing is about being present with oneself and with others. Holistic nursing encompasses all facets of healing and is an ongoing process. It does not occur only with patients or clients because it is not doing; it is a way of being. It is not a magical cure although I have seen miracles happen. Holistic nursing is truly a journey, one that co-exists and embraces the self, the persons for whom we care, and the Universe.

In 1983, I began working at the Medical Center Hospital of Vermont, and in the hospital newsletter I found the following quote which I have clipped and taped on my refrigerator.

Come Walk Among the Stars

And as my life has been gently touched by other lives
It follows that I have touched theirs too
One cannot always know the time of greatest need
Perhaps it is as it should be
Perhaps it is only for me to light
one darkened corner of the path
To place a hand upon your shoulder
as a symbol of my kinship and my love
Perhaps I came this way
As did you
To fill some special need
But this is not always given to us to know.

—Winston O. Abbott

—Nancy Lukas Perrault, RN, MS
Holistic Nurse Certified
Certified Healing Touch Practitioner

NOTES

1. M. A. Newman, *Health as Expanding Consciousness* (New York: National League for Nursing, 1994).
2. Florence F. Nightingale, *Notes on Nursing* (Philadelphia: Lippincott, 1859), 76.

The Role of the Breast Health Specialist

My assignment in contributing to this volume was to document the evolution of my particular field of nursing, and to compare it with those nurses who have gone before. My entertaining but ultimately fruitless search of the archives of the Vermont State Nurses' Association (VSNA) underscored the emergence of positions such as mine, and kindled my curiosity about what other types of nursing may have sprung up in the past fifty years. In my survey of the literature in the archives, I was unable to locate any specific information on oncology nursing, much less on the role of the Breast Health Specialist, which is my title. In a report of a state survey of nursing needs and resources from 1952, the categories of nurses in Vermont were listed as: nursing in general hospitals, psych nursing, TB nursing, public health, industrial, private practice, and office nursing.[1]

The role of the nurse as breast health specialist evolved as the sophistication of the medical consumer developed in the 1980s and 1990s. In her 1981 VSNA keynote address, Jean Steel noted, "The purchaser of care has, along with the rest of the world, learned to assert himself and his rights."[2] This is a position not created by nurses, but by breast cancer patients who felt lost and overwhelmed with the crisis of diagnosis. They wanted a health care professional who could answer their questions; guide them through the maze of surgical, radiation, and medical oncologists, and reconstructive surgeons; and provide the education and support necessary to assist them in making decisions around their treatment. As Karen Stabiner notes in her book *To Dance with the Devil*, "Any university medical center tends to attract patients who are more aggressive about their health than most people—they ask more questions, they demand the best and have the insurance to pay for it."[3] (Stabiner xiii) Thus the role of breast health specialist was created (1995 in Vermont) as a response to these needs, conjuring the image of the nurse, literally and figuratively monitoring the pulse of those in her care and providing the necessary treatment and education.

The breast health specialist is pivotal to the care of any patient in the Breast Care Center at Fletcher Allen Health Care, Burlington, Vermont. This clinic houses primarily surgical oncologists, but twice weekly multidisciplinary clinics are held for clients newly diagnosed with breast cancer. An opportunity is thus offered to meet with surgical, radiation, and medical oncologists, a psychologist, and the breast health specialist all at the same appointment; and to know their specialists are talking with each other, as well as communicating with the client, family, and referring provider. The breast health specialist coordinates these clinics, acts as interpreter, and is the identified educator and support person for these clients facing the crisis of their lives.

Before the process of education can begin, it is necessary to assess the needs of the newly diagnosed patient. Clearly, most are overwhelmed and desperate. Facing the possibility of loss of a breast, loss of hair, loss of life, certainly loss of the security of their former lives, they are frequently cracked open emotionally, and require honesty and compassion—care that is comprehensive, accessible, and accountable. What they most want is the assurance that they will be okay, that this will all soon be behind them.

> And yet no one can promise them a cure. No one can even promise them a consensus, since treatment is an exasperatingly imprecise art. All their doctors can do is make sure they get what those doctors define as comprehensive treatment. This is how bad it is: Every breast cancer patient, even women who could buy a solution if there was one, faces a lifetime of apprehension.[4]

Those with ultimately benign findings are also cared for by the breast health specialist. The job entails educating these clients about their palpable and/or breast imaging abnormalities, about the types of biopsy available, calling them pre- and post-biopsy, notifying them of biopsy results, instructing them on treatment recommendations, and coordinating their follow-up among their providers. Another important aspect of the job is community education.

As the awareness of breast cancer swells into panic of the disease, it is common to find that many women greatly overestimate their chance of developing breast cancer. The oftquoted statistic "one woman in eight" has women glancing surreptitiously around the room wondering which one or more are currently experiencing it. But when the statistic is explained, that the number reflects a lifetime risk, that by the age of 80 one woman in eight will have breast cancer, the group visibly relaxes. However, the goal is not to lull women into complacency about their risks, rather to give them a realistic view of their chances of developing breast cancer, and to teach them about the vital importance of early detection. It is all we have as of now, with no certain tools for absolute prevention. As careful as we are with our diets and exercise, as lucky as we can be with our family histories, there is no sure way to avoid breast cancer.

> . . . and a generation spoiled by easy medical answers comes face to face with a foe that has so far defied the doctors. In a culture obsessed with a woman's beauty and youthfulness, they face the specter of treatments that would dismantle their physical and sexual identity, bit by bit: the removal of a breast; possibility of premature menopause from chemo-therapeutic drugs. The media told us we would be vibrant well into middle age, even beyond, while breast cancer snickered and plucked women off that path at random.[5]

Therein lies the need for nurses to become breast health specialists. As yet, we can only dream of the time when this position is obsolete, when research advances us to the place where breast cancer is only the memory of a disease that exacted its terrible price. When that day comes, other new positions will be created and other venues for nursing practice will appear. This has been the history of nursing. This is our legacy. This is our challenge.

—JOHANNA SHEEHEY-JONES, RN, BSN

NOTES

1. James Bates, "A Report on the Nursing Journey in Vermont," *Vermont Health* XXXV (Spring 1952): 2. Vermont State Nurses' Association Special Collection, Library Research Annex, The University of Vermont, Burlington.
2. Jean Steele, keynote address at the Vermont State Nurses' Association annual meeting, October 1981.
3. Karen Stabiner, *To Dance With the Devil: The New War on Breast Cancer* (Delacorte Press, 1997), xiii.
4. Ibid., xii.
5. Ibid.

Continence Nursing in Northern Vermont

A Personal Account

MANY PEOPLE have asked me why (and how) I became a continence specialist. The answer is not hard for me to explain . . . incontinence seemed like a bad problem, and I didn't see a crowd of other nurses heading for this speciality area. Choosing to work with incontinent clients is something that I have never regretted, and perhaps my story will help another nurse have an idea or goal that will be as fulfilling to attain.

My first realization that I might want to become a nurse came not when I was eight or eighteen years old but rather, four years after I had graduated from college with a degree in physical education. Luckily, I found a graduate nursing program at Massachusetts General Hospital Institute of Health Professions for students like myself who had previous college degrees. At the end of three long years, my visions of the excitement of the emergency room or the intensive care unit had dimmed, and I was happily enjoying my student experience as a gerontological nurse practitioner. I liked the nursing-home rotation, my experience with the hospital consultation, and the home health work. Most of all, I was intrigued by the dementia and incontinence clinics and the nurse practitioner roles that I observed there. The seed was planted; I would move to Vermont with my husband and start an incontinence clinic. What I didn't know was that this seed would take about six years to grow.

The climate was not particularly ripe for nurse practitioners in Northern Vermont in 1985. I began to get that impression after interviewing with many doctors who could not see the need for my services, or couldn't find the funding to support a new initiative like an incontinence clinic. I took a job as an RN on the night shift at Copley Hospital in Morrisville, and as my unplanned pregnancy blossomed, I felt more like the subject of a country-western song ("Pregnant on the Night Shift") than a master's-prepared gerontological nurse practitioner. I must have known that things would come together if I was patient and did my homework. In 1987, a teaching job opened up at The University of Vermont, and I was able to interface my previous teaching background with my nursing skills.

I needed to keep my clinical skills current as I taught, so I began looking for opportunities to start an incontinence clinic. A helpful mentor at this time was Diane Smith, a nurse practitioner with a continence practice in Philadelphia. Diane was employing other nurse practitioners to work with her, doing assessment and treatment of urinary incontinence in the clinic, home, and nursing-home settings. Diane convinced me that I could purchase biofeedback equipment for teaching pelvic muscle exercises and start my own practice rather than waiting for an opportunity to come along with a physician. I also took a certifying course in biofeedback to help build my credentials. Learning about starting up a business was perhaps the most challenging. I found the resources at The University of Vermont Extension Service to be very helpful, and I wrote my business plan using this guidance.

In 1991, I approached Lamoille Home Health and Hospice (LHH&H) about contract work doing home visits for assessing and treating urinary incontinence. Anne Mallet, RN, executive director of LHH&H, accepted my offer although some of the staff were skeptical that frail, rural elders would be accepting of biofeedback-assisted pelvic muscle exercises. I worked with the staff to increase understanding of all the potential interventions for urinary incontinence, once it was correctly diagnosed. My practice was now a reality.

I remember one of my first patients was an octogenarian status post-radical prostatectomy. He wore large overalls, chewed tobacco, and spit constantly. I had to move his gun to plug in my biofeedback equipment in his bedroom. He responded well to seeing the light bar change as he contracted the pelvic floor muscles. His compliance with the prescribed audiotaped exercise routine was great. Soon he was able to feel enough control to go out and work in his garden without having a leaking accident. I learned never to assume an intervention wouldn't be acceptable to someone until you try.

I wanted to expand to an office-based practice in 1993 and studied in preparation for negotiating with business managers. (Reviewing and revising the business plan was also useful.) I was successful at negotiating a contract to work out of the offices of a urologist and geriatrician on a part-time basis. In 1994, I started monthly continence rounds at Starr Farm Nursing Center in Burlington. I worked with the nursing staff to help them plan appropriate care for their incontinent residents based on their assessments.

Continence nursing was growing as my practice was growing. I now have wonderful groups of peers to network with through organizations like the Society for Urological Nursing and the Wound, Ostomy, and Continence Nurses Society. Being the only continence specialist in Northern Vermont was great, but I was always hungry for trading experiences with my peers. Certification opportunities became available for

Continence Care Nurse and Urology Advance Practice Nurse. More and more nurses were finding the rewards of helping men, women, and children regain continence in a variety of practice settings.

In 1996, I needed to make an important decision. I could no longer contain my practice to the hours that the School of Nursing allowed for clinical practice. I could either grow an independent practice or join a urogynecologist at Fletcher Allen Health Care. It was a difficult time for an independent practice. Managed care was making more and more demands, and working with groups of providers rather than individuals. Medicare was strictly enforcing rules which required that a physician be in the suite when billing collaboratively. Nurse practitioners could not bill Medicare except in rural areas and nursing homes. I decided that I could continue my practice with nursing home and home health work, while I joined Anne Viselli, MD, in her urogynecology practice. Leaving The University of Vermont School of Nursing was hard, but it was the right decision.

Looking ahead, I see a promising future for advance practice nurses and entrepreneurs in Vermont. In 1998, federal legislation changed Medicare reimbursement guidelines to accept nurse practitioners as billing providers in all settings. Nurse practitioners who are developing practices in rural and urban Vermont will be able to set up direct computerized Medicare billing. This change, and the growth in acceptance of nurse practitioners in Vermont, will mean that consumers will have more choices. Advance practice nurses and nurse practitioners need only to step forward with vision and determination to meet emerging needs.

—Mary Val Palumbo, RN, MSN, GNP

Geriatrics and Long-Term Care

THE YEARS FOLLOWING World War II brought changes in the manner in which elder care was provided in our country. During the war many women were working out of the home. The extended family helped care for children, and many homes had three or four generations living under the same roof. Geriatric nursing—specialization in the care of the elderly—was in its infancy during this time. Life expectancy in Vermont for males and females was late sixties and early seventies, respectively. Nursing homes, for the care of the elderly, were usually large converted homes, often operated by an individual who was either a registered or practical nurse. There was no formalized nursing education that offered a specialized curriculum in geriatrics. The elderly received medical nursing care primarily in hospitals.

In 1963, Holiday House Nursing Home in St. Albans was the first facility built as a nursing home in the state of Vermont. Cultural changes were creating a need for the deliverance of custodial and medical care within an institution. Two progressive nurses, Ardelle Rich, RN, and her sister Helen Hibbard, RN, worked tirelessly to develop standards of nursing care in this new type of facility. Charting, medication administration, nursing care, and other procedures had to be meticulously created.

Twenty-four hour nursing care was provided with an emphasis on caring for the medical, social, and physical needs of the patient. Nursing in this environment was practiced in an independent manner. Unlike the hospital setting where physicians were available daily, nursing home nurses had to be very astute at evaluating and assessing their patients. The standards of practice were patterned after those in the hospital; however, because of the long-term stay of patients, there were many care issues that needed to be addressed in a different manner. The emphasis of nursing needed to be on prevention of complications. Vermont nurses working in this field joined together through the Vermont Nursing Home Association, and through this arena encouraged the education of all professionals working in this rapidly growing field.

The inception of Medicare and Medicaid in the 1960s and early 1970s helped to spur a tremendous growth in the development of formalized geriatric care. The custodial care of long-term patients was converted into "extended care" with the stroke of a pen. The new mission of Vermont nurses in this field emphasized recuperative and rehabilitative care. Many new facilities were built, and nursing positions in this specialty expanded rapidly. Historically, postsurgery or medical episode patients were cared for in one of the Vermont-based hospitals. Medicare encouraged the rapid growth of geriatric facilities where the care was directed by nurses. The name "*nursing* home" in essence denotes the driving force of nurses within this area of practice.

Medicare revolutionized the type of care provided. Nurses cared for individuals with complex medical and surgical episodes. Individuals moved from hospitals still requiring intravenous therapy, stroke rehabilitation, orthopedic care, wound care, and other complex treatments. Medicaid, the medical insurance for the impoverished, extended the time that people could stay in long-term care after their skilled coverage had ended. Nurses were then challenged with the care of individuals with a multitude of medical needs who remained in these facilities after their Medicare stay was completed. The nursing standards during this time mirrored those of hospital nursing, with the challenge magnified to prevent the complications of bedrest, immobilization, and depression. Rehabilitation nursing became the philosophy and method of preventing contractures, decubitus, and other complications of disuse.

In 1989, the federal government once again revolutionized nursing standards in long-term care. The Omnibus Reconciliation Act would redefine nursing practice. Methods of care from the previous decades of geriatric nursing practice no longer seemed appropriate. For example, the utilization of physical and chemical restraints for the protection of the patient was once seen as paramount in the care of the frail elderly: restraints were used on nearly fifty percent of patients in long-term care. Long-term care nurses in Vermont and New Hampshire lead the country in changing this standard of practice. Today, this practice is only minimally used.

Other practices were also revisited and changed. Catheterization for incontinence gave way to bladder training. Nursing assessment became the priority for all nurses.

One of the most important changes in long-term care nursing came about in the late 1980s through the requirement of formal education for nursing assistants. Prior to this, individuals were trained on-the-job to give patient care that was custodial in nature. Training and licensure improved the quality of care received by long-term patients.

Responding to the technological and information revolution was the mission of geriatric nursing in the nineties. Nursing care was assessed through the computerization of all care on Minimum Data Sets. Registered nurses were trained to assess patients and to fill out this nineteen-

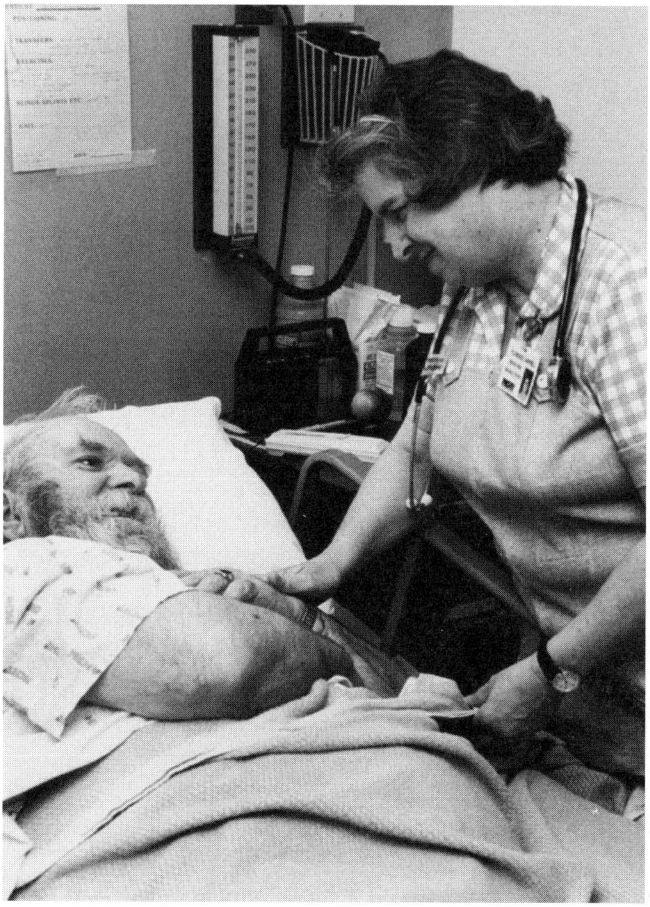

Courtesy Public Relations Office, Fletcher Allen Health Care

Nursing care at the bedside

page form. With the data collected in this document, the computer gives a list of problems that must be addressed by nursing. This information is shared by federal and state governments. Nursing care is now evaluated by "quality indicators" that review the outcome of patients with similar conditions.

Revolutionary new bio-tech equipment has enhanced the practice of nursing. Included in this are glucometers, oxymeters, pacemakers, portable X-ray and EKG (electrocardiogram), MRI (magnetic resonance imaging), and CAT (computed axial tomography) scans. Many of these life-saving devices have been created in bio-tech firms in Vermont.

As we approach the millennium, Vermont nurses in geriatric care are facing many challenges. Care that they are providing is now subacute, high-tech and limited in time. Medical care has improved the aging process. Life expectancy has increased rapidly. Nursing care of an individual who is 70 varies from an individual who is 100. As the life span increases, so do the challenges that geriatric nurses face. Patient education is a daily requirement. Vermont nurses have seen the potential care issues that are being born out of the development of "megabugs"; the challenge of caring for individuals who are being infected with resistant strains of bacteria will effect nursing care into the next century. The AIDS epidemic creates another challenge that will impact the long-term care nurse. Individuals requiring long-term nursing care will be very different than those in care during the fifties and sixties.

Long-term care nursing is a rapidly changing field that will continue to develop and grow as strides are made in the care and cure of Alzheimer's disease and other chronically debilitating diseases. Vermont is very fortunate to have the multitude of nurses who specialize in and enjoy long-term care.

Vermont has led the nation in innovative care of its elderly or frail populace by creating options for receiving nursing care, including remaining in their homes utilizing "care without walls." Vermont geriatric nurses are offering leadership through this experiment.

Vermont long-term care nurses are revolutionizing the manner in which care is given. During the forty-year evolution of this specialty in Vermont, nurses have witnessed a major change in their role. Specialization in this field, along with the ability to achieve certification, provides the impetus to increase the number of practitioners in Vermont today.

—TRESSA CONDON, RN, BSPA, NHA

Evolution of a Nurse to a Nurse Practitioner

A Personal Account

As I VOLUNTEERED in the Planned Parenthood Clinic in the late sixties, I was struck by how many women would come into the clinic with so little knowledge of the options for birth control. There were no easy answers for those women with unplanned pregnancies. The clinic, held in the lower-level clinic rooms of the original Mary Fletcher Hospital, was run by Planned Parenthood of Vermont (PPV). Residents in OB-GYN and several volunteers attended to the women who came for low-cost birth control. The volunteers took a history, performed simple laboratory tests, helped the women get ready to see "the doctor," and provided some basic information about available birth control methods.

Out of this rather top-heavy medical atmosphere, came the beginning of the woman-oriented, informed choice clinics of today. The volunteers and the administration of PPV in those early years were committed to patient education, respect for a woman's decision, and providing safe and efficient birth control methods. Much of this basic patient care in the early clinics came from the dedicated volunteers, physicians, and lay people, and the basic support of Planned Parenthood Federation of America (PPFA).

After receiving a diploma in nursing, I graduated in 1972 with a BSN. Following graduation, I was part of the group of women (and men) who started the Vermont Women's Health Center. With another nurse, June Aschenbach, I helped assure that the new clinic would have trained personnel, simple and safe medical procedures, accurate laboratory tests, and lots of education, with options fully explained. Volunteering at the PPV clinics helped me to appreciate how difficult it was for most women to get to the clinics in Burlington. The founders of PPV were active in gaining the help of folks in the small towns of Vermont, where clinics could be started so that it would be easy for those in rural areas to get women's health care.

While leafing through one of the 1972 issues of the *American Journal of Nursing*, I discovered an advertisement for a program for educating

"Nurse Practitioners in Family Planning." I was intrigued by the short article about what these nurses could do. After applying, I got a letter from Miriam Manisoff, the director of PPFA's Nurse Practitioner Program, indicating that I needed sponsorship by the local Planned Parenthood organization. She suggested that I meet with the director of PPV, David Wagner, and the clinic supervisor, Theresa S. King, and get a commitment that PPV would use nurse practitioners to deliver services. It was incumbent upon the local affiliate to develop this new role for nurses to work in the clinics—to see more patients, provide all methods of birth control, and improve the delivery of health care.

After doing a thorough study of PPV and the needs of the women who used the services, I was ready to meet with these leaders. My preparation helped me to be very certain that they would approve my becoming part of the Third Class of the Nurse Practitioner Program. Little did I know when I set up the meeting that I was going to meet the most compassionate, concerned, and flexible but firm, obstetrician and gynecologist, the part-time medical director for PPV, Ralph Gause. All three asked sharp questions, tested my ability to stand tough, and really seemed interested—but were not sure what kind of employment they could offer at the end of the training. They did approve my official application to the training program and promised to prepare PPV for the role of nurse practitioner.

Immediately after Christmas, I was off to Newark, New Jersey, to begin one of the most important experiences of my life. Several of the Third Class of ten were black women, many were from larger cities, and some had clinic experience. Most of the patients were black, as were the women on the floor of the YMCA (Broad Street) where we lived. Our teachers, the OB-GYN physicians from the New Jersey College of Medicine and Dentistry, lectured, demonstrated, and supervised techniques in clinical practice. The residents were also our "teachers," but many had definite sexist and racist views. We took one very obnoxious doctor-to-be, told him to "strip from the waist down" (words all the clinic patients heard frequently), and put him on the exam table. Then, everyone was called into the exam room (by yelling down the hall) to look at him. This is what he did to many of the women who came to the clinic.

We had much to learn about male and female bodies, pap smears, wet smears, ovulation, pregnancy tests, pelvic exams, observation of mucus, and breast exams. The custom of doing first exams on black women who were going to have a hysterectomy, without asking permission, was an accepted procedure in that clinic. Several of us refused to do these examinations (especially when the women were awake because of spinal anesthesia). Clay Burchell, MD, medical school professor and director of the training program was incredulous at our refusal, but listened when we suggested that we would do exams on each other and learn from each other. Thus, for the Third Class of Ten, most of us being feminists, began a transformation of ourselves, our group, and some of the program's directions. This support of the group helped each of us to see how we could change our philosophy concerning health care for women. For some of us, the experiences helped cement plans for women's health programs that are founded on listening, lots of information, and choices.

As we moved into our courses on history taking, examinations, and diagnosis of various conditions and diseases, as well as gynecological pharmacology, it was obvious that we had to have a protocol in which we could function when we returned home. In the programs where the medical director was dedicated to the emerging role of the nurse practitioner, the trainee had awesome support. The medical directors (or clinic directors) who came to Newark, worked with us to develop protocols, to outline future medical practice collaboration, and to start the process of the prescription writing procedures. The "male midwife" (as Dr. Gause called himself) was not afraid to support and promote all the new medical procedures, the changing attitudes, and the philosophy of advanced practice of nursing.

Many of us had come into this new knowledge and awareness of women's health care through our own experiences, by helping other women, and in founding reproductive and health centers. By having these past experiences, we brought new ideas and different goals to the training program planned by the PPFA, the affiliates of Planned Parenthood Essex County and Montclair, plus the New Jersey College of Medicine and Dentistry. Besides changing the way pelvic exams were learned in the programs, we started teaching small classes on sexuality, birth control, and pregnancy prevention at the Broad Street YMCA (on the floors where we lived). Members of the group went into the schools and churches for the first time with influential community people. We even got the interns and residents to sit down with some of the women who used the hospital clinic and discuss their feelings about the care they received.

Our months in Newark were spent studying, doing work in the classroom, and practicing in the clinics and offices of the Martland Medical Center (formerly Newark City Hospital), the Planned Parenthood clinics of Essex County (in the city) and Montclair (in the suburban areas). We did pelvic exams, pap smears, pregnancy tests, and diagnostic exams; provided birth control methods by prescribing birth control pills, providing condoms and spermatocides with instruction, fitting diaphragms, inserting IUDs, and describing "natural birth control" to a few women. We were awed by the decision of the Supreme Court on January 22, 1973, to legalize abortion, leaving this decision between the woman and her health care provider, who most of us knew would be one of us.

Travel included a weekly Friday evening trip to Vermont on the "Montrealer,"* and return ride on the Sunday overnighter which brought some of us back just in time to run to class Monday morning. Cars were handy to get around, but parking and the high incidence of theft was a real concern. Study on the train, study at home, and study every free moment seemed to be the way we used our time for the months we were in the training program. We were all encouraged to practice our new skills by using all the experiences possible. The instructors of the program were firm in helping us to develop the new role, to practice all the procedures often, and to articulate how we would function in our agencies or health centers.

Following an exciting graduation (and all the activities that went along with that celebration), we headed back to our home clinics, health centers, and medical offices with the promise that Miriam Manisoff and other instructors would come to visit each of us and see how things were going. I met with Dr. Gause and the administration of PPV and found out that they could only use my new knowledge and skills as a part-time nurse practitioner. I was warned that there were medical people as well as some clinic volunteers who were very concerned about this new role. The doctors (especially the OB-GYN Department of The University of Vermont Medical School) indicated that they doubted that the nurse practitioner could perform the procedures that were necessary for Planned Parenthood clinics. The volunteers were worried that the "patients" would not want a woman taking care of them.

My introduction as a nurse practitioner was at the clinics in Burlington (both at the hospital clinic and the Church Street office/clinic). The residents asked me many questions, challenged my decisions, and wanted to see every one of my charts. I was thankful that Dr. Gause was at those clinics and was the teacher for all of us. He provided assurances to the local physicians, the administration of PPV, and the patients that my practice was legitimate, medically sound, and very practical for the women who came into the clinic. He made the trip from Grafton, Vermont, many times to support my function and role as nurse practitioner in PPV.

As the hours of work increased for me as nurse practitioner, Dr. Gause accompanied me to most of the clinics around the state. All the folks were glad to see him, to confer with him about unusual medical problems, and to listen as he reassured them concerning my role. It was then up to me

* Train route from Washington, D.C., to Montreal, Canada.

to do the things that I had learned in Newark for the women who came to those clinics. Most of the clinic volunteers accepted my new role because they could ask me questions and "not feel dumb." The older clinic directors, many volunteer nurses among them, seemed to hold their thoughts and judgments for several clinics. The visit of the trainers and teachers from the training program in Newark was helpful in showing PPV that we were developing the new role of nurse practitioner well.

I truly believed that women who came to PPV would wholeheartedly accept the role of nurse practitioner. One evening, after being at the Rutland Clinic for the third time, my belief was affirmed. After finishing the pelvic examination of a young farm woman who was seeking birth control, I observed that the woman was softly weeping. Very concerned that I had done something terribly wrong, I asked if I had done something to hurt her. She said through her tears that she had never had such a "wonderful exam" and she would be back again. I asked what would have happened if I had not been there. She said she would have left because she did not want an exam from a "male doctor" ever again.

In the first year as a nurse practitioner, I traveled all over the state to clinics in St. Albans, Rutland, St. Johnsbury, Middlebury, Brattleboro, Barre, Enosburg, Morrisville, and Springfield. We had clinic training sessions in Woodstock, St. Albans, Bridport, Castleton, Stowe, Waitsfield, and Randolph, plus many other meetings with the administrators and the staff of the clinics around the state. I carried a folding exam table in my car, plus a life-size model; these allowed me to teach staff, teachers, and others who talked to women, about pelvic exams, pap smears, and other women's health issues. My job at PPV included activities that assured that we had high standards of clinic health care and an exceptional level of teaching and benefit/risk instruction for each of the birth control methods. I attended the Grand Rounds of the OB-GYN Department of the Mary Fletcher Hospital (later the Medical Center of Vermont) to increase my knowledge and to make contacts with the medical profession to whom I would be making referrals.

Along with the work at the clinics at PPV, I rejoined the Vermont Women's Health Center (VWHC) as their first nurse practitioner. My role in the VWHC was to provide the high level of women's health care and provision of birth control methods that I had learned at the training program in Newark. I had a particular challenge in that I had to develop two protocols for the two organizations and two medical directors. Each of the organizations used the basic protocol that we had developed in Newark, and each clinic used similar therapies, but had slightly different procedures and activities. Because of the volatility and politics of abortion, it was not included in my protocols for either PPV or VWHC. I took histories, performed tests and pregnancy sizing for pregnancy determination, and provided clear, unbiased options for women coming into either organization for help with an unplanned pregnancy.

There were various bumps along the road toward introducing the role of nurse practitioner to the state of Vermont. Some of the areas of concern were:

- functioning with the other medical providers, physicians, and other practitioners, plus the professional societies
- networking with other medical providers in order to learn and to make medically sound referrals
- developing working relationships with the pharmacies that would accept our prescriptions
- beginning the process of getting the Nurse Practice Act changed to legalize the role of nurse practitioner
- securing financial compensation for the increased responsibilities

Looking back on all these activities, many of them seemed impossible at the time. But, with the help of many other nurse practitioners who were soon coming on the scene in Vermont, these tasks got done in due time.

The next nurse from Vermont to go to the Nurse Practitioner Training Program was Marge Hoyt from St. Johnsbury. As my work increased from part-time to full-time, the expectations of the role of nurse practitioner in PPV increased. We had responsibilities in doing complete clinics (without the local physician), teaching the staff about delivering services, introducing new procedures, interpreting required standards, and introducing a new medical record. With the help of Dr. Gause, and with Larry Weed, MD, as consultant, we were able to introduce the Problem Oriented Medical Record (POMR). It helped a great deal to have a standard patient record with a problem list and organized medical information that could be transferred easily to any clinic in which the woman (man or couple) might make an appointment.

By the third year of full-time work as the first nurse practitioner, the role was firmly established in PPV. We could see more women, provide more clinic appointment slots at convenient hours, increase the services of contraceptive care for working women and teens, plus, cover the clinic services for vasectomy. Another nurse (Eileen Dick from Rutland) went to the University of Colorado for a nurse practitioner program in reproductive health. She came back to function as a nurse practitioner and manager in the Rutland PPV clinic, thus increasing the services in the mid-portion of the state. Ann Fielder, from Brattleboro, joined the team of nurse practitioners at PPV after she went to the program in Newark in the fourth year of using the nurse practitioners.

The role of the nurse practitioner as teacher became more apparent as time moved along. The reputation of PPV was growing as a place to learn about women's health, to receive comprehensive contraception information, and to gain awareness in providing compassionate medical care. First, individual physicians and nurses seeking increased skills in providing contraception requested training and education. Next, the family practice residents of The University of Vermont (UVM) Medical School, along with medical residents and internal medicine, were slowly integrated into training programs, which I taught each year. Each would spend about a four-week rotation in the clinics at the Burlington Center (and other clinics if possible). Each learned how to take a sensitive medical history, to provide unbiased contraception information, to do a gentle, teaching exam, and to prescribe a method of contraception that would be used successfully by the woman and her partner.

Connections with the wider medical world—both locally and worldwide—were important for the role of the nurse practitioner to grow and meet the needs of patients and society. Attendance at annual meetings of nurse practitioners where practical information as well as legal status and protocols were discussed was a must for professional development. As the first nurse practitioner in women's health care, an invitation to be on the committee to pick the chairperson of the OB-GYN Department of the UVM Medical School was an honor—and a tremendous responsibility. Also, I was invited to teach in the human sexuality class for undergraduates at the university. It was the first time pelvic exams, pap smears, and STD (sexually transmitted disease) tests were discussed while seeing a slide show, which was developed to be shown in a large classroom. Knowledge of various levels of sexuality of women and men were necessary in order to assist the people who came into the clinics.

Planned Parenthood was maturing, as were the women (and men) who came in for services. For the older woman who came to PPV for help, we were able to start a program that was developed with the help of PPV Medical Director, Dr. Judy Tyson, who took over for Dr. Gause. In the early 1980s, our "Midlife Program" provided services and information for women in the perimenopausal phase of their lives. PPV had grown to include New Hampshire, Maine, and Vermont, and was now known as Planned Parenthood of Northern New England (PPNNE). Many of the women had been coming to Planned Parenthood for many years, and some were bringing their daughters to the clinic for their first pelvic exams. Programs about teen sexuality, STDs and herpes, decision making in sexuality, practice in saying "no" to sex in relationships, and natural family planning were all part of the teaching role of the nurse practitioner.

Couples having problems getting pregnant began to seek information from PPNNE. Learning about their bodies, what happened during ovulation in the woman's cycle, and how sperm fertilized the ovum was the beginning of information that was provided for folks who were having difficulties in getting pregnant. Judy Tyson, MD, and I, in consultation with Mark Gibson, professor of OB-GYN at the UVM Medical School and an infertility specialist, planned and implemented the infertility program for PPNNE. Couples could go through their whole work-up at the Burlington Clinic of PPNNE, including the final test, the hysterosalpingogram (done at the hospital by one of the infertility specialists and accompanied by me). After making a major presentation at the Medical Committee of PPFA in New York City (to the sub-committee for New Services), I was able to start a program for treatment of infertility. In the clinic, injections of Clomid were given, checks for effectiveness were done, and tests for determining pregnancy were part of the protocol. Over a period of several years, PPNNE could record results of normal pregnancy, adoption, and induced (via Clomid and in vitro fertilization) pregnancies.

As you can see, the role of the nurse practitioner has evolved from those early years. In the beginning when the role was new, we had to find out how we could function in the established medical field as a nurse practitioner where the physician was "god" . . . the Gatekeeper to medical care. We had to gain knowledge, use our new skills well, and become clinically competent. Laws and nurse practice acts had to be changed to fit the functioning of our new role. Protocols had to be constantly reviewed and changed as nursing and medical practice changed. Health assessments, patho-physiology, therapeutics, pharmacology, disease prevention, laboratory tests, prescription writing, and health teaching were all areas where the nurse practitioner had to keep studying, attending conferences, and getting continuing education at the level of our clinical practice.

For those of us who had to create a new role and new functioning for nurse practitioners, we created our place in expanded health care services, and in high quality patient care demanded by patients and HMOs. We have been able to provide sensible assessments, compassion and understanding of life styles, comfortable and thorough examinations, an education concerning the management of therapies, clear instructions for the individual, and, if necessary, referral to a known specialist who is interested and concerned. Over time the nurse practitioner has uniquely demonstrated the ability and the skills to serve the unmet needs of primary health, women's health, and family health. We have provided a personalized service, encouraged continuum of care for women and families, promoted health and wellness, and developed choices for women and their families.

—Janet C. Patterson, RN, BSN

Oncology Nursing in Vermont: A Specialty Practice Emerges

Oncology nursing began in Vermont in the 1970s, with the development of the medical oncology service at the Medical Center Hospital of Vermont (MCHV) and the Vermont Regional Cancer Center at The University of Vermont (UVM). At that time, Dr. Jerome Yates, a medical oncologist from Roswell Park Cancer Center, arrived to establish the service. A Cancer Care and Rehabilitation Grant was written in 1974 and was funded in 1975 by the National Cancer Institute. Dr. Irwin Krakoff from Sloan Kettering Hospital also arrived in 1975 to direct the Vermont Regional Cancer Center.

Marie Kassakian, RN, was the first oncology nurse to join the group in 1974. She had previous oncology experience in Boston. Later that year, she was joined by Carole Wood, RN, who brought extensive experience as a community health nurse with the Visiting Nurse Association. Both Carol and Marie completed the first family nurse practitioner program at The University of Vermont in 1975. In 1975, Alan Sousie, RN, Lin Bailey, RN, and the rest of the interdisciplinary team were hired. Marilyn Rinker, RN, joined the team in 1976, bringing extensive hospital experience.

At that time, the concept of caring for oncology patients using an interdisciplinary team of health professionals was considered state-of-the-art cancer care. Nurses were a part of the team following cancer patients in the hospital and clinic. In addition to nurses, the team included physicians—internists, oncologists, surgeons, and psychiatrists—as well as enterostomy specialists, social workers, physical therapists, occupational therapists, nutritionists, statisticians, and members of the clergy.

The oncology clinic was located in the Burgess Building at MCHV. It consisted of patient examination rooms, a large chemotherapy room, a private room for sick patients, conference rooms, and office space for staff. Patient care included physical examinations, consultations with members of the interdisciplinary team, and various interventions such as pain and symptom management and procedures particular to care management: blood transfusions, paracentesis, thoracentesis, lumbar puncture, or any other care or procedure which was indicated. Patients received laboratory work, X-rays, and other diagnostic procedures at the

Mary Fletcher and DeGoesbriand units of MCHV. In 1979, the clinic moved to the DeGoesbriand unit. It is presently located at the Mary Fletcher unit of MCHV.

Patients also received care in radiation oncology, which continues to be located at the Mary Fletcher unit of FAHC. In 1979, Maura McLure, RN, was the nurse in radiation oncology. Other nurses in this area included Elizabeth McGrath, Sandie Cote, RN, and Sue Guillan, RN. (The latter two are currently practicing in radiation oncology.) These nurses managed patient care and supported patients and their families through treatment. Patients were often seen in both medical oncology and radiation oncology, and were managed concurrently as care was delivered through protocols combining treatment modalities such as radiation, medical oncology, and surgery.

The Cancer Care and Rehabilitation Grant added another dimension to the care of patients with cancer: case management and home visits by oncology nurse practitioners. All patients enrolled in the grant program would continue to receive oncology care, but were randomized into one of two groups: a control group, or an experimental group that would receive home visits by oncology nurse practitioners. The goal for the experimental group was better coordination of care, improved pain and symptom management, earlier problem intervention, and better tolerance of the disease and its treatments. It was thought that this focus on care in their homes would help family members become more involved in patient care, resulting in increased support for the patients.

Many patients lived in rural areas of Vermont; sometimes nurse practitioners traveled ninety miles one way to see them. Patients received home visits weekly or more often if necessary. Home visits consisted of a physical examination, a functional assessment, and an assessment of pain control, appetite, toxicities and other side effects from therapy, and other issues confronting the patient.

Flow sheets were used for documentation of data in a standardized, organized manner. Nurses' notes regarding followup were sent to physicians and other health care providers. Patients were discussed with attending physicians and others who followed these patients. Adjustments were made in areas of concern. Relationships were built between the nurses and patients and families, as well as with physicians and other care givers. Nurses working in this extended role found it to be a very satisfying practice environment.

Patients enrolled in the grant program also received workups by members of the interdisciplinary team who were present at weekly rehabilitation rounds held at the oncology clinic. Team members had input into the plan of care at this time. Both patients in the control group and in the experimental group received visits from data collectors who gathered information regarding vital signs, issues of pain control, symptom control, activities of daily living, and quality of life.

In addition to introducing a team approach and specialized oncology nurses, this new concept of cancer care included comprehensive involvement with patients and their families. Patients seen in radiation and medical oncology clinics and the inpatient areas were encouraged to have their families present for discussions in order to provide emotional support and to keep everyone informed. This was especially important at times of diagnosis and disease progression.

Prior to this time, information was often kept from cancer patients, to the point of withholding diagnoses. In the 1950s and 1960s, nurses were not permitted to discuss diagnosis, treatment, or prognosis with patients. This could leave patients alone, fearful, and afraid to ask questions. Patients and families often did not discuss the disease or know the prognosis. This resulted in isolation for patients and families at a time when information as well as comfort and support was needed.

As a student nurse, the author remembers caring for an oncology patient in 1954 who was receiving radiation therapy and experiencing severe diarrhea and abdominal pain. She was thirty-nine years old, the mother of a high school classmate. No discussion of her disease or the debilitating side effects of inadequate control of pain or symptoms was permitted.

In the early 1970s, cancer began to be approached in a different manner. Care givers were beginning to be educated in oncology as a specialty. It became apparent that patients and families needed to be fully informed and educated about prognosis, treatment options, goals, and expectations before making decisions; and that patients who were part of the decision making process had better outcomes. In the 1970s, patients seen by the oncology team received detailed explanations of their disease and the treatment options open to them, including necessary procedures, tests, and followup. Prognosis, side effects, and toxicities were also discussed.

The oncology nurses, then and now, play an important role in patient education, and in helping patients and families understand the disease process and treatment options. In most cases, it is the oncologist who gives the patient the diagnosis and discusses treatment options. It is the oncology nurse, however, who follows up with the patient and family to determine their understanding and knowledge regarding the situation. This may happen when the patient begins the first radiation or chemotherapy treatment, or when the patient is preparing for surgery. Patients and families have received information from the physician and are now able to ask questions or voice concerns and feelings they might have to the nurse. The oncology nurse becomes the patient's advocate and helps patients and families through many difficult times. This approach requires intense education of care givers.

Founded in 1975, the Vermont Regional Cancer Center's mission became patient care, education, and research. Education was delivered in many ways. Experts in the field of cancer care were brought in to teach members of the cancer team. Case histories were reviewed at weekly oncology rounds, where the type of cancer, its therapies, and management were discussed. Radiation rounds were held weekly by that department. This allowed a forum for physicians to present patient cases and conduct discussions regarding care. Physicians from MCHV, UVM, and private practice attended, as well as nurses, medical students, residents, and other health care providers engaged in cancer care.

The Vermont Regional Cancer Center presented oncology grand rounds weekly in Austin Auditorium at MCHV. These offerings included presentations by Cancer Center staff, scientists from UVM, the VRCC lab, and visiting oncology experts from other centers. Oncology nurses presented on pain and symptom management strategies in anti-emetic therapy. The Cancer Center staff also traveled for educational presentations, including tumor boards in St. Johnsbury and Rutland. Oncology nurses have educated student nurses, medical students, house staff, oncology fellows, and attending physicians.

These tumor boards served a dual purpose—consultation and followup for patients, as well as education of medical and nursing staff. Local physicians referred patients to these boards to be seen by the oncology team. This included consultations with various specialists in medicine, gynecology, radiology, or surgery. Plans of care were then proposed which might include chemotherapy, radiation therapy, or surgery. The educational presentations at these tumor boards could be on specific types of cancer or therapies. They were held at hospitals and open to all hospital staff.

Professional and public education was often a joint venture carried out with the American Cancer Society. Oncology nurses, physicians, and other care givers served on state and local committees as officers and board members. Presentations on types of cancer, followup treatment, and patient care were presented to local organizations such as women's auxiliary groups, church groups, and Home Demonstration groups by members of the oncology team. The goal was education about recognition of cancer signs and symptoms, its treatment and its prevention.

Smoking cessation was an important component of the educational program. Health fairs in grammar schools, high schools, colleges, and work sites were places to have exhibits and health professionals available to impart information. Breast and testicular self-exams were educational

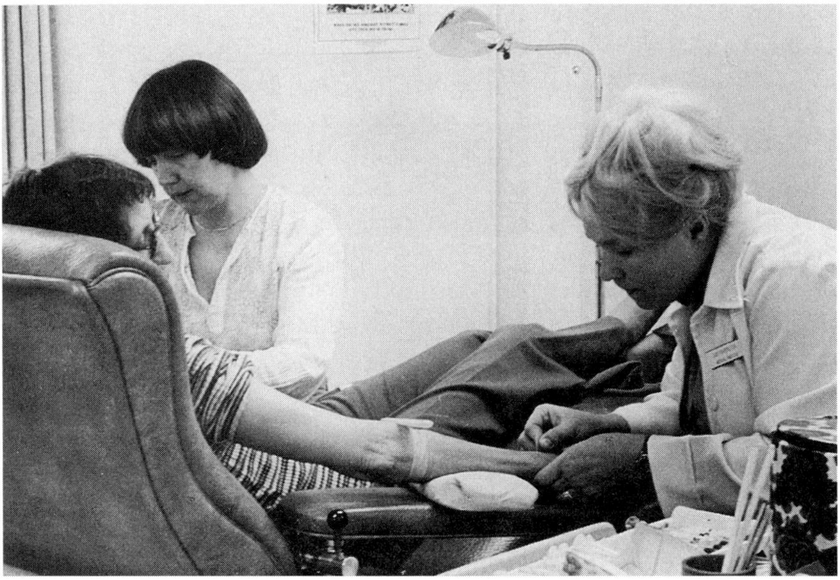

Courtesy Fletcher Allen Health Care

Judy Rivers, RN, and Marilyn Rinker, RN, administering chemotherapy, Vermont Regional Cancer Center, 1982.

focuses. Colorectal cancer was also the focus of screening clinics which were sponsored by businesses and service organizations.

The cervical screening project was a nurse practitioner VRCC endeavor in conjunction with the American Cancer Society (ACS). During the mid 1970s, ACS volunteers such as Sally Lanphear from Jericho set up clinics at churches, schools, and service organizations. Many women were seen that had not had a pap smear for many years. These clinics were also times for other education on cancer prevention, breast self-exam, nutrition, etc.

Other patient and family services began to emerge as part of total cancer care. The first cancer support group sponsored by the Vermont Regional Cancer Center was organized in 1982. It centered on spouses of cancer patients. An observation had been made that spouses would often accompany patients for visits to radiation or medical oncology and spend time speaking together informally in the waiting room. It was felt that a more organized approach might be helpful. Jane Wolfe, MD, a medical resident, and Marilyn Rinker, RN, oncology clinic coordinator, met weekly with Sam Dietzel, PhD, the director of Counseling and Testing at The University of Vermont, to learn how to lead a support group. The group met for twelve weeks, and among its members was a unique couple—the husband was a cancer survivor who had been followed by the Rehabilitation Grant, and his wife was a patient currently receiving therapy for Hodgkin's disease.

Cancer Center Medical Oncology, and the Medical Center Hospital of Vermont continued to sponsor support groups over the years. Nurses, social workers, and physicians participated as facilitators. The American Cancer Society sponsored "I Can Cope," a programmed approach covering various topics. There are currently groups for breast cancer and prostate survivors. The Visiting Nurse Association has sponsored bereavement groups. Participants—including patients, families, and professionals in health care—have all spoken of the support and comfort these groups have offered.

In addition to the educational mission of the Cancer Center, there was the research mission. Nurses played a large role in this phase and continue to work in various areas of research today. Patients in the oncology clinic and radiation therapy were being cared for under conventional protocols and studies. Oncology nurses in the clinic and on the oncology unit were administering chemotherapy. In 1988 and 1989, the interleukin therapy protocol was coordinated by Neva Cunningham, RN. Another group of oncology patients received chemotherapy in the clinical research unit at MCHV. There nurses managed research protocols including those of the National Surgical Adjuvant Breast Protocol Group (NSABP). Patient education was an important part of followup. Data collected from NSABP protocols was accumulated nationally and internationally, and has contributed to current strides in breast cancer therapy.

In addition to monitoring patients on conventional protocols, clinical research nurses followed patients on cancer research studies that needed extensive monitoring regarding sampling for blood work, cardiac and other studies. Patients who needed twenty-four-hour followup and monitoring were also followed on the clinical research unit.

The development of new therapeutic agents and the testing of combinations of conventional chemotherapeutic agents was carried out in clinical trials by the Vermont Regional Cancer Center in its laboratory at UVM, in oncology clinic, and in the hospital. Oncology clinical research nurses played an important role following patients throughout the studies, administering chemotherapy, managing toxicities and side effects, and most importantly providing support and education to patients and families.

In addition to participation in National Protocol Groups, nurses worked on protocols for symptom management, including anti-emetic control. Protocols which covered oncology nurses in extended practice were also developed by oncology nurses and attending physicians. Oncology nurses in this role included Judy Rivers, Stella Miner, Joyce Silveira,

Marilyn Rinker in medical oncology, and Elizabeth McGrath in radiation oncology. The development of these protocols has furthered the safe and competent practice of oncology nursing.

While participating in the mission of the Department of Medical Oncology and the Vermont Regional Cancer Center, oncology nurses have had an influence on many people. Nurses have helped patients and families cope with cancer through administering therapy, managing side effects, helping provide adequate pain control, and in some cases providing end-of-life care, enabling patients and families to face death with comfort and dignity.

Initially, patients positive for HIV were treated in medical oncology, and nurses developed protocols while learning on the job. Oncology nurses were also active in gathering data to ascertain the safe preparation and administration of chemotherapy. Studies that examined blood and urine to assess the effects of chemotherapy administration were done by oncology nurses. Oncology nurses served on a committee with the oncology pharmacist and oncologists to set up the chemotherapy administration program for the Medical Center Hospital of Vermont.

From the beginning, Dr. Yates and Dr. Krakoff were very supportive of nursing. To quote Dr. Yates, "Listen to the oncology nurses; they will teach you much about oncology care." Nurses who were employed in medical oncology and at the Cancer Center were fortunate to be participants in an innovative approach to cancer care.

Many nurses have been part of the oncology team throughout the years: Judy Rivers in 1979, Stella Miner in 1980, Joyce Silveia and Jane Silman in 198l, Elaine Owens and Trish Cummings in 1984, Ellen Flanagan in 1989, and at present Anne Ireland, Neva Cunningham, Angie Hill, Sandy Shubel, Deb Clark, Joanne Neilson, and Laurie Chassereau. Each has brought a special aspect of nursing expertise to cancer care.

As the specialty of oncology nursing evolved during the 1970s and as it continues today, nurses are the care givers closest to patients and families as they travel the course of this serious and sometimes devastating disease. Patients and families get to know their nurses well and benefit from their expertise in pain control, symptom control, and management of other problems which impact on their quality of life. The oncology nurse has developed the skills necessary to provide care and caring to patients and families faced with the diagnosis of cancer.

—Marilyn Rinker, RN, MSN, APN, OCN

Psychiatric Nursing in Vermont: In Hospital

THE PROBABILITY of predicting the future of events and trends is plagued by low rates of accuracy. Likewise, historical descriptions can only come approximately close to what actually occurred. Particularly, the assignment of significance to historical events is colored by the worldview and opinions of each historian. With this in mind, I offer my view of a piece of nursing history in Vermont.

In 1941, psychiatric nursing was synonymous with inpatient care at the Brattleboro Retreat, the Brandon Training School, and the Vermont State Hospital (in Waterbury).

The Brattleboro Retreat, a private psychiatric institution, was founded in 1834 as the Vermont Asylum for the Insane at Brattleboro, and at that time was one of only ten mental hospitals in the country.[1] By 1891, it was very overcrowded and the Vermont State Asylum for the Insane was built in Waterbury, which later became the Vermont State Hospital. A somewhat simplified characterization (still true today), is that wealthy patients were cared for at Brattleboro retreat, and mentally ill Vermonters with no resources went to the State Hospital. Consequently, there has always been a social stigma associated with being a patient, or a nurse, at Vermont State Hospital.

The Brandon Training School was founded by the Vermont Legislature in 1915 as the Vermont State School for the Feeble Minded. At its peak in the 1960s, it cared for 700 children and adults with severe mental retardation, later defined as developmental disabilities.[2] The nursing role was primarily one of parenting, plus meeting the medical nursing needs associated with severe brain dysfunction. The fifty years post World War II saw Brandon's services evolve from total institutional care to complete family services and foster home placement, so that the Department of Developmental and Mental Health Services was able to close Brandon in 1993. Afterward, the nursing needs of this population were met by home health nurses, public health nurses, school nurses, and wrap-around services in home settings provided through community mental health centers.

The attempt, in a small space, to describe a history of broad topics and the actions of a large number of people, who themselves changed over time, is a task similar to an artist painting a panorama of events on one canvas. Faced with several choices of paint pots and a multitude of ideas, the painter daubs a little here and a little there. By making choices to create a picture, the painter rejects many forms, colors, textures, images, and styles. But if the painting is successful, it will evoke in the imagination of the viewer everything that was left off of the canvas, and stimulate thoughts about the present and future. I will attempt the story of Vermont inpatient psychiatric nursing by focusing primarily on Vermont State Hospital, and will try to weave a picture of the issues for nursing in each decade.

Vermont State Hospital in the 1940s

In 1941, Vermont State Hospital (VSH) was a total psychiatric care institution, with a thousand patients, a farm, geriatrics, a laundry, sewing rooms, doctors' dining rooms, live-in staff, separate buildings for men and women, hydrotherapy, alcoholics, homeless poor people, unwed mothers, and the beginning of shortages caused by World War II.[3]

The living conditions for patients were bare, crowded, and not clean. There were huge problems with lice, scabies, rats, bed bugs, and cockroaches. There were insufficient toilets, and five-gallon cans were used as urinals on the wards at night because there were not enough staff to allow patients to be up at night to go to the toilet.

Because of the war, there were shortages of soap, towels, nails, paint, and staff. Patients wore nightclothes all day, or plain cotton dresses with buttons in the back so they would not strip them off. There were no medications and many patients screamed all night. There was no Dilantin for seizures, and often patients were put in camisoles and tied to benches and chairs.

For some, there was no exercise. Others contributed to the work of the institution in the kitchen, laundry, and the farm. Patients with wheelbarrows shoveled and wheeled as much as 35–40 tons of coal every day into the four big boilers in the heating plant. There were large lawns to be mowed and privileged patients were chained to the lawnmowers so that they would not run away.

Staff lived at the hospital and devoted their whole lives to it. A nightwatch attendant slept on the ward. The official shifts were twelve hours and a sixty-hour workweek, but often much longer.

World War II revealed an appreciation for the value of nurses in the care of the wounded, and they were included in the military.* In 1944, Mildred Murphy, RN, resigned as Superintendent of Nurses and Matron

---

*Funds were provided for nursing education, and by 1947 the Army–Navy Nurse Act provided commissioned rank for women nurses (but not men nurses until 1955).[4]

at Vermont State Hospital and entered the Army Nurse Corp, as did many staff before the war was over. Also in 1944, Dr. Rupert Chittick became superintendent, and was one of three doctors for 1,076 patients. There were no registered nurses on any of the wards. There was an RN supervisor for the North side (women patients) and one for the medical patients. There were 106 attendants. By contrast, fifty years later in 1994, there were 80 patients, 25 registered nurses, and 100 psychiatric technicians/LPNs.

Between 1944 and 1950, thirty-six people had been added to the staff and 348 had left. Chittick was determined to establish a training program for attendants, raise their pay and status, hire more nurses, and put nurses in charge of the attendants. Attempts to employ a qualified psychiatric nurse educator failed.

Finally, Vera A. Hanks, RN, agreed to go to the McLean Hospital in Waverley, Massachusetts, where Chittick had been on the staff for several years just prior to coming to Vermont. She participated in McLean's three-month affiliate nurse's psychiatric training course; visited with some of the instructors of neighboring state hospitals; and then returned to set up a program at Waterbury.

Hanks had joined the Vermont State Hospital staff soon after Chittick arrived, and had taken over the charge of the men's infirmary where the need was urgent. There were no nurses on any of the wards at that time, but the women were coping better than the men. On her return to Waterbury, she organized the primary training program and taught it herself, repeating it at least twelve times to small groups until every ward employee and supervisor had participated. This was the start of the program which later expanded into one of the best psychiatric technician training schools in the country.[5,6]

In January 1945, electric shock treatment was made available and proved successful in certain types of mental illness. However, there were no muscle relaxant medications, and convulsions resulted in many broken bones. About the same time, the use of malaria fever was instituted in the treatment of those patients with a syphilitic infection of the brain. Those patients responded well, and several were able to return to their normal lives. Penicillin began to be used in the acute treatment of first stage syphilis, so that, while in the 1940s half of the VSH patient population had general paresis due to third stage syphilis, this disappeared as a diagnosis category as years went by. Advances in the treatment of tuberculosis, also, over time, eliminated the need for tuberculosis wards.[7]

A new nurses residence (Stanley Hall) was completed in June 1948, but even this did not fill the need, and staff began to be hired who were willing to live in their own homes away from the hospital.

A new medical-surgical building opened on February 6, 1949, for 124

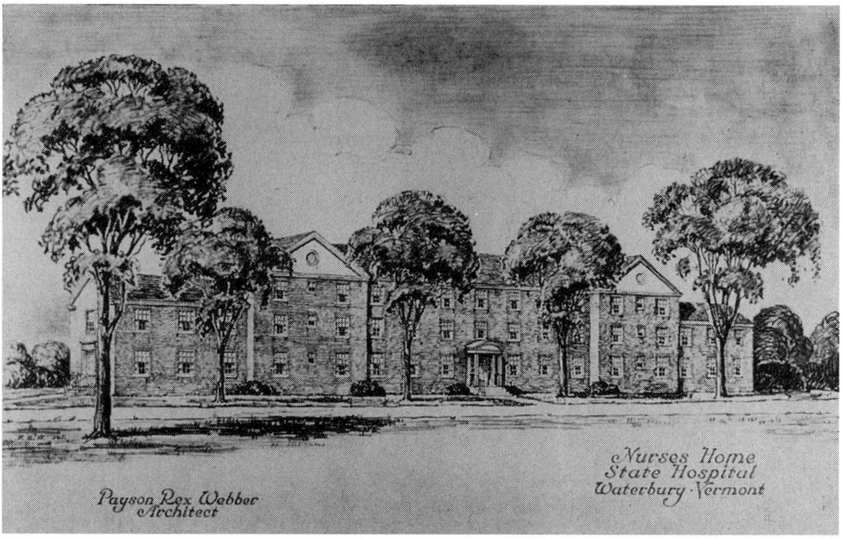

Courtesy Vermont State Hospital Archives

Stanley Hall architect drawing, 1946

patients. Besides the patient care wards, the building contained a section room, pathologist's office and laboratory, an incinerator, a large classroom, a nursing demonstration room, an office for the director of nurses, operating room, surgeons' dressing rooms and showers, a minor surgery room, nurses' utility room and supply room, pharmacy, dental office, X-ray room, electrocardiography room, electro-therapy room, as well as a large medical library, and two doctors' offices. All types of major surgeries were done here, and this was a complete general hospital for the village that Vermont State Hospital had become. It was the crowning piece in a self-sufficiency that was already beginning to end.

Public Interest in Psychiatric Care: The 1950s

1950 saw the beginning of the Korean War, and the beginning of a breakdown of VSH isolation. Dr. Chittick met resistance in the Vermont Legislature to his requests for money, and gained the support of the press.

On April 4, 1951, Miss Mary Spargo, news analyst at radio station WCAX, visited the State Hospital. On April 7, she gave a report on the overcrowding.

> I have to report that at Waterbury I saw our fellow human beings, our fellow Vermonters herded together closer than a Vermont farmer would think of keeping cattle in a barn. The hospital has had to take in 1300 patients in quarters only large enough for 982. This overcrowding is seri-

> ous and delays the recovery of the patients. Under proper conditions many more would recover. In many wards the beds are less than a foot apart and beds line some of the corridors. Tiny rooms hardly large enough for one single bed have two. There is no privacy and women are herded into a single bathroom facility, which does nothing to maintain dignity and self-respect. Dr. Chittick feels that private bathroom facilities alone would contribute very considerably to the rehabilitation of the patients. Every precaution against fire is taken, but the hazard remains. The imagination of the listener can function better than any words of mine to visualize what a fire at the State Hospital would mean.[8]

On July 24, a special commission made its first report to the governor, recommending the construction of one new dormitory to accommodate 180 patients, using the two old round wards to take care of 70 patients, the transfer of 60 patients to the Brattleboro Retreat, and the crowding of 20 more into the new building (over its rated capacity), when it was completed. These recommendations were based on the fact that there was a slight drop in the population at the hospital over the previous year. The committee believed that it might be the beginning of a trend. It also requested that the American Psychiatric Association (APA) survey the facilities and conditions at the hospital.

The report of the APA was released on January 1, 1952,[9] and recommended a fifteen-point building program covering every area of the hospital operation—from recreation to surgery. It found that the hospital had 473 beds over its rated capacity, according to APA standards. The report also recommended the renovation and modernization of the buildings in the main group as soon as possible, and the abandonment of some wards entirely. The Legislature began to approve money for various building projects and fire sprinkler systems.

An attendant education program was firmly established in 1950, taught primarily by nurses. A nursing education staff was developed. Gertrude Blake, RN, became a staff instructor (1950–74). In December 1955, Beverly Brown, RN, joined Blake and Hanks to help with the supervision of procedures being done on patients rather than just the demonstration doll in the classroom.[10]

In 1952, the federal Public Health Service released a national nursing needs and resources report.[11] The Vermont section reported that there were 1,291 active RNs and 592 other nursing personnel employed in Vermont. Only 3% of Vermont RNs were working in Vermont's mental hospitals, caring for one-and-a-half times more patients than were in general hospitals. The 1952 guidelines of both the American Nurses' Association and the American Medical Association, for inpatient care, was one RN for 25 patients and one aide for four patients; the recommendation of the

Health Service report was that Vermont had a deficit of 55 RNs and 214 aides engaged in psychiatric care.

Another observation of the report was that Vermont schools of nursing sent their students out of state for their psychiatric nursing affiliations. It was recommended that funds be provided to Vermont State Hospital by the Legislature to host student nurse affiliations. This would create a potential pool of new graduates wanting to work at VSH, improved patient care while students were at VSH, and include state psychiatric hospital care as an essential part of a nurse's education.

A Director of Nursing Education joined the VSH staff in 1956, Alice Robinson, RN, MS.[12] This allowed Director of Nursing Hanks to concentrate on developing the nursing department, and made it possible to establish a psychiatric nursing affiliation for student nurses. Diploma students came from Heaton Hospital in Montpelier, Gifford Memorial Hospital in Randolph, and Bishop DeGoesbriand and Mary Fletcher Hospitals in Burlington. Board and room were free at Stanley and Wasson Halls. Robinson and two instructors were directly responsible for students, and did all of the clinical supervision and most of the teaching. In return, student nurses stayed for twelve weeks and provided many hours of direct nursing care. Janet (Barrett) Perkins was one of those student nurses, and in 1960 she returned as an RN, remaining at VSH as a teacher in the psychiatric technician program until her retirement in 1994.

There was a burgeoning recognition that kindness, good staff intentions, and a safe haven in a clean environment were not enough; rather, it was the application of knowledge about human behavior in a kind, clean, safe environment that produced good patient care and helped with recovery. It became fully recognized that nurses and ancillary staff, who were with patients twenty-four hours a day, could develop therapeutic relationships with patients that were conducive to marked improvement.[13] There was still an emphasis on highly polished floors, but it also became a priority for nursing staff to lead groups, work with individual patients, and pay attention to a therapeutic ward atmosphere.

While she was director of nursing service and nursing education at Boston State Hospital, Alice Robinson had written the first textbook specifically for psychiatric aides.[14] When she came to VSH in 1956, her teaching emphasized attitudes of care that promoted growth and rehabilitation.

Hope of recovery entered the scene in 1954, when George Brooks, MD, began controlled experiments with chlorpromazine (Thorazine) and reserpine. Lobotomy and insulin coma disappeared, and the use of electroconvulsive therapy (ECT), seclusion, and restraint dropped. There was a decrease in the destruction of property by patients, and an increase in the number of patients able to engage in occupational therapy and other self-care activities.[15] Prior to these medications, a nurse's duties revolved around treatments with hydrotherapy, electric shock, restraints, seclusion, and rigid routines to control filth, nudity, assaultiveness, and the provision of life's bare essentials.[16]

Also in 1954, television was introduced to the wards by an attendant during the World Series baseball games. Television became a way to combat the isolation of being in an institution.[17]

With the swirling changes in patient care and staff education, it was also the beginning of changes in working conditions for VSH employees. The first chapter of the Vermont State Employees' Association* was established.[18] Dr. Brooks was president, and Vera Hanks, RN, was also an officer. Peer and administrative pressure was high to be a member.†

In 1957, the workweek changed from sixty to forty hours, and to eight-hour shifts with no loss in pay. There were twenty RNs and 252 attendants for 1,175 patients. Ninety-seven attendants were in nine sections of the first year of the training program; twenty-six in two sections of the second year of the program; and 121 were in five sections of the advanced program.[19] In 1959, in the United States, 50% of all hospitalized patients were mental patients, yet only 4% of registered nurses worked with them.[20] To fill the need for a much larger work force, the VSH attendant programs taught principles and procedures of nursing care, and the curriculum was similar to that of the affiliating student nurses. It also emphasized the interpersonal and rehabilitation skills necessary for the planned discharge of patients who were responding to the new medications.

Dr. Brooks headed a research project concerned with patients who had been ill and institutionalized for a long time. It involved rebuilding productive work skills, social reorientation, and finally job placement and independent living outside the hospital. The focus of daily nursing care switched from comforting and controlling the incurable, to rehabilitation and life outside of a hospital. A rehabilitation house was established in Montpelier in 1957, and two more in Burlington in 1958.[21]

With the cooperation of the Vermont Department of Education, a program of elementary education was provided for the child patients. Part of nursing care became getting the kids to the hospital school and helping profoundly autistic and schizophrenic children with homework and the normal activities of childhood in order to maximize their growth and development.

Apprenticeship was still an avenue for becoming a nurse. VSH staff who passed two years of VSH nursing classes wore a nurse's cap with one

---

* Labor union representing employees of the State of Vermont.

† It is interesting to contrast this with the atmosphere of disapproval toward union membership that existed in the 1990s at many hospitals in Vermont.

stripe and were called "class girls." In 1960, the Legislature passed a law that gave an eighteen-month window, which for VSH nonnurses practicing nursing meant that they could take an additional course at Heaton Hospital in Montpelier or Barre City Hospital, pass a state board examination, and become Registered Nurses. After the eighteen-month deadline, people had to graduate from an accredited school of nursing in order to obtain permission to take the state board licensing examination for nurses.[22]

During this period, a housekeeping department was established at VSH. Prior to this time, domestics were under the supervision of a "matron" in nursing service. The control of dirt has always been a big part of nursing, but the shift to organized housekeeping departments in hospitals was a welcome relief to nurses and patient care aides.

In the late 1950s, a new kind of patient appeared in increasing numbers. The courts quadrupled the number of people sent to the State Hospital after an opinion regarding legal responsibility for criminal acts. The evaluation periods were often several months, and the care needs were usually very different from other patients at VSH. These patients had many legal issues and treatment was complicated. The blend of a rehabilitative atmosphere with the need to protect the public safety became a constant theme.[23]

The 1960s: Growing Outward

The Cultural Revolution in the 1960s was not only in music, dress, Vietnam War protests, and re-definitions of acceptable social deviance. There were also health care revolutions. New mothers still were hospitalized several days after delivery, but they began demanding to be with their babies instead of creeping to the nursery window for a peek. Rooming-in was invented, and hundreds of articles were written on the importance of newborn bonding with the new mother. Surgery and orthopedic patients were allowed out of bed as soon as they could stand it, as more and more evidence emerged that activity speeded the healing process.

In mental health, a strength developed for the idea that hospitalization itself was a traumatic experience, and that people would be better helped if they could receive services while living in their own homes and communities. As early as 1948, Vermont had developed a statewide community mental health clinic system, and there were therapeutic residential communities such as Spring Lake Ranch near Rutland.[24] Federal legislation was passed in 1963, that provided funding for the building of thousands of Community Mental Health Centers nationally, and nine were initially established in Vermont, located in Bennington, Brattleboro, Burlington, Middlebury, Montpelier, Newport, Rutland, St. Albans and Springfield.[25] As time went by, these centers prevented many admissions to VSH, helped people who would never have gone to VSH at all, and provided followup care for people discharged from VSH.

In 1964, a Department of Mental Health (DMH) was created by the Vermont Legislature, giving it a commissioner and an independence from previous assignments to the Department of Health, Department of Corrections, and Department of Institutions. The new DMH included VSH, the Brandon Training School, and the Division of Community Mental Health Services. Rupert Chittick, MD, superintendent of VSH, became acting commissioner until Jonathan Leopold, MD, was appointed in January 1965.[26]

In 1961, *The Vermont Story: Rehabilitation of Chronic Schizophrenic Patients* was published, and ushered in an era of hope and national attention.[27] The 1960s became a time of open wards, bars removed from windows, normal and personal clothing for patients, a rehabilitation atmosphere, patient education, outings, discussion groups, psychodrama, and the Homer S. Murray summer camp for the children (later named Father Louis Logue's Camp).

The total hospital population was twelve hundred, of whom five hundred were defined as schizophrenic. At least one hundred of these were working full-time at jobs in the hospital, and they were included in the intensive rehabilitation effort described in *The Vermont Story.* Led by Rupert Chittick, MD, George Brooks, MD, William Deane, sociologist, and Francis Irons, vocational rehabilitation, the VSH staff and 253 schizophrenic patients were part of a ground-breaking rehabilitation effort. The patients received medication to control psychosis, social skills training to make up for years of institutionalization, and massive doses of cheerleading and hope from nursing and activity staff. The Vermont project became a landmark guide for many similar efforts across the nation. The way for it to be successful was to engage in a period of preparation where individuals could rehearse the situations they were likely to encounter. Patients were given detailed, concrete information in an instructional fashion by the staff. Halfway houses or some form of graduated return to the community were established.

In 1965, Brooks and Deane reported that nine years of work had led to the successful placement of 500 severely disabled chronic mental patients into the surrounding communities. There were 12,000 supportive contacts each year, and this seemed likely to increase indefinitely.[28]*

---

*In a twenty-year follow-up in 1977, 89% of the original cohort was located and many were substantially improved and doing well. Less than half were still classified as schizophrenic.[29] This was exciting proof against the beliefs that a person could never recover from schizophrenia, and that being sent to Vermont State Hospital was a life-time sentence.

In view of these changes, the State Hospital was faced with a redefinition of goals. It seemed that VSH would return to custodialism of the remaining patients, and be the prolonged care facility for the failures of the various community centers. However, it was not in Dr. Chitticks' nature to contemplate such a goal. He applied for another grant.

The Hospital Improvement Project (HIP) Grant was received April 1, 1965, for the establishment of "A State Hospital for Education Therapy."[30] The aims of this project were to provide rehabilitation, training, and re-education for long-term patients, increase community contacts, and increase staff education.

HIP Education Therapy Coordinators were located squarely in the nursing department, and were responsible to the director of nursing service (Vera Hanks) who met with them daily in planning conferences. Being solidly a part of nursing service meant they were not disruptive or competitive to other activities in nursing service. This structure isolated them slightly from other staff positions, such as the school department, occupational therapy, social service, and hospital industries, but kept their functions close to the wards.

Ivan Belknap's book, *Human Problems of a State Mental Hospital,*[31] was a detailed sociological analysis of the many levels of social organization within a large institution, and a poignant description of the gulfs between the administrative/executive system, the clinician system (physicians, specialty services, therapists), and the 24-hour ward system (nursing staff). Each of these three groups thinks they run a hospital, and that the other two are helping or interfering. When one group wants to make changes in another group, it is often a dismal failure.

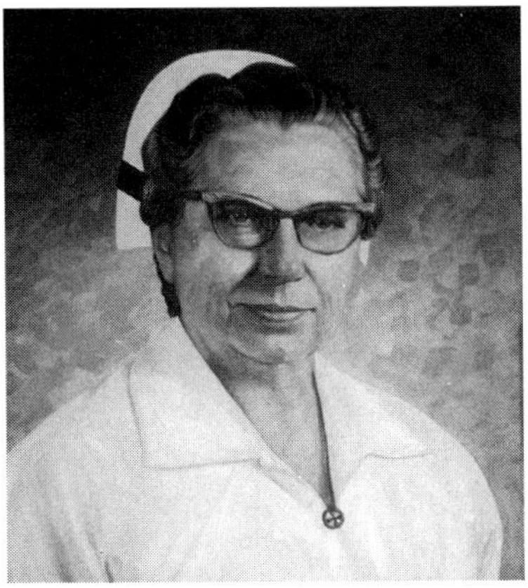

Vera A. Hanks, RN
Director of Nursing Services, 1957–1980
Vermont State Hospital
Portrait at Vermont State Hospital Archives

Chittick and his colleagues fully realized that if they, as one system, wanted to achieve the goal of the project—"to assure that all the education activities resulted in direct improvement to patient care at the ward level"[32]—then the coordinators had to be located in the same system they were trying to change. Because of this wise decision on the part of the planners, the ward nursing staff took ownership of this project, breathed life into it, and developed it beyond anyone's expectations. Ward occupational therapy, games and entertainment to heighten social skills, remotivation groups, and patient government were in existence before the project, but, because of the heightened emphasis, the number of daily patient contacts rose from 341 to 1,132.[33]

Just a few years earlier, in 1962, there had been 1,414 occupied beds, which was 268 more than the rated capacity. Discharges were rising, but so were admissions. The increases in volume taxed the patient care system greatly.[34] As a result of the many facets and activities of H.I.P., from July 1, 1965 through June 30, 1967, the hospital population reduced at an accelerating rate, and showed every sign of continuing this trend.

In June 1968, Dr. Chittick noted that in spite of the increase in admissions, the average daily census had decreased. He attributed this to the effectiveness of treatment programs, and to the impact of the Title XIX Program which enabled the placement of many patients in boarding homes and nursing homes. He also noted that the increase in deaths—from 120 in 1967 to 161 in 1968—was largely due to an influenza epidemic, which greatly weakened many of the elderly patients. The number of cases of alcoholism, drug addiction, and people sent by the court for observation after a plea of "not guilty by reason of insanity," were growing categories in 1968.[35]

In his 1969 "Fourteen Year Projection," Brooks noted that the rise in admissions since 1966 had been dramatic. In spite of this, the improved treatment and rehabilitation services resulted in a steady decrease in the patient census compared to the previous decade. The inpatient caseload dropped to under 1,000, but, with the aftercare responsibilities to ensure rehabilitation success and prevent re-admissions, the total case responsibilities were in excess of 3,000.[36] The new community mental health centers had not yet taken over all the responsibility for post-hospital care.

In addition to funding community mental health centers, in 1963 the National Institute of Mental Health expanded their training grants to allow juniors and seniors in baccalaureate degree nursing programs to receive stipends of tuition, plus $1,800 annually to finish the baccalaureate and continue on in graduate programs in psychiatric nursing. Psychiatric nursing had begun to develop as a specialty after World War II, when many nurses used the G.I. Bill to obtain a Bachelor of Science on the way toward a specialization in psychiatric nursing.[37] The Nurse Training Act of 1964 (Title VIII of the Public Health Service Act) provided money for nursing school construction, faculty development, student grants, and loans. Master's education for nurses became firmly established, which produced a pool of doctoral candidates. At first only an EdD in nursing or a PhD in a related field were available. A doctorate in nursing science

(DNS) was developed in the 1970s.[38] The concept of clinical nurse specialist was developed, and these nurses began to consult with other nurses in general hospitals who were dealing with "psych" patients who had been admitted for a medical problem.[39]

The next three directors of nursing at the Vermont State Hospital had graduate nursing education, and it became a requirement for the position: Lois Sabin, RN, MA, director of nurses, 1978; Barbara Boisse, RN, PhD, nursing administrator, 1984; Marsha Kincheloe, RN, MS, MA, CS, nursing administrator, 1985.

In the 1960s, there was a shift in all mental health disciplines from intra-psychic explanations of mental illness toward an emphasis on interpersonal relationships as the greatest single factor in mental, emotional, and spiritual health. This was a phase of double-bind theories of communication and ambivalent mothering as a cause of schizophrenia.[40] Psychiatric nurses were expected to be comfortable with patients with psychosis, errant behavior, delusions, and intense moods; and cure them with warmth, consistency, firm limit setting, and tolerance.[41] Alice Robinson, in her role as chairperson of the American Nurses' Association Conference Group on Psychiatric Nursing, gave a speech in which she described mental illness as an illness like any other; psychiatric patients, like most other sick persons, most frequently needed nothing more than the removal of environmental stresses and sympathetic psychiatric counseling to restore the person to economic, social, and family capabilities.[42]

Nationally, Hildegard Peplau's work had brought interpersonal theories from psychiatry firmly into nursing to be used as a basis for the analysis of nurse–patient interactions in terms of therapeutic quality.[43,44] At the same time, Virginia Henderson's description of a nurse's role was taught in all nursing programs: The unique function of the nurse was to assist the individual (sick or well) in the performance of those activities contributing to health or recovery (or to peaceful death) that the person would perform unaided if the person had the necessary strength or knowledge; and to do this in such a way as to help the patient gain independence as rapidly as possible.[45] These philosophies pervaded the VSH nursing programs, and continued when Frances Magee, RN, replaced Robinson as director of nursing education in 1966.[46] Magee had graduated in 1942 from Heaton Hospital in Montpelier with a diploma in nursing.

The education program for psychiatric technicians, the elementary and secondary education program for young patients, and the rehabilitation programs developed at the Vermont State Hospital gained such international attention that each year several workers in this field from other states and from foreign countries visited the hospital, after being referred to it by the World Health organization or by the National Institute of Mental Health.[47]

Grant money from the NIMH in 1964 made it possible to expand the psychiatric technician program to a four-year curriculum, and develop a strong faculty to teach it. The basic philosophy was to develop the 274 aides as clinical team members, to broaden an understanding of mental illness, and to teach the concept of the importance of the patient as a person with needs for respect, dignity, recognition, and individuality. By 1968, a recognition system, with associated salaries, was established. In the fall of 1968, graduation ceremonies were held for sixty-five psychiatric technicians. Another seventy received diplomas in the spring of 1969.

The VSH psychiatric technician program was developed during the same time that the American Nurses' Association adopted the position that a minimum preparation for a professional nurse should be a baccalaureate degree; minimum preparation for technical nursing practice should be an associate degree in nursing; and education for assistants in health service occupations should be short, intensive preservice programs in vocational education rather than on-the-job training.[48]

Rupert Chittick retired in 1968, and George Brooks left the research department to become superintendent. Brooks agreed with Chittick: "the objective of the Vermont State Hospital is to restore the patient to the level of health and function that will allow him to leave the hospital to continue his convalescence elsewhere."[49] Brooks maintained that deinstitutionalization was merely taking the patient out of the institution, but that rehabilitation was the more difficult task of taking the institution out of the patient.

Brooks was to later summarize what he considered were the four most important events which expedited the extensive rehabilitation and deinstitutionalization of severely mentally ill patients at Vermont State Hospital.[50]

1. The initiation of comprehensive training in psychiatric technology for the attendants, taught by the registered nurses.
2. The implementation of the Barden-Lafollette Act of 1943 by Vermont's Vocational Rehabilitation Agency. In 1948, Donald M. Eldred, a clinical psychologist, was transferred from Vocational Rehabilitation to become the chief psychologist at the hospital, and began what later became the Eldred School.
3. The 1952 controversy between VSH and the state government over the advisability of a building program to relieve overcrowding. Community groups and a friendly press rallied to publicize and arouse interest in the meaning of the overcrowding and the fire hazards that existed. The end result was a com-

plete victory for the hospital's building program, but also the way was paved for community acceptance of rehabilitation programs and the return of patients to ordinary community life. In their report to the General Assembly of 1953, the commission to study conditions at the Vermont State Hospital gave a strong opinion that the State of Vermont must invest in chronic care alternatives—particularly for the elderly—other than state hospitalization. The Commission argued against the advisability of continued growth of a central state institution, and instead recommended that the state support community programs.

4. The initiation of modern drug treatment with chlorpromazine (Thorazine) and reserpine in May of 1954, and its extensive study in the fall of 1954 and throughout 1955. These early drug treatment efforts, as so often happens with new and untried treatments, were initiated with long-term, profoundly disabled patients. The results were dramatic for the subjects, but the effect on the staff was more profound as they saw the changes in patient behavior. The door had been opened on limitless possibilities, and care of the mentally ill entered the era of hope, energy, belief, and available money, all of which made the rehabilitation efforts of the 1960s possible.

Four more events set the stage for a rehabilitation revolution that was to occurr in the 1970s, and the end of isolating people with mental illness into one self-contained village-like institution.

1. The creation of Medicare and Medicaid by the passage of P.L. 89–97 in 1964.
2. The 1966 Fair Labor Standards Act requiring patient labor to be paid.
3. The introduction of lithium carbonate in 1968 for the effective treatment of manic/depressive psychosis.
4. The public acceptance of the idea that not all mentally ill people were dangerous.

Changes for Hospital Staff: The 1970s

The decade of the 1970s was marked by changes in nursing education, labor organization, and further deinstitutionalization of patient care.

At VSH in 1972, the medical recordkeeping changed from a source-oriented system to a problem-oriented system. Nurse's notes were no longer kept in a separate section of the chart. This reflected a philosophical change, putting the patient at the center of a multidisciplinary team approach, with nursing staff as treatment team members, and not just caretakers and observers/recorders of patient behavior.

The diploma RN schools had been closing one by one, and by 1970 most of these programs had been phased out, so that RNs obtained a two-year Associate Degree in Nursing or a four-year Bachelor of Science in Nursing. More than 1,000 diploma student nurses did affiliations at Vermont State Hospital between 1957 and 1970.[51] The three VSH nursing education directors during this period were Alice Robinson, Francis Magee, and, beginning in 1967, Lois Sabin.

In 1971, affiliations were made with Vermont College in Montpelier and The University of Vermont. Student nurses no longer provided direct service, their rotations were shorter and primarily observational, and they brought their own instructors with them. Louise Davis, RN, from Vermont College, had a lengthy assignment covering the clinical rotations at VSH, and was a source of up-to-date educational materials for the VSH nurses and the psychiatric technician program. In exchange for the student placement, each semester a VSH Nursing Department member was allowed free enrollment in one three-credit course at Vermont College.

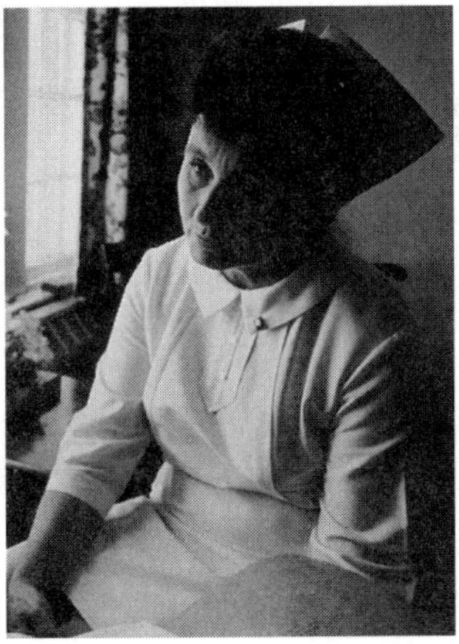

Courtesy Vermont State Hospital Archives

Lois Sabin, RN, MA
Chief of Nursing Education, 1967–1975
Director of Nursing, 1978–1984
Vermont State Hospital

The move from hospital-based diploma schools to academic institutions was an effort to upgrade the educational status of nurses. Likewise, an attempt was made to upgrade and formally recognize the status of psychiatric technicians.

VSH Superintendent George Brooks sought state licensure for psychiatric technicians through the Vermont State Board of Nursing in 1968.[52] He presented the rationale that just as the licensed practical nurse was created to fill the shortage of nursing personnel in general hospitals, the psychiatric technician filled the same need in mental hospitals.

He believed, as did Dr. Chittick before him, that there would never come a time when there were enough college-trained RNs to fill the nursing staff needs of Vermont State Hospital or any mental hospital. References were made to the technician licensure systems in Colorado and California, and Brooks proposed that the Vermont State Board of Nursing similarly administer standardized state examinations and control licensure, to both protect the public and protect the integrity of the Psychiatric Technician title.[53]

On December 6, 1968, Mental Health Commissioner Leopold, Helen Penna, RN, MA, Lois Sabin, RN, MS, Geneva Shand, RN, Marian Segale, RN, and Vera Hanks, RN, attended a meeting of the Vermont State Board of Nursing in Montpelier to discuss licensure of psychiatric technicians. Dr. Leopold explained,

> The Department of Mental Health employs non-professional personnel in addition to the professional staff to provide care, custody, treatment, training and rehabilitation of mentally ill and mentally retarded Vermonters who are institutionalized at Vermont State Hospital and Brandon Training School. Both institutions have inservice training programs that provide pertinent instruction for non-professional personnel so that they can give safe, effective and efficient care to the patient and residents.[54]

There were two proposals: 1) psychiatric aides and mental retardation aides would be eligible for certification after successfully completing basic training, and 2) psychiatric technicians and mental retardation technicians who completed advanced training and passed Board of Nursing examinations would be eligible for licensure. Certification and licensure were considered to be necessary and beneficial for:

1. The protection of those receiving care, by establishing standards of training.
2. The elevation of the status of workers involved in the treatment and care of the mentally ill and mentally retarded.
3. Job mobility to other states that recognize such positions.
4. The improvement of compensation, thereby attracting capable people.
5. The establishment of career ladders that would allow entry into college and university programs.

Dr. Leopold also presented three alternatives if the Board of Nursing did not want control over technicians: 1) The Department of Education could be approached to oversee training programs, certification, and licensure; 2) Legislation could be introduced to allow the Department of Mental Health to grant certification and licensure; or 3) A new state board could be established that would function as the licensing body for psychiatric and mental retardation aides.

The delegation returned from the two-hour discussion with the Board of Nursing mystified at their reluctance to accept this responsibility or to see merit in the justification.

Over the next year, there was considerable debate within the Vermont

State Nurses' Association (VSNA) regarding the proposed licensure of psychiatric technicians. The American Nurses' Association (ANA) philosophically opposed the licensure of specialty groups. VSNA invited Lois Sabin, to attend a March 28, 1969, meeting at Gifford Memorial Hospital in Randolph to speak on the issue.[55] Subsequently, VSNA took the same formal stand against licensure as did the ANA

The November 1970 issue of *Vermont Registered Nurse* (the official publication of the Vermont State Nurses' Association) published an article by Jeanette Folta, RN, PhD, Chairperson of the VSNA Legislative Committee, outlining the pros and cons of licensure.[56] She listed the points presented two years earlier by Dr. Leopold, and also VSNA's arguments against the proposal. One of these was that since technicians were less expensive than RNs, hospitals would never employ enough RNs if they could employ technicians instead. The end of the article invited reactions. Lois Sabin wasted no time in responding, and wrote a six-page point-by-point rebuttal of VSNA's assertions, a critique of the logic, a correction of erroneous statements, and a restatement of the request and rationale for the Vermont State Board of Nursing to oversee psychiatric technician licensure.[57]

The effort was to no avail, and the State Board of Nursing continued to take no action on the issue. Meanwhile, the Vermont State Hospital Technicians developed the Vermont Psychiatric Technicians Association, and were recognized by the National Psychiatric Technicians Association in 1971. They applied to the Legislature for licensure under their own Board in 1975. The bill went to committee but was not acted upon. The bill did not get to a committee in 1976 due to reevaluation of all licensing boards, including the Board of Nursing.[58]

The Vermont State Nurses' Association actively campaigned against a separate board for technician licensure on the premise that 1) the technician role was a combination of nursing, recreational therapy, occupational therapy, art therapy, and vocational rehabilitation and not unique, therefore should not be licensed separately; and 2) all nursing care givers should be under the Board of Nursing.[59] After begging for six years to be under the Board of Nursing, this was the ultimate irony.

Even though Vermont State Hospital RNs were not part of VSNA's opposition, and actively taught, encouraged, and supported the technicians, this battle produced a long-lasting bitterness and a feeling that registered nurses in general did not appreciate the talents and knowledge of psychiatric technicians, and how technicians could be of great assistance to them. It appeared to them that most RNs only saw them as competition, and that some RNs hadn't studied as long as they had.

Despite the problems of trying to obtain licensure, George Brooks and Lois Sabin were able to negotiate for advanced education for technicians. In 1972, the psychiatric technician program became affiliated with the Community College of Vermont. Thirty-three credits from the VSH program were recognized toward a sixty-credit curriculum for an Associate Degree in Mental Health Technology. Many students availed themselves of this opportunity and were able to qualify for jobs in the growing community mental health centers as a result of this education.[60]

As the philosophy in the care of the mentally ill began to focus on patients remaining in or returning to the communities, the VSH nursing education faculty started classes for boarding home operators under the IMPAC (Improvements in Alternate Care Program).[61] The same goal of development of enrichment activities occurred with boarding house operators as had occurred in-hospital under the 1960s HIP grants, in order to avoid creating miniature "back wards" and improve the quality of life for boarding home residents.[62]

In June 1971, when IMPAC workers first began, there were seventy-six alternate care facilities. In June 1974, there were 161, and the client population in these facilities had risen from 268 to 516. Return rates from alternate care facilities to the hospital were cut in half.[63]

Admission rates to VSH remained high: 1,657 admissions in 1972.[64] More resources were needed in community care to prevent re-admissions, and to provide alternatives for people in an acute crisis other than VSH hospitalization.

Another grant supported the Rural Community Screening Program (RCSP), which began in October 1974.[65] The RCSP goal was to reduce hospital admission rates from the three nearest counties (Orange, Washington, and Lamoille). The staff included crisis workers (many of whom had worked at VSH) who developed a thorough knowledge of alternative resources, and who responded in person anywhere, any time. They received formal training in assessment of suicide potential, early symptoms of alcohol DTs, psychotropic medications, and legal aspects of screening. As a result of the project, yearly admissions to VSH were reduced to 632 in fiscal year 1976–77.[66]

Success had changed the very nature of the institution. The fifteen years of rehabilitation effort had resulted in the discharge of most of the patients who provided useful labor at the hospital. This was good for them, but up to 1954, two-thirds of all the manual work in the hospital had been performed by unpaid patients.[67] The loss of nearly 90% of this labor force meant that, as the hospital grew smaller, it became more expensive to operate—people had to be hired to perform functions that had once been done for free. This was hard for the public and the legislature to understand. They saw shrinking populations at the hospital, accompanied by mushrooming budget requests from both VSH and the community mental health centers.

The Fair Labor Standards Act of 1966 was interpreted to mean that patient labor could no longer go unpaid, and that a great deal of what had been called Industrial Therapy was straight-out exploitation. In 1968, even with an already reduced supply of patient labor, it would have cost the state $800,000 annually to pay these workers the minimum wage.

In 1971, it became no longer economically feasible to operate the hospital farm. It was sold, and the dairy herd auctioned. The laundry closed when it became cheaper and more efficient to contract with a laundry service. The medical/surgical building was closed as it became more economical to transfer patients to Central Vermont Hospital in Berlin and the Medical Center Hospital in Burlington for medical procedures, and hire nursing staff to stay with until they were able to return to VSH. Groundskeeping was completely taken over by the State Buildings and Grounds Division. Reductions in patient labor required the addition of ten building custodians, and twenty-seven psychiatric aides were re-assigned to housekeeping duties.

Nursing staff began to demand better working conditions, higher pay, better schedules, overtime policies, grievance procedures, and rules regarding lay-offs, as the hospital became smaller. The Vermont State Employees' Association became the official bargaining agent for all state employees.[68]

VSH nurses and psychiatric technicians entered the 1970s with the women wearing white dresses, white shoes, white stockings, and hospital caps; the men wore white pants, white shirts, and black ties. They exited the decade with a very eclectic dress code of ordinary clothing, symbolic of the effort to normalize all aspects of patient care.

By 1979, the Vermont State Hospital patient population had further reduced to 300, with the highest admission rates being from Chittenden and Windham counties, and there was a continuing need for more and better community residential alternatives.

The 1980s: Regionalization of Psychiatric Care

The early 1980s brought a continuation of regionalization of mental health care, with further decreases in the size of the State Hospital and the establishment of psychiatric units in general hospitals—such as the opening in 1981 of a nine-bed psychiatric unit at Central Vermont Hospital, with Jean Axten, RN, MS, as head nurse (later called nurse manager). In the 1960s, general hospitals did not see a role for a psychiatric nurse, although those skills were a nice add-on to other types of nursing and the value was seen in primary prevention work with patients in medical crisis or in childbirth, or in handling an impending death for patients and relatives. Psychiatric nursing was viewed as a part of every nursing role. It wasn't until the psychiatric treatment units began to appear in general hospitals that psychiatric nurses developed a specific role in direct service and in consultation to other nurses.

Treatment units at the Medical Center Hospital of Vermont (later named Fletcher Allen Health Care) in Burlington, Central Vermont Hospital, and Rutland Hospital were voluntary and anyone who was a danger to themselves or others, as a result of mental illness, and who refused treatment, still went to Vermont State Hospital. The increasing variety of outpatient services and sheltered living situations offered through community mental health centers matched a burgeoning growth in outpatient care, same-day surgery, and one-day baby deliveries that was occurring in all aspects of health care. Nurses in schools, emergency rooms, public health, home health, nursing homes, and general hospitals increasingly cared for people with major mental illness diagnoses. This was the beginning of a shift in thinking in Vermont from providing holistic inpatient care to a mentally ill person in a self-contained separate mental hospital, to providing all services, including mental ones, through the local general hospital.

"De-institutionalization" became an old-fashioned and unpopular term in mental health circles, and "reorganization of services" became the major goal of the Department of Mental Health.[69]

The concept of "regionalization" actually began in 1957 with the Vermont Project and gained momentum in 1965 with the VSH Hospital Improvement Project (HIP). Part of the HIP grant was to develop regional teams wherein the education therapy coordinators, social workers, team nurses, psychologists, and physicians were assigned regions of the state. Each regional team met regularly with representatives of the mental health clinics of the patients from a particular region.[70]

As the community mental health centers continued to grow, so did their ability to provide rehabilitation and alternatives to hospitalization. As a result, by 1984, the hospital census dropped to 150 patients, and the legislature was faced with declining federal funds, mental health centers in great need of more money, and a small, expensive state hospital that was going to require an even greater investment to pass the standards of both the Joint Commission on Accreditation of Hospitals (JCAH) and Medicare.

The Vermont Department of Mental Health, under Commissioner Sutherland Miller, commissioned a study by the Center of Psychiatric Rehabilitation of Boston University, with Paul Carling, PhD, as the principal investigator. The purpose was to study the feasibility of providing all of the services of the State Hospital at the regional level through general hospitals, emergency residential beds, and a wide variety of crisis and rehabilitative services at the community mental health center. VSH patients and state resources were studied from July through October, 1985.

1985 was a low year for Vermont State Hospital. George Brooks had retired the year before. Vera Hanks and Lois Sabin were both gone. Social worker Claudia Stone had been named interim director while a search for an executive director was conducted. There was no medical director, nor any applicants. The nursing administrator, Barbara Boisse, left. During her two-year stay, the Vera Hanks School of Psychiatric Technology was dismantled and classes discontinued, based on the belief that all nursing staff should be college educated prior to employment. Morale in the nursing department was very low, with most staff thinking it was a short time before the hospital would close. A full-scale JCAH survey was upcoming, and the strong opinion was that decertification would result. Medicare was also threatening to discredit the hospital as a reimbursable provider. The legislature placed credibility on newspaper stories about an expensive albatross that provided not only poor care, but awful conditions for patients. What had been the shining star of state hospitals was now a mess, and the future of VSH looked very gloomy.

Claudia Stone was appointed permanent executive officer of VSH, and reorganized the hospital from a medical superintendent's model to a model of chiefs of clinical service (nursing being one) as an executive committee to set hospital policies. Marsha Kincheloe, RN, MS, MA, CS, was hired as nursing administrator.

By 1986, the Vermont State Hospital passed the JCAH inspection, but was decertified as an approved facility to receive Medicare reimbursement because of not enough doctors, not enough nurses, and poor medical recordkeeping.[71]

It was a political dilemma: whether to close the state hospital or bring it up to standards. The latter was chosen, and by 1987 recertification was achieved.

VSH always suffered from overcrowding. Every time the census went down, wards were converted to state offices, perpetuating the lack of privacy for patients and insufficient room for staff to work. From 1985 to 1987, VSH had room for eight fire-safe wards and was staffed for 150 patients, but actually operated nine wards and had 190 patients.[73] During this period, a new emphasis on regionalization began, and a concerted effort was made to find community placements for chronic but stable patients living at VSH. Media publicity about the needs of the State Hospital, urging by Department of Mental Health Commissioner William

Dalton, legislative tours of VSH, plus public pressure to support mental health, inspired the Legislature to appropriate money to make VSH improvements, as well as additional money to back regionalization efforts.

Regionalization efforts intensified in 1987, when a special discharge project began with funding from the Robert Wood Johnson Foundation.[73] Opinions were high for and against regionalization, and the accompanying staff reductions were a controversial subject.

In June 1987, *Hospital and Community Psychiatry* published a study by Paul Carling, PhD, and associates under the title, "A State Mental Health System with No State Hospital: The Vermont Feasibility Study."[74] This was somewhat of a dramatic mis-title, since the study itself proposed that the forensic population would continue to be treated at the State Hospital. By the time the study was published, however, the Vermont State Hospital had pulled itself up by its bootstraps with Medicare, JCAH, the Vermont Health Department, the Legislature, and advocates—taking the "oomph" out of the idea to close it.

In the same *Hospital and Community Psychiatry* issue, a commentary on the Carling study appeared by Marsha Kincheloe and Trudee Ettlinger, RN, MS, calling it a false dichotomy to talk about funding a community care system *or* a state hospital, and that a good, small, community-oriented state hospital could be the backbone of a community mental health system. The two were not mutually exclusive, and each was inadequate without the other.[75]

The Department of Mental Health and advocate groups began pushing for more money for the whole mental health system,[76–78] so that the quality of the State Hospital could be maintained, plus every alternative to state hospitalization could be developed—such as step down units, home intervention crisis teams, wrap-around programs, and 72-hour inventory holds in general hospitals.

The Role of Vermont State Hospital in the 1990s

As the numbers at Vermont State Hospital reduced to less than 65 patients by 1996 (273 admissions per year), the psychiatric units in general hospitals grew: Central Vermont Medical Center, Fletcher Allen Health Care Center, Rutland Regional Hospital. As VSH grew smaller, the nature of the general hospital units changed from totally voluntary, to also being able to hold someone involuntarily for seventy-two hours for their own safety. By 1996, two-thirds of the 72-hour holds converted to voluntary care, and one-third continued on to Vermont State Hospital.

The general hospitals struggled with the need to effectively care for an increasing amount of psychotic behaviors, destructiveness, aggression/

violence, involuntary medications, and longer stays. In the 1990s, many of VSH's nursing staff also held part-time jobs on the psychiatric units at Fletcher Allen Health Care in Burlington, and Central Vermont Medical Center in Berlin. As VSH becomes smaller, or is closed, the general hospital will be the location for inpatient care when it is needed. However, they currently are prepared to treat short-term mostly nonviolent admissions.

Over the last twenty years, long-term, nonacute inpatient care has increasingly shifted to nursing homes. In 1996, almost all people with organic brain conditions needing 24-hour care—who would have gone to VSH in 1946—went to a nursing home or foster family care. For example, Alzheimer's dementia produces behaviors that in past years would have resulted in a VSH admission. As AIDS dementias begin to appear in numbers beyond the capacity of hospice, nursing homes will see this group, too. Most RNS, LPNs, and aides who currently staff nursing homes will agree that there are not enough staff to do much more than custodial care. For most, nursing homes have an "end-of-the-line" atmosphere rather that one of rehabilitation and recovery toward community living. The advantage over a central state hospital is that a nursing home is usually smaller and located near the person's community.

The role of VSH has become treatment and care for people who do not fit into the services offered by the current mental health care system. For example, consider three elderly patients at VSH in 1996: one with paranoid schizophrenia whose violence had kept him on the most secure ward for twenty years; one with Parkinson's disease; and one with brain trauma from an alcohol-related accident thirty years previous. The patient with schizophrenia responded to Clozaril, one of a new generation of anti-psychotic medications, and, although still delusional, became manageable and was successfully placed in a foster home operated by a VSH nurse. The other two patients continued to be at VSH, because they were still physically fit enough to produce staff injuries with their violence. A nursing home would not accept them until they became too physically feeble to be aggressive. Even within VSH, they each required a constant personal care technician to prevent them from hurting themselves or someone else.

The cost of this level of care at VSH in 1996 was about $164,250 per year per person ($450 per day). The cost of nursing home care, if calculated at $200/day (some are less), is around $73,000 a year, more than most families can afford, but considerably less than VSH. A general hospital psychiatric unit costs more than VSH: $600–800 a day or $219,000–292,000 a year.[79]

In 1996, the groundwork was being laid to present the Vermont Legislature with a parity bill that would require insurance companies to provide coverage for mental illness on a par with physical illness. While this is a good change in many ways—moving further to reduce the stigma of mental illness and increase the access to treatment for acute situations—it will also increase the involvement of managed care companies in deciding what is active reimbursable treatment and what is denied coverage because it is long-term care. There is likelihood that mental illness parity coverage will not help the chronic severely mentally ill with access to treatment and care.

As state government becomes more and more committed to reducing its role in direct service through the State Hospital, and more committed to contracting with private health care providers, the severely long-term mentally ill will be increasingly served in community residential treatment facilities, step-down units, and foster care homes operated by the community mental health centers; nursing homes; general hospital psychiatric units for acute crises; and prisons. Psychiatric nurses have found their place in all of these settings and especially in crisis intervention, as members of outpatient group practices with other clinicians, and long-term monitoring of medications and concomitant physical illnesses.

There is a growing population of mentally ill people in Vermont prisons. A psychiatric unit for psychotic inmates was established at the Northwestern Correctional Center in St. Albans. A 45-bed women's prison is slated to open in Waterbury in 1999, with a heavy emphasis on psychiatric services. In the past, a prisoner in need of psychiatric care was sent to the secure units of Vermont State Hospital. Currently, with VSH capabilities greatly reduced and a disinterest on the part of general hospital psychiatric units to treat the mentally ill criminal population, there is likely to be an increasing need for psychiatric nursing in Vermont's prisons. The ultimate goal for any prisoner is rehabilitation by the time of release; but the goal of incarceration is also punishment, which sets a different atmosphere than a hospital. Vermont prisons are large, overcrowded, located at distances from the prisoner's community, and staffed primarily with correctional officers (not nurses and psychiatric technicians). The therapeutic problems the correctional system faces are very similar to those faced by the Vermont State Hospital in the 1950s.

—Marsha Kincheloe, RN, MS, MA, CS

NOTES

1. M. Kincheloe and H. Hunt, *Empty Beds: A History of Vermont State Hospital* (Barre, Vt.: author, 1988).
2. Ibid.

3. Ibid. All details regarding the Vermont State Hospital in the 1940s are from Kincheloe and Hunt unless otherwise noted.
4. Patricia Donahue, *Nursing, The Finest Art. An Illustrated History* (C.V. Mosby, 1985).
5. R. A. Chittick, "The Rebuilding of the Vermont State Hospital" (paper written for the Bicentennial Committee, 20 May 1975). Vermont State Hospital Archives, Waterbury, Vermont; hereafter referred to as VSH Archives.
6. Vera Hanks, "History of the Training Program for Attendants," 1957. VSH Archives.
7. Kincheloe and Hunt, *Empty Beds.*
8. Ibid.
9. Ibid.
10. Ibid.
11. Edyth Barnes, ed., "Report of the Vermont Survey of Nursing Needs and Resources," U.S. Public Health Service, 1952.
12. Lois Sabin, "Waterbury and the Vermont State Hospital," in *History of Waterbury, Vermont, 1915–1991*, James Sabin, ed. (Waterbury Historical Society, 1991), 89–98.
13. Alice Robinson, ed., "The Role of the Head Nurse in a Large Public Mental Hospital," *American Journal of Nursing* (April, May, June, 1955).
14. Alice Robinson, *The Psychiatric Aide* (J. B. Lippincott, 1954).
15. Kincheloe and Hunt, *Empty Beds.*
16. Alice Robinson, "Communicating with Schizophrenic Patients, " *American Journal of Nursing* (August 1960).
17. Kincheloe and Hunt, *Empty Beds.*
18. Ibid.
19. Ibid.
20. Robinson, "Communicating with Schizophrenic Patients."
21. Kincheloe and Hunt, *Empty Beds.*
22. Ibid.
23. Ibid.
24. Hans Huessy, "Deinstitutionalization in a Rural State: The Vermont Experience," in *New Directions for Mental Health Services: Perspectives on Rural Mental Health*, no. 9 (Jossey-Bass, 1981), 33–38.
25. Vermont Biennial Report to the Legislature, Department of Mental Health, 1966.
26. Kincheloe and Hunt, *Empty Beds.*
27. R. A. Chittick, G. W. Brooks, F. S. Irons, and W. N. Deane, *The Vermont Story: Rehabilitation of Chronic Schizophrenic Patients* (1961).
28. G. W. Brooks and W. N. Deane, "The Chronic Mental Patient in the Community," *Diseases of the Nervous System* XXVI, no. 2 (February 1965): 85–90.
29. C. M. (Daum) Harding, G. W. Brooks, and Albee, "Twenty Year Follow-Up of 253 Schizophrenic Patients Originally Selected for Chronic Disability: Pilot Study," *Psychiatric Journal of the University of Ottawa* 2, no. 3 (September, 1977).
30. G. W. Brooks and R. Hyde, "Progress Report of Hospital Improvement Project: A State Hospital Center for Education Therapy," Public Health Service Demonstration NH15162-04 from the Department of Health, Education and Welfare, Washington, D.C., 1 July 1967 to 1 November 1968.
31. Ivan Belknap, *Human Problems of a State Mental Hospital* (New York: McGraw-Hill, 1956).

32. Kincheloe and Hunt, *Empty Beds.*
33. Ibid.
34. Ibid.
35. Ibid.
36. G. W. Brooks, "Fourteen Year Projection," 1969. VSH Archives.
37. Ibid.
38. Donahue, *Nursing.*
39. Alice Robinson, "Action for Mental Health: The Implications for Nursing" (paper presented at the American Nurses' Association Convention, Los Angeles, California, 1962).
40. S. Arieti, *Interpretation of Schizophrenia*, 2nd ed. (Basic Books, 1974).
41. Belknap, *Human Problems of a State Mental Hospital.*
42. Robinson, "Action for Mental Health."
43. Hildegard Peplau, *Interpersonal Relations in Nursing* (G.T. Putnam, 1952).
44. Robinson, *The Psychiatric Aide.*
45. Donahue, *Nursing.*
46. R. Magee, "In-Service Staff Development at the Vermont State Hospital: A Dynamic Process in the Teaching of Psychiatric Aides," in *Mental Health with Limited Resources*, Hans Huessy, ed. (Grune and Stratton, 1966), 106–112.
47. Kincheloe and Hunt, *Empty Beds.*
48. Donahue, *Nursing.*
49. G. W. Brooks, William Deane, and Peter Laqueur, "Fifteen Years of Work Therapy," *Diseases of the Nervous System*, GWAN Supp. vol. 31 (November 1970): 161–65.
50. G. W. Brooks and V. R. Graham, "Rehabilitation and De-institutionalization of the Mentally Ill. Vermont State Hospital, A Brief Historical Summary," April 1975, revised May 1981. VSH Archives.
51. Lois Sabin, "The History of Nursing Education at Vermont State Hospital, 1903–1976." VSH Archives.
52. Kincheloe and Hunt, *Empty Beds.*
53. Ibid.
54. Vermont State Board of Nursing, Minutes from Meeting of 6 December 1968. VSH Archives.
55. Jeanette Folta, "Licensure of Psychiatric Aides," *Vermont Registered Nurse* (newsletter of the Vermont State Nurses' Association), November 1970, 5–7.
56. Ibid.
57. Lois Sabin, "Letter of Response to VSNA Regarding Licensure of Psychiatric Technicians," January 1971. VSH Archives.
58. Sabin, "The History of Nursing Education at Vermont State Hospital."
59. Vermont State Nurses' Association, "Statement on H.261, A Bill to License Mental Health Technicians, to the Vermont Health and Welfare Committee." Vermont State Nurses' Association Special Collection, Library Research Annex, The University of Vermont, Burlington, Box #9.
60. Sabin, "The History of Nursing Education at Vermont State Hospital."
61. Suzanne Fields, "Rethinking Rehabilitation, Breaking Through the Boarding House Blues. An Interview with Dr. George Brooks," *Innovations* 2, no. 2 (Summer 1975).
62. Ibid.
63. G. W. Brooks, "Rural Community Screening Program for a State Hospital,"

Grant Application to Department of Health, Education, and Welfare, Public Health Service and Mental Health Administration. Progress Report, 29 January, 1974, 27, 29.

64. Kincheloe and Hunt, *Empty Beds.*
65. Linnea Taylor and G. W. Brooks, "A Screening Program to Reduce Admissions to a State Hospital," *Hospital and Community Psychiatry* 31, no. 1 (January 1980): 50–60.
66. Ibid.
67. Kincheloe and Hunt, *Empty Beds.*
68. Ibid.
69. Ibid.
70. G. W. Brooks, "Reflections on the Impact of the April, 1978, Reorganization Plan at the Vermont State Hospital" [introduction to a graphic display], March 1979. VSH Archives.
71. Kincheloe and Hunt, *Empty Beds.*
72. Ibid.
73. Lois Sabin, "Waterbury and the Vermont State Hospital," 89–98.
74. P. Carling, S. Miller, L. Daniels, and F. Randolph, "A State Mental Health System With No State Hospital: The Vermont Feasibility Study," *Hospital and Community Psychiatry* (1987): 616–23.
75. M. Kincheloe and T. Ettlinger, "A False Dichotomy," *Hospital and Community Psychiatry* (June 1987): 623–24.
76. Y. Daley, "Patients Claim that 'Warehousing' Exists at VSH: Increased Population Means Less Therapy, Even Longer Stays," *The Times Argus* (Barre, Vermont), 12 July 1987.
77. J. Dillon, "Mental Health Advocates Say Tightened Funding Taking Toll on Programs," *The Times Argus*, 28 June 1987.
78. N. J. Donnelly, "Mental Health Programs Cite 'Crisis in Funding'," *The Times Argus*, 21 August 1987.
79. M. Kincheloe, "A State Mental Health System With No State Hospital: The Vermont Plan Ten Years Later," *Psychiatric Services* (August 1997): 1078–80.

Psychiatric Nursing: A Nurse Perspective

A Personal Account

The voices of women arise from a range of life experiences. Some early experiences pave the way for the great empathic qualities that connect nurses with the person for whom they care. The story that is presented here gives voice to a nurse who reminds us of our own life experiences from which we mold our professional beings. On one level, this is a story of one's courage to share a personal, frightening time in youth when the struggle to find "place" in the world was difficult. The story, however, is one of victory over circumstances that could defeat us. This story reminds us of the indubitable nature of the human spirit. The spirit allows us to seek our destiny even though some environments are hostile. We do continue our journey, carrying our burden with us until we find those places that permit us to succeed. With that success we go forth and live quiet but truly heroic lives.

—Loraine M. Welch, RN, EdD

To record for history my participation in the field of psychiatric nursing seems insignificant, as the story of one; yet a formidable task, exposing a personal journey. As with most journeys there are steps we take with ease, and others that require maximum effort.

As a girl, I answered the "What-would-you-like-to-be-when-you-grow-up?" question with "A nurse." In junior high, being a nurse apparently wasn't a steadfast commitment, because I recall being distraught over choosing an academic path. At that time, my parents who had very little money, invested in an extensive two days of testing to help determine where my strengths lay. I remember being told, on completion, that I had very good manual dexterity, and therefore laboratory technician was the suggested career choice. I also remember feeling that something was askew in the summary equation, because wouldn't that require a background in science and math? My poorest subjects. As high school graduation neared, my mother discussed my future with a guidance counselor. I did not want to go to college, because it was such a relief to be getting out of high school. But my sister, a year older, was in college and my mother was determined I should have an equal opportunity.

At age sixteen I graduated from high school and that fall, barely seventeen, I found myself enrolled at a five-year nursing program. Within a very short time I was overwhelmed by chemistry, which was more than difficult in high school and impossible now. I transferred to the three-year hospital-based nursing program. Even there, I had an awful time because—try as I would—I could not conquer the sciences, and felt such a failure. It was during this time that I looked with envy at the group of girls enjoying their cigarettes in the lounge, and worked hard to join the smokers in spite of all the admonitions, rules, and regulations. We had to cover our uniforms, then brush our teeth and air our hair before returning to duty and the bedside.

I begged my mother to allow me to return home. Her response was to stick it out, that I would be glad I had. In those days we had affiliations, training in specialties in hospitals at other sites. My first was to New York Hospital for pediatrics for three months. Next was Johns Hopkins Hospital in Baltimore for psychiatry. Though filled with self-doubt, I plodded on, working first on a Women's Unit where I recall two things. The first was witnessing insulin shock therapy, which was dramatic indeed, and the patient we observed showed a remarkable improvement after each treatment. The difficulty was that the improvement could not be sustained. The second memory had to do with an attempt to communicate in Spanish with a young woman lying huddled in bed. I had studied Spanish in high school and, full of optimism, embarked upon my assignment, using all the appropriate Spanish I could muster. The encounter was brief. What I got for my effort was a surprise swift kick in my gut which signaled the end of the interaction!

I continued to be depressed, and sought out a staff psychiatrist available to students. I recall that his surname and mine, though uncommon, sounded alike, different spelling. In the cafeteria I chose one chocolate milk and one orange three times a day. I could determine no reason to live. A beautiful sunset did not hold much meaning for me.

My assignment shifted to the Men's Unit, where I felt even more inadequate. The keys to the medicine cupboard were at my disposal, and one day I simply helped myself to two full bottles of little white pills. Next, I recall being in our dorm lavatory, swallowing by handfuls the entire contents of both bottles, disposing of the bottles in the hall incinerator drop before returning to my room. I went to bed thinking nothing was happening and that I had bungled this, as well.

After eleven days, I awakened. There was a folding white screen outside my door, and a large attendant in a corner chair eating ice cream. The addiction to nicotine had not disappeared and the urge promptly returned; only now I exhaled through a tracheostomy tube. I continued to recover, and soon was accompanied on a train by an RN who was paid the princely sum of one hundred dollars for the journey. I was deposited at the then-called Boston Psychopathic Hospital.

In due time, I was interviewed by two outside psychiatrists, and I can still vividly recall the plaid blouse and black skirt I wore, disheveled now from the long train ride and several days' wear, no longer the good-looking outfit I saved for "best." I was utterly and naïvely truthful in acknowledging my disappointment that the suicide attempt had not succeeded, and it was therefore deemed appropriate that I remain in the hospital for treatment. It was an excruciating time for my family—and that is another story, but one silly thing I remember was that they brought me both ice cream and fried clams from Howard Johnson's, an unheard-of extravagance!

This was 1948 and I was eighteen years old. Treatment was ECT, electroshock therapy. Work-up then was skeletal films, because risk of broken bones during the procedure was the legal caveat at the time, before anesthesia and curare derivatives. There was a line-up for treatment, and I don't recall being given any premedication. Asked to "hop up here" on the gurney, there were sandbags and an attendant for each limb. Electrode jelly was placed at the temples and a wide elastic held two electrodes which had been soaked in salt water. Then I was asked to bite on the flat mouthstick. I received a series of twenty treatments, and soon began being prepared for discharge.

After consultation with a social worker, I enrolled at a secretarial school, taking the medical-secretarial course and found it to be a breeze. On one occasion a friend and I were smoking after lunchbreak when the director approached and urged us to go outside, instead, because the healthy fresh air would contribute to better grades. It was a moot point, though, because as she looked up my grades and saw straight As she said no more. That was a sweet, if fleeting, moment.

I completed the two-year course and got a job at a high-priced internist's office where I was the junior secretary. After a year and a half, I was becoming indignant that no raise was offered and I would have to seek it myself. The good doctor agreed that I certainly deserved a raise and he would so like to give it, but he could not possibly afford it. That was my initiation to the method of keeping low overhead by always employing new-hires at starting salaries.

Then I got a job closer to my home working for a neuropsychiatrist who had two offices, one urban, the other suburban. I worked there for six years, becoming proficient not only in secretarial skills, but with assisting in ECT treatments done in the office. It was my job to have everything ready and to assist in the procedure and recovery. At home on my portable singer sewing machine I made plastic covers for the felt bite sticks. On days the doctor spent in his Boston office, it was my job to wash and wax the floors and clean the blinds and windows layered with nicotine smoke. Of course, I served coffee, too. A vivid recollection is of a rather high-sounding lecture about the attributes of menial labor, a la Gandhi, being convinced to revel in the nobility of the tasks. That motivation was short-lived, however, and I resented it, especially after noting that other secretaries in the building enjoyed professional cleaning and seemed not to lack in nobility!

Along came a major technical advancement in the ECT procedure to include a short-acting anesthesia and curare derivative to dramatically reduce the musculoskeletal stress. The work-up included an EEG as well as spine films. The treatment site moved from the office to the out-patient section of the local hospital, where on treatment days I would arrive carrying the medications and "the box." I remained with the patients(s) throughout, including recovery and discharge. On one memorable occasion, the boss was away and his friend was covering for him when an emergency OD (overdose) at the hospital needed care. I spoke to the covering psychiatrist about a journal article I read, suggesting the possibility of using intermittent sustained low voltage ECT in such situations. Imagine my amazement when that idea was put into action and the patient recovered nicely! Heady stuff!

There was more irony. My boss was one of two examining psychiatrists at the State Hospital, and other facilities, where persons could be held no longer than ten days without review and a court order. We used to go on Sundays, and I would take notes during interviews and then, back at the office, prepare the legal forms for presentation at Court. How often I was reminded of sitting on the other side of the interview in my plaid blouse and black skirt. Another aspect of my job was to accompany the boss during consultations for the Parole Board at a State Prison. My budding feminism noted that entering security-tight prison areas was the only time "ladies first" was honored.

There was a period of time when I hoped to complete my nursing studies, and went to speak with the nursing director to discuss the possibility. She was not at all interested in entertaining that thought after the considerable trouble I had caused her.

In 1956, marriage and moving concluded six years of work for the neuropsychiatrist. I had several part-time positions in various locations before children arrived. Our sixth move was to Vermont in 1965.

Another suicide attempt in 1968 resulted in hospitalization, during which I again received ECT—fifteen this time—each preceded by Seconal administered by the night RN. Two daughters, eight and ten years old, were in grammar school. Gradually, my isolation decreased, beginning with my identification with the staff nurses who, in turn, felt comfortable to come to my room to chat. After six weeks or so I was discharged. In 1969, I saw an article in the local newspaper announcing the formation of a two-year associate degree program in nursing at The University of Vermont (UVM). Could this be for me? Intrigued, I made a tenative inquiry—apparently one of the first to do so, because when I met Virginia Allen, the new chairperson, she herself was orienting to her office and had to inquire about use of the telephone. Twenty-three years after high school, I was asked to take a test of some kind. It was at first mind-boggling, then numbing, and finally, ridiculous—marking, certainly, the end of a short excursion into an attempt to conquer the unfinished. With the idea put long behind me, a letter of acceptance arrived from UVM. I can still vividly feel how completely stunned I was. How could they possibly accept me after that test performance? A mistake? Desperate for enrollees? Intrigued by the "older student" phenomenon?

But it was true. After I got used to the idea, I realized that a great deal of reading would be required, especially since nursing education had shifted from a hospital-based setting to a university setting. A poor reader with poor retention, I enrolled in UVM's remedial reading course, an essential fifty-dollar investment. I completed the course with a score just below the one that I earned when I entered. No further intervention or suggestion was offered other than to "keep reading." Next, I needed to work on math skills, and asked a neighborhood friend if he would help. At the time I did not appreciate how overqualified he was. He was so young, only twenty-six, after all. I learned later that he had worried about his ability to respond to my request, but was quickly relieved of his concern when, in disbelief, he realized how truly basic my needs were. He was a PhD full Professor in Math!

Buoyed by great fanfare and support from family and friends, I embarked into a new world. The majority of classmates were just out of high school, but the group was peppered with LPNs and others of different backgrounds. I veered toward the only other married student, and though much younger and two heads shorter, we became friends and have remained so to this time. There was one male student. This educational experience resembled not at all that of twenty-three years earlier. There was a minimum of demonstration by faculty. Instead, individual instruction by film or cassette and slides while sitting at a work station was in vogue. We also took advantage of audiovisual references at the UVM library as well as the Dana Medical Library. We had lectures and study guides. My home, not far from campus, became a gathering place for study sessions with endless pots of coffee.

There was good physical exercise, too, because nursing was located five floors up in the Waterman Building. Some lectures were held at UVM's Given Building, where the innovative Basic Integrated Science course was taught by medical school personnel. I was entirely out of my league. But I tried to compensate with my secretarial skills and took copious notes, and taped the lectures as well. Late into the night I transcribed all the notes, blackboard illustrations, and cassettes into a magnificent representation in a well-ordered notebook of knowledge which belonged in my head, but seldom reached there. The day of the final exam in Basic Integrated Science happened to be an official day of mourning for Kent State students who had been shot (May 4, 1970). In solidarity, classes were canceled. There would be no exam, and we received whatever grade we had earned on the last quiz. Thus, I passed!!

Psychiatric nursing was taught during our second year. Lectures were coordinated with experience at the Vermont State Hospital. We gathered in a small group with our clinical supervisor prior to meeting with clients to identify folks we would work with, hopefully for the length of our course. We received guidance in outlining our goals, short-term and long-term, and discussed methods of interaction we might find useful in building trust, which was essential to working toward goals set. In addition, we kept careful records of this process. Following our sessions with selected clients, we again came together as a group to process our experiences and evaluate effectiveness of our interactions. Throughout the course we also kept a personal journal to record our feelings and responses to the day's events. This was a valuable tool for assessing growth and confidence. The contrast between my first psychiatric exposure and the second was significant. My role had changed from unwitting caretaker to one of purposeful learning with goals, and supervision for achieving those goals.

During our final semester it was impressed on us that membership and active involvement in our professional organization, the Vermont State Nurses' Association (VSNA), was a privilege and a responsibility—the only group to speak directly for nursing in the state. Looking up to our instructor as role model and mentor, I took that to heart and joined, keeping my membership for twenty-five years, until a year ago, four years after I retired. I am still an avid enthusiast for this fine professional group which works diligently and painstakingly to contribute to the betterment of nurses and nursing. It has been my impression that the level of work is even more noteworthy given the small numbers of active participants and the budget restraints which prevail. With my first hospital employment we were given time off with pay to attend VSNA functions, to encourage membership and involvement in our professional organization. Through the years I held several minor posts at the district level and became completely immersed every third year when it was our turn to host convention. Finally, I served two terms at the state level as delegate-at-large. It was a wonderful exposure to the breadth and function of the organization and its parent organization, the American Nurses' Association.

I am ahead of myself. After graduation, I couldn't believe I really had graduated, because "I still don't know anything." Everyone at our celebration dinner laughed, but I knew it was true. The new status did not make me a competent, but rather a minimally safe, practitioner.

That first summer I was the nurse at a camp in Enosburg Falls. My girls could be with me and take part. Filled with anxiety that I would be faced with events for which I was totally unprepared, I armed myself with a *Merck Manual* and several texts on emergency procedures. I was lucky and escaped unchallenged. My girls soon tired of the novelty, as the program and campers had just a one-week cycle.

That fall I began work at the UVM Student Health Service. This was a rather bizarre experience with a health care setting and policies of a bygone era. There were inane expectations of nurses, such as staffing an empty building on an empty campus on Christmas Eve in full white uniform, and spending my time sorting pills from samples to small envelopes, and handwriting directions to be dispensed during cold and flu season. It was hard to think I could not spend that night with my children because of such priorities. The "tight budget" did not allow the purchase of a new extension cord badly needed, and the older staff nurses had a routine of taking the ace bandages to their homes to launder, roll, and recycle.

My goal was a part-time night job so I could be available to my family during after-school and evening hours. I applied at the Medical Center in response to an ad in the paper for a night RN on a 32-bed psychiatric unit. Twice I was turned down because they really wanted a full-time person. Finally, it was agreed to hire me for a 24-hour permanent part-time position. I was certain I could do it well, though there was a nagging feeling that the recommended year of med/surg experience after graduation would be the wiser course. It was two aides and me, doing 30-minute checks on everyone, and 15-minute checks on others. There were one-to-one constant observations, and at times door watch. Some clients were up very late, some never slept, others woke very early. Documentation revealed a rare black line indicating all asleep at one time. We had to be on our toes, often using a sixth sense in response to remarkable, sadly utilized, ingenuity on the part of patients. It was NEVER dull! We poured our own medications from stock supplies, and I felt no compunctions about holding a nose, as for a child, to get the medicine down, knowing how much better the person would soon feel, and that it was the illness itself that was the resistant motivator.

Still haunted by my lack of clinical nursing experience, I made an appointment with the assistant director of nursing, asking for guidance. In response, she was delighted to transfer me to a respiratory unit that, in retrospect, was in desperate need of a night RN. Their staffing requirement, on paper, was now filled, and I would get some needed bedside experience. There was an LPN and an aide. I was in charge position, with my teachers being the staff who had a right to look to me for leadership. Instead, they were showing me how things were done on that unit. It was a literal nightmare, and I transferred back to psych as soon as a year had passed. Soon, a day position opened on psych and I was ready. My optimism about working nights and being a functioning family member in good standing had gradually paled as reality evidenced itself to affirm that there is no substitute for a real eight hours of uninterrupted sleep.

There was an entirely different aspect to learn on days. There were regularly-scheduled gatherings of all team members, including patients, in the large TV room. Residents, medical students, nurses, social workers, occupational therapists, and drama staff were all present. It was standing-room only, many patients gamely trying to function despite medication effects, and staff clutching their treasured cups of coffee. General questions were responded to, requests for passes were discussed, as well as plans for the day or weekend. There were family meetings when many family members came to participate and learn. All pertinent members of the patient's treatment team were present and involved to better understand the family dynamics and treatment options were explained to the family. Often these were conducted with family consent, to include observation behind a one-way mirror which provided an excellent teaching opportunity. Average length of stay was six weeks. There were evolving attempts to provide consistent care by the same personnel. Attendings offered their individual strengths for instruction to interested staff. During team rounds to discuss and plan for each patient, it was most gratifying to me that not only were nurses permitted to speak, but their observations were welcomed and respected in recognition of relative time spent with the patients.

Again, I assisted in ECT treatments. There were many refinements in its administration and monitoring. Work-up continued to include an EEG and an EKG. Anesthesia was fine-tuned by that department, providing the least medication for effectiveness and smooth recovery. During the procedure there was continuous EKG and EEG recording. As I relate the advancing technologies which provide a safer treatment modality, I cannot resist also relating that as an office secretary and assistant with ECT treatments in the 1950s, I would collect the fees. For a series of ten ECT treatments the fee was $150, and that was considered costly!

Then came the big move from one 32-bed unit to two smaller units, and a division of staff. One unit, where I worked, became a locked unit, eliminating the need for labor-intensive "door watches." Soon there were two psych intensive care rooms, camera and sound monitored, adjacent to the nurses' station. The ECT treatment room was on this unit. Over the years, the debate continued from many corners concerning attitudes and ethics toward ECT as a method of treatment. It seemed not to be an effective treatment in all cases. In my experience, every effort was made to be wise about the candidate selection; it was NOT a course of last resort. Often ECT is considered the safest treatment of choice, especially considering the time lapse for medication to be effective. Sometimes results are very dramatic, as in the story of Mary (not real name) who came to our unit from another floor, totally unmanageable, disoriented, and hallucinating, with a diagnosis of postpartum psychosis. ECT was deemed the most appropriate option for relief of her symptoms. However, the patient was over 18 and not married, unable to make a rational decision on her own behalf. She had a loving boyfriend and doting parents, but legally it was necessary to present the case in Court in order to obtain permission to proceed. Most vividly I recall the angst produced by the seemingly interminable legal proceedings, resulting in the prolonged need for restraints, tube feedings, and her dreadful struggle with her demons. Finally, treatment could proceed. There was definite improvement even after the second and third treatment, and there was steady improvement in the clearing of her sensorium. Her parents and boyfriend rejoiced, as did the staff. In time, Mary was reunited with her baby and proved fully capable to function well with her. The series of ECT was completed and she was discharged to her family. Some time later, pushing a stroller, Mary stopped to say "hello," proud of her growing child, and reported she had continued to do well. Instances such as this, and others, maintain my support, though I do understand reservations held by some. On rare occasions I shared my story with a patient and/or family to help allay fears and apprehension. I have often wished the treatment had a different name. Would *Franklin Therapy*, for instance, conjure up such a repugnant response?

In comparison, the second unit of the patient care units became humorously described as the place for the "worried well." Though requiring hospitalization, the patient was not violent or a danger to self or others, was better able to benefit from talk therapies and group processes, and could be relied on to come and go according to the treatment schedule. If a locked-door environment became necessary, the patient could then be transferred downstairs. My work involved a concentration of interaction with the most severely distraught and disabled. Laws reflected a change in attitude, and no longer would I even dream of "holding a nose." Medications also improved, so results could be had without the possibility of the severe side effects of the earlier psychotropic drugs. Also, drugs were delivered to the units in single doses, prepared by the pharmacy, largely eliminating a great amount of preparation time.

Although there were groups designed to foster socialization and self-esteem, and to reflect reality-based thinking while increasing function and self-care and appropriate behaviors, the continued pressure to shorten hospital stays altered the approach to treatment. At its core was the determination of the correct diagnosis, and when applicable, medication. The nurse's role was to astutely observe, measure, guide, document, and intervene when necessary. Gone were the routine family meetings with team members present. This became the purview of the social worker and, perhaps, a medical student, though I continued to have a major personal acknowledgment for the pain and confusion of the family as well as their hospitalized member. Though many of the folks we dealt with caused great challenges to staff, I often felt awe and respect for those who cared for such troubled persons on a long-term basis. Perhaps hospitalization for the patient also provided respite for the caregivers.

I took the examination given by the American Nurses' Association's Committee of Examiners for Psychiatric and Mental Health Nursing Practice, which conferred on me Certification as a Psychiatric and Mental Health Nurse.

Requirements for documentation increased as society became ever more litigious. The advent of the computer demanded a minimum of familiarity. For some it became a wonderful new toy, opening up grand vistas; for others, familiarity with the word *cyberphobia* evolved. Initially untroubled, because of the presence of the familiar keyboard, I soon discovered that my earlier secretarial skills were of little use when dealing with the box that seemed to have a mind of its own which I could not read, nor could it read mine! Except for the simplest maneuvers, the computer remained a challenge, despite courses offered and taken. I did continue to avail myself of many learning opportunities offered on and off the campus for continuing education that enhanced my nursing practice.

Shortened hospitalizations also brought a quick end to passes as we knew them, and trial periods for a patient to go home to assess progress and readiness for discharge. The goal became to get the patient stabilized on medication and discharged to some form of out-patient care. The once-popular myth of entering a hospital psychiatric unit expecting a complete analysis of inner workings and a general mental overhaul to result in a "new person" at the end of a conveyer belt, persisted for a very short time. At the same time it was sad that so much had been thrown out with the bathwater due to the shorter hospital stay. In addition, the Vermont State Hospital was determined to decrease its numbers dramatically, causing the option of transfer there from our unit to become exceedingly rare. I understand that at times mentally impaired persons were arrested and sent to Vermont State Hospital from jail, and admission could not be refused via that route. This recourse, I believe, was short-lived, as was the hospitalization.

As experience increased and years passed, the "revolving door" phenomenon evidenced itself. More and more we recognized the next admission. I believe this was true in other specialities as well. Medical, surgical, orthopedic specialities—all had repeaters. This did not mean we had not done our job; rather, that persons generally respond to stresses with difficulties in already-weakened body systems. Also, time lapses between admissions tended to increase; it is always rewarding to appreciate how well people can function when homeostasis returns.

My long-range planning became closer as I worked into my sixties(!), and I anticipated sixty-five would be an appropriate age to end my hospital working life. Times and events have a way of altering plans, however. A "buyout" was offered just a year before I became sixty-five, and after careful thought I opted for it. It happened quickly and was completed in July 1993. It was a strange feeling when, in April 1997, I decided not to renew the license that meant so very much to me.

A Nurse's Journey to Improve the Environment

A Personal Account

I GRADUATED from nursing school in 1976 from Gloucester County College in Sewell, New Jersey. Prior to that I had worked as a nurse's aide in a community hospital, a nurse's aide in a nursing home, and a candy striper at Hahnemann Hospital. I remember looking up to the RNs everywhere that I worked. They always seemed to have a command of situations and knew just how to make things right.

My first job as an RN was at Graduate Hospital in Philadelphia, Pennsylvania. I worked on an alcoholic detox unit, and then on a medical surgical unit, and also did some floating assignments. Wishing a quieter pace, I worked at Underwood Memorial Hospital in Woodbury, New Jersey. I took a critical care course and began working nights in an ICU-CCU unit. In addition, I started working for an air ambulance, transporting patients all over the country. I picked up another part-time job for a surgeon in Philadelphia, working a couple of afternoons a week.

In 1978, I moved to Burlington, Vermont, when my husband was transferred and I started work at the Medical Center Hospital of Vermont's ICU unit. The eight-week orientation was a terrific learning experience. After a year of rotating shifts and getting tired of seeing so many critically injured people, I transferred to the renal dialysis unit, which offered a more sane work schedule and a chance to really work with patients over the long term. I spent as much as fifteen hours per week or more with some patients during their dialysis.

At about this time, though, I was getting a little tired of "nursing" and wondering if I had made the right career choice. The long hours, rotating shifts, and exposures to toxic substances (formaldehyde, mercury, etc.) in the workplace was taking its toll. I visited a career counselor, and decided to go back to school and get my bachelor's degree. The University of Vermont (UVM) nursing program at the time didn't meet my needs, so I opted for a degree in psychology from UVM. I did my senior research project on coping skills in dialysis patients and their families.

In 1982, I was pregnant with twins and life took a slowdown. Due to complications in my pregnancy, I was put on bedrest in December 1982, until the babies were born in May 1983. That was a challenging experience, indeed. After the twins were born, I went back to work part-time for our pediatricians in November 1983. That experience was very different from my previous clinical assignments, and introduced me to the process of telephone triage, family/child assessments, and a less hectic pace.

In addition to the part-time work at the pediatrician's office, I began doing some part-time consulting for a local attorney, evaluating medical records. After several years of these assignments, I went back to nursing part-time (per diem) as a float pool nurse at the Medical Center Hospital of Vermont. The float pool was a perfect arrangement for me, as they were willing to have me at odd hours and for "cross shifts"—so I could work in any department, come in when I had childcare available, etc. I worked very nontraditional hours, and enjoyed the diversity of working in all different areas. Staff in every department seemed grateful for the help, and gave me challenging assignments, which broadened my set of nursing skills. In 1987, I moved to Pennsylvania for a year while my husband was engaged in obtaining a graduate degree in a fast-track program. We returned to Vermont in 1988, and eventually were divorced. I continued to work as a nurse, and was grateful for having a profession that could support a family as a single parent.

In 1990, I signed on for a full-time position in the recovery room, after having floated there often and finding I liked the staff and the work. It was in this environment, that I had time to reflect on my role as a nurse and on environmental issues. In 1990, after a vacation with my children, I realized that the amount of trash waste each of us creates does make a difference on the environment. I changed my practices at home, began recycling, purchased less toxic products, and started composting. It was during a busy night at work that I realized that I was creating a lot of excess wastes in the workplace, and if my children could see what "a mess" I made at work, they would be ashamed of my behavior. So I started to try and get my hospital to start recycling. Through months of ongoing badgering, the hospital was finally willing to get programs started to recycle paper and cardboard, and they gratefully accepted my help.

I linked up with the Association of Vermont Recyclers for information to help with my recycling project at the hospital. It was through that project that I met my current husband, Glenn McRae, the executive director of the Association of Vermont Recyclers, who has been instrumental in helping me pursue my environmental interests. Later the same year, I got together with Connie Leach-Bisson, an avid recycler and president of the "ReStore," a reuse nonprofit. We explored hospital wastes, and eventually wrote a grant to the State of Vermont for a hospital waste reduction study. The project was a big success, and we ended up collecting most of the waste from the operating room for a month, or 3,565 pounds of packaging wastes. We proceeded to sort the waste by category, and published our findings in a paper dubbed MedCycle. The story was picked up by the Associated Press wire service and made national news.

I continued to work on expanding hospital recycling efforts, and eventually was offered a position to be the full-time clinical waste reduction coordinator. I worked in that capacity at MCHV until 1996. In 1991, I married Glen McRae. Later that year, Glenn, Connie, and I formed an independent consulting company, CGH Environmental Strategies, Inc. We co-authored a book for the American Hospital Association entitled, *An Ounce of Prevention: Waste Reduction Strategies for Healthcare Facilities.*

I continued my dual role as hospital waste reduction coordinator and entrepreneur/president of CGH Environmental Strategies, Inc. for several years. I had the opportunity to present at more than 100 conferences and workshops around the country, in the U.S. Virgin Islands, New Zealand, India, and Canada. I was able to help dozens of hospitals implement waste reduction, recycling, and pollution prevention programs to improve their environmental performance. Glenn and I wrote another book on hospital wastes for the American Hospital Association in 1995, entitled *The Hospital Guidebook for Waste Reduction Program Planning and Implementation.*

During this time, I was continuing to work on getting my master's in administration at St. Michael's College. In 1996, I shifted my career focus and began doing more environmental health project work. My role at Fletcher Allen Health Care (the former MCHV) became Environmental Health Coordinator. I continued to work through CGH doing consulting. In 1998, I cofounded The Nightingale Institute for Health and Environment, a nonprofit focused on educating healthcare professionals about the environmental impact of health care in the world.

Throughout all these work projects, I have remained connected to the Vermont State Nurses' Association (VSNA) and the American Nurses' Association (ANA). At one point, I served as a vice president of district I, and as a director. While I am not always able to attend meetings, I try to do things to help VSNA be a thriving organization. One of the best things about VSNA is the relationships I have had the blessing of having with other nurses who are willing to share their experiences. In particular, Faith Emerson, Ellen Ceppetelli, Laura Nosek, Sally Sample, Judy Mara, Katie Geran, Lynn Dapice, Betty Carney, and others, have always had time to work on projects and help uplift the station and image of nursing in Vermont. Through VSNA, I helped introduce an environmental resolution in the early 1990s, and also helped draft a resolution to introduce an environmental resolution to the ANA in 1997. The ANA resolution passed, and in 1998, the ANA hired me through The Nightingale Institute for Health and the Environment to create a Nurses Pollution Prevention Kit. Throughout all the work in which I have been involved, I continue to draw strength and inspiration from the writings of Florence Nightingale. She wrote at length about the importance of the environment to human health. I am most proud of the fact that Florence Nightingale's vast wisdom can be a guiding light today.

One of the most thrilling moments of my nursing career was in 1997 in Washington, DC, at the ANA House of Delegates meeting when VSNA President Betty Carney introduced the environmental resolution. There were nine microphones around a massive conference room. Each microphone had a nurse standing by it, prepared to testify as to the importance of this resolution and advocate for support of it. Nurse colleagues from Association of Operating Room Nurses from California, nurses from Oregon, Washington, Vermont, Massachusetts, and other states were all supportive. When the resolution passed, that was indeed a high moment. ANA earmarked $86,000 toward the resolution and the development of tools so nurses throughout the country would learn about what they can do to reduce pollution in healthcare.

In closing, I feel very blessed to have so many "hats" to wear to express my nursing practice. I also enjoy being an adjunct faculty at The University of Vermont School of Nursing, as well as pioneering the role of environmental health coordinator at Fletcher Allen Health Care. My involvement as a Visiting Scientist at the Harvard School of Public Health has broadened my knowledge and understanding of environmental health issues.

—Hollie Shaner, RN, MSA

Reflections on Nursing Administration

A Personal Account

I WAS BORN and raised in the rural town of St. Albans, Vermont, during the thirties and forties, and graduated from St. Mary's High School in 1949. My decision to go to Bradford Junior College in Massachusetts was one of three possible choices: work in the dime store, become a lifelong secretary for the railroad, or go to college. Given those choices by my mother, I chose to go to college. Two years later, an even greater challenge faced me in trying to choose what to do with the rest of my life. I chose nursing. I had probably been influenced in some part by the fact that my father was a successful surgeon and our household ran on his practice schedule; or by the fact that I spent time at the local hospital where the nurses spoiled me as my father made rounds; or that his office nurse was an early role model of a nurse practitioner, and I loved to hang out around the office after school and get an ice cream cone. In any event, I was accepted for nursing school at Johns Hopkins Hospital in Baltimore and Northwestern Hospital School of Nursing in Chicago. My choices were to go south or west—obviously my geography was a bit narrow in scope.

Living and learning at Johns Hopkins was a series of challenges. It was my first contact with segregation. All patient care wards were organized by sex and race. It was my first contact with violence—one of my classmates was attacked and raped. It was my first experience in living in a different culture with different value systems as the majority of the students came from the south. All the students were housed in Hampton House, which was connected to the hospital by a long underground tunnel. It was always a challenge to walk through it at night, which was supposed to be safer than exiting across the street. Our uniforms were pale blue with white collars and cuffs, beige hose, and brown sturdy oxfords. White winged caps perched on our heads. We received ten uniforms for the entire three years, which were laundered by the hospital. The collars were starched so crisply that you lined them with cotton balls to preserve your neck. Students were scheduled forty-four hours/week, frequently with split shifts from 7 to 12, 3:30 to 7 PM to cover the wards.

In the fifties, Hopkins was perceived as one of the "meccas," so that your clinical experience was a challenging one. My fond memories are of patients who were so grateful for any attention to their needs. All of us hoped to get scheduled on the black male wards where the patients were not only tolerant but caring of us. There were no intensive care units. Critically ill patients were cared for in private side rooms off the wards. Oxygen was delivered by huge oxygen tubes, and oxygen tents were often in use.

The new wonder drugs were penicillin and streptomycin. I remember preparing trays of "pen and strep" to be given IM q 3 hours into the arms and buttocks of these poor patients. All needles and syringes were boiled up on the wards. IV solutions were in glass flasks with rubber stoppers, into which you inserted a glass connector with rubber tubing. One of the joys of night duty was to boil up all the IV equipment. Many a student smelled the acrid smoke of burning rubber when the pot boiled dry. As students we became charge nurses on evening and night shifts by our second year, and learned to appreciate the helpfulness of the supervisors who would come to your rescue in problem solving. I am certain these supervisors had a subtle influence on my administrative career.

Following a candlelight graduation in 1954, I attended Johns Hopkins University summer school to complete nine credits required for my baccalaureate degree . . . this was the five-year nursing program that was still in vogue. I returned to Vermont where I worked for three months at the small rural hospital in St. Albans before a planned trip to Mexico over the holidays. I worked nights and was nurtured by the night supervisor, Gertrude Catlin, who presided over Kerbs hospital and all its night-time activities. Coming from Hopkins, where interns and residents prevailed on all the wards, it was a culture shock to find that our physicians were home asleep, as all of them were in private practice and on call at all times. It was the nursing supervisor who assessed situations and made management decisions and clinical decisions within unwritten but well-known medical protocols. The night shift was a stable environment in which to learn and grow. Most of the nurses knew their patients as neighbors in the community. The nursing policies and procedures that were a part of my practice were hardly referenced by these experienced nurses, and soon I became more skilled and independent in my practice. There were no ICUs—instead, there was an active private duty registry. My father would schedule his cases around the availability of specific nurses whom he believed were the most competent to care for his patients. During these three months I began to understand the concepts of trust and respect, caring and accountability, and the pure pleasure of having a fun time with a great group of nurses who mentored me.

In 1955, I went to work at Mary Hitchcock Memorial Hospital in Hanover, New Hampshire, where I began as a staff nurse on a small twenty-bed isolation ward. Within six weeks, I was its head nurse, and later was the head nurse of West Ward, a twenty-five bed medical-surgical ward plus private rooms for the critically ill and dying. During the summertime, I was relief supervisor on evenings and nights; and so began my career in nursing administration. As a head nurse you were clinically competent. Frequently you passed all the medications and fluids to patients, helped with feeding and ambulating patients, and were actively engaged in assessing and communicating with patients. I recall my favorite patient, Elizabeth, who was frequently admitted with congestive heart failure. We used rotating tourniquets as a treatment modality! I had a great mentor during these days who helped me learn how to influence the system. Between us, we developed a new organizational approach for the department of nursing service, which at that time had a single nurse leader for both the School of Nursing and the hospital, not an uncommon design. However it was our firm belief that more attention needed to be given to the issues of hospital nursing, and were able to convince the hospital administrator of the need for a separate Nursing Service Department. This was my first experience in making a difference in a large organization, and that became one of the tenets of my career; making a difference in an organization requires diligence, creativity, and the skills of influence and negotiation.

After five wonderful years at Mary Hitchcock Hospital, I journeyed to the West coast where the new University Hospital was opening in Seattle. Much to my dismay, the hospital was not ready when I arrived and I had to seek different employment. I joined the staff at Harborview Medical Center in the emergency department—and what a culture shock. This was the receiving area in the county where the battered, neglected, homeless came for care. I had never witnessed such needy folk. Within six weeks, I was promoted to head nurse of a 36-bed surgical unit composed of four wards. Here I learned the attitude of "making do," for this was a county facility being managed by the university. Its source of funding was always in jeopardy, so one learned how to adapt different IV tubing to the prevailing source of IV fluids, to break thermometers into smaller pieces (so you could claim more breakage, hence getting an increased supply for your unit), and to work with social service workers on a daily basis for this patient population. I was beginning to develop an interest in and a flair for nursing administration, so I decided to return to the east and enter the master's program in nursing administration at Teachers College in New York City. However, it was not to be. I was not excited by the bureaucratic admissions process, so made a decision to return to Mary Hitchcock on the faculty for a few months while I sorted out my choices, once again. The opportunity came to interview at the Mary Fletcher Hospital in Burlington, Vermont, for the Associate Director for Nursing position and on a wintry icy day in 1961, I drove to Burlington, interviewed, and accepted the position.

For the decade of the sixties, I was privileged to be a part of the leadership team at Mary Fletcher. It was a time of great expansion of hospital facilities, of the development of coronary care units and intensive care units, of nursing shortages and organizational change. It was a time of caring and a time of coping. It was a time of great social unrest and great national pride as man walked on the moon. It was the decade when the historic Medicare/Medicaid legislation was enacted that would forever change how health care would be financed in this country.

There was a nursing shortage in Vermont; it was similar to that which was occurring throughout the country in the sixties. The shortage was in direct relation to the growth of hospital beds as hospitals expanded, and to the development of critical care units. The change in the utilization of nursing students from staffing the hospital to having more controlled time on the units with faculty supervision affected staffing patterns too. The response to the nursing shortage was to work with the schools of nursing to produce more nurses, to offer financial incentives for nurses to work on evenings and nights and to be in charge, and to advertise for nurses throughout New England and in targeted locales where it was thought that nurses might be attracted to Vermont.

As Associate Director for Nursing, I literally managed the nursing services on a daily basis in conjunction with supervisory staff who had been there for many, many years. I learned once again the value of developing teamwork amongst your peers, in spite of differences in age or stage of one's career. I was the newcomer and I was not yet thirty. One of my mentors was Dr. E. L. Amidon, the medical director, whose office was next to mine. He guided me and supported me and essentially resolved any issue with house staff or medical staff. On the other side of my office was the admitting office, managed by Nurse Petit, who ruled admissions by her criteria. Many times there were no beds and one had to negotiate well with Nurse Petit to place patients where nurses were available to provide care.

The changes in nursing uniforms coincided with the social changes taking place throughout the country. Medical students were wearing beads and headbands. Nurses' hemlines rose, followed by the pantsuits and clogs. This dress style was clearly of the young, and the dress code was debated in committee to achieve consensus on policy of nurses' dress. The older nurses continued to wear the classic white uniform, shoes, and cap during this time period. Throughout my time at Mary Fletcher I made rounds daily, dressed in white uniform and cap.

To truly learn what was happening within the organization, one visited the operating room and labor and delivery suites for the latest rumor or best information. I worked hard to communicate directly with the staff not only in my rounds but by monthly newsletters: my famous "Sandwich Sessions with SAS" which were an attempt to bring together the nurse managers and supervisors to learn from other administrative departments or guest lecturers. I also established a journal club which was held in the evenings in someone's home. This was a very scary concept that had to be nurtured to engage the managers in reviewing and discussing articles from nursing journals. We learned to have a good time in the process.

Although we were busy expanding the facilities, some traditions remained constant. Every year the organization gave a box of chocolates to employees with less than a year of service and a dollar for every year of service to the remaining employees. As nursing had the largest number of employees, this was an annual challenge. I determined that every employee who received cash would receive a personalized letter from me, thanking them for their contribution to nursing care throughout the year. We would gather in the boardroom with stacks of letters, and organize a system to provide the correct name, money, and supervisor whose duty it was to deliver these letters with a cheery Christmas smile. Every manager and supervisor received a personalized letter, focusing specifically on their contribution to the goals of the department. This effort describes the opportunity to make a tradition become a team effort and to provide employees with a personalized message that makes a difference in their lives.

In 1968, the historic merger of the Mary Fletcher and the Bishop DeGoesbriand hospitals took place. The official ceremony was held at the Hotel Vermont with the members of the board of each hospital present, plus major community leaders. I was privileged to be part of that evening's celebration, and still have the brochure of the event in my memorabilia.

My counterpart at the DeGoesbriand, Sr. Mary Cassell had made a decision to leave both the order and the organization. At this time I was the Director of Nursing Service at Mary Fletcher and now had the opportunity to become the director for the newly merged organization, the Medical Center Hospital of Vermont. My first challenge came when I brought the nursing management staff from both organizations together for the first time. The issue that sparked debate was the Nursing Kardex. Each organization had one, each had a different color, each was organized differently. If I had available the number of books today on organizational change, I would have recognized that this was merely the symptom of the underlying concern by the nurses relative to their role and control in this new organization. As it was, I organized and supported a process to resolve this issue and moved on to the larger issues at hand—the realignment of clinical services between the two hospital units.

In my annual report of 1970 to the nursing staff, I noted there had been eighteen different moves and consolidations of clinical units between the two hospitals! With every consolidation there had to be a choice between two head nurses. This was especially challenging, as we consolidated OB, Peds, Labor and Delivery, ER, and ICU at the Mary Fletcher site. Most of the nurses had a strong allegiance to their respective hospital; many of them graduates from its school of nursing. During this time period, both hospital schools of nursing closed, which was another loss for those nurses who proudly wore nursing caps from these school. The University of Vermont (UVM) was expanding its baccalaureate program, and opened an associate degree program to meet the continuing need for more nurse manpower. The national salary goal for nurses was $6,500. As I recall, we did not achieve that goal in the sixties. I worked closely with the UVM faculty in trying to "bridge the gap" between nursing service and education, a goal which I have consistently tried to reach throughout my career. Many of the faculty were good friends, and we developed a professional network that exists today.

Midst the challenges of organizational and cultural change, I helped the nursing leadership group to envision the future of nursing as we moved toward the seventies. When I review annual reports and newsletters which I had written in the sixties, I find that many of today's concerns were voiced at that time. There was consistent support for a professional department of nursing, for improved support services, for more education, for better relationships with physicians. I employed the first clinical nurse specialist, Bobbie Lambert, whose role was to improve nursing practice in respiratory care. She was the courageous nurse who was not on anyone's staffing pattern, and so had to demonstrate her skills in patient care to the skeptics who wondered why she didn't have to rotate shifts. I appointed the first UVM graduate nurse to a head nurse position on pediatrics. She had the "sixties" persona; she was young, smart, wore her long blond hair in a pony tail, her uniform was short, her name badge read Rhoda, and she wore clogs. She was also a survivor, and became one of the most respected leaders we had till she went off to graduate school.

During this time, leadership development for nurses was being provided under a grant-approved project sponsored by the New England Council for Higher Education in Nursing (NECHEN). The University of Vermont School of Nursing was one of its sites, and I was invited to serve as one of its faculty. I was highly influenced by a mentor and role model, Winifred Griffin, who was the overall project director. On each of her trips to Vermont, the faculty developed under her guidance and inspiration. This was the beginning of my role as a teacher, which I developed in giving countless workshops and speeches in Vermont and later around the country.

With guidance from my friend and colleague, Norma Woodruff, the dean of the UVM School of Nursing, I made a decision to go to graduate school. My choices were to stay on in a position I loved, where I was respected and successful, or to seek graduate education. It took the dean to help me believe I needed to take the opportunity to advance my education, so I did. In 1971, I left for the University of Washington, where I received my master's in nursing administration. I was fairly successfully in graduate school, receiving the Nursing Education Award from the faculty upon my graduation. My professors were intrigued with my paper, "The Mandate is the Merger," for what I had experienced in Vermont was literally unique in the country at that time.

As I concluded graduate studies, I knew that I wanted a senior leadership position in an academic medical center with an opportunity to collaborate with a school of nursing. Two fine opportunities presented, one at the Good Samaritan Hospital in Phoenix, Arizona, and one at Vanderbilt University Hospital in Nashville, Tennessee. The home of country music was my choice, and I accepted the position as Assistant Hospital Director for Nursing Service and Assistant Dean in the School of Nursing. At Vanderbilt, they were experimenting with the concept of joint-appointment of clinical nurse specialists who would teach in the senior courses of the curriculum and be responsible as the manager of a clinical unit. I felt this was a perfect opportunity for me to enhance collaboration with the school and provide professional leadership within the hospital. My first challenge was in learning that the nursing shortage was severe and of long duration. Vanderbilt technicians had been trained to relieve the shortages, and I discovered these unlicensed individuals were frequently in charge on nights. Needless to say, I increased my malpractice insurance and devised strategies with the clinical nursing specialist to revise staffing patterns. As the newcomer to the south, I had to assess and understand the southern pace and culture. I was frequently admonished to "slow down, Sally Ann, you are going to wear yourself out." I thought I was going at my slowest pace.

Working with a critical mass of clinical nurse specialists was a privilege and a joy. These nurses were committed to making the joint-appointment concept work, and I spent many hours with them—sharing their vision and dreams and helping them to sort out priorities in the realities of this setting. With their leadership on the units, patients, staff, and students benefitted from their intelligence, their caring, and their astute problem-solving. It was not easy. I organized a series of leadership retreats for all the head nurses and specialists on a regular basis, in locales that allowed for building new relationships and respect. The symptom of unrest midst organizational change in this setting was the issue of nurses' caps! The head nurses were in impeccable white uniforms with caps, the clinical nurse specialist looked equally professional but wore no cap. I chose not to debate this issue and made my rounds in white uniform, sometimes with cap, other times without cap, and soon an acceptable double standard existed.

It was with regret that I left Vanderbilt after five years to return to the great Northwest. At the time of my departure, all the clinical units had the leadership of clinical nurse specialists, including the ambulatory clinics. The energy, enthusiasm, and commitment of the cadre of professional nurses was one that sustained me and gave me great insight into the advancement of professional practice and education. Their greatest gift to me was their work on shared governance that would undergird their practice model that was dedicated to me. I shall always treasure it.

In Seattle, I had accepted the position of Associate Hospital Director at Harborview Medical Center and Assistant Professor at the University of Washington School of Nursing. It is here that I integrated all my experience and education into the development of the Nursing Service Department. Harborview served as the major trauma center for the state. Eight of ten admissions came through the Emergency Trauma Center. It had both surgical and medical intensive care units and a regional burn center. To staff these units in the seventies was a major challenge. To have the majority of your staff be young, smart, feisty critical care nurses was another type of challenge. Medical care was provided mostly by young, smart, and feisty house staff that added to the challenge.

The development of nursing by-laws with the staff began the process of change to a more professionally focused organization. Creative and courageous nurse leaders were supported in reshaping nursing practice midst acute nursing shortages. In my first summer, I experienced a city-wide nurses' strike with only Harborview and the children's hospital remaining fully operative to meet emergency needs of the community. This was a true challenge, not only in the provision of patient care, but in supporting one's colleagues who were directly engaged in the negotiation.

With each step forward, another staffing crisis would emerge that required limiting admissions for short periods of time. To keep sane, we developed Code Pink that returned all the leaders to the nursing office for yet another juggling of staff to meet the latest trauma admission. In spite of the daily staffing concerns, creative new joint appointments were developed, even to the exchange of a faculty member from the school of nursing as an interim head nurse while I paid for the faculty member's replacement. There was a tremendous spirit of caring and responsiveness to the clinical challenges, but eventually fatigue and frustration with staffing would create "burn-out" within the critical care staffs. Eventually, my decision to curtail admissions for limited times due to staffing shortage provided a conflict with the medical staff that culminated in my being asked to resign from my leadership position. I was devastated. I had not assessed the tension between administration and medical staff correctly, and was unable to turn the situation around. It was one of my best efforts in developing a nursing department, yet it was one of my worst moments.

During those seven years I had been very active in the Washington State Nurses' Association and was encouraged to run for national office, which I did. I was elected to the American Nurses' Association (ANA) Commission of Nursing Services, and subsequently was elected its chairperson. These professional pursuits had me away from Harborview, which was not perceived by the administrator as an essential part of my development. Lessons learned: Relationships between the administrator and the medical staff need to be continuously assessed, particularly when decisions are made that are conflicting to their goals. Participation in professional organizations must be supported during the tough times as well as when all is going well. When I left this position, the Seattle nursing community gave me a magnificent party, during which the executive director of the university hospital system which included Harborview said he had no idea of my contribution to nursing. I always like to think perhaps he regretted supporting the decision for my termination.

Participation in my professional organization has always been a part of my career. While I was chairperson of the Commission on Nursing Service I had the opportunity to participate in the first Sino-American Nurses' conference in Beijing, China. All of the Commission Chairpersons of Practice, Research, Education, Economic and General Welfare, and Nursing Service were invited as faculty to make a presentation relative to the focus of nursing in the United States from our Commission's perspective. To stand in one of the conference rooms in the Great Hall and deliver a speech to an audience of Asian nurses, clad in simple dark blue outfits, with eyes downcast yet attentive, was the thrill of a lifetime. It was a time and a trip that I will never forget. I was able to successfully run for a seat on the ANA Board of Directors, campaigning when the convention was in Hawaii. Another exciting and thrilling experience. While on the Board, I was mentored by "mama Dear," Dean Norma Lang. She taught me a great deal about how to be effective on a National Board and we continue our colleague-ship with equal admiration for each other's contribution in nursing.

As I pondered my choices at this stage of my career, once again an opportunity presented itself from a colleague on the East coast. She called to ask if I would be interested in the Corporate Executive Nurse position at the University of Michigan. I was, I interviewed, and was accepted for yet another great challenge in my career. This was a staff position, not a line position. This position was being operationalized for the first time following a six-week nurses' strike which had demoralized both nursing and administration. Staffing shortages were extreme, with high utilization of supplemental nurses from national agencies . . . and over a million dollars expense line. Nurse manager positions had a turnover rate of over fifty percent. University of Michigan Hospitals was a complex of 900 beds with four separate buildings for the children's hospital, women's pavilion, adult medical-surgical, and psychiatric facilities. As a tertiary referral hospital for the state, it had extensive ambulatory care services plus home health care. The hospitals functioned at ninety percent occupancy, and plans for a new medical center complex were in the process of being funded.

Again, a cadre of clinical nurse specialists provided leadership, even though they were part of the union. Learning to work within the constraints of an extensive union contract was a new experience for me, but learning to understand and appreciate the attitudes of unionized nurses was extremely tough to do. It was necessary to seek respect and trust of the nurses in the rebuilding of this nursing department, and I utilized every experience and strategy to enhance relationships. I was viewed as the nursing leader who sat at the corporate table and would speak for nursing. With the support of key nursing leaders within the system, we strategized together in reshaping the spirit and the structure that would enable nurses to be more satisfied in their professional roles and to improve the quality of care.

Amidst that effort I assumed the role of hospital administrator of the 650 bed Med-Surgical Adult Hospital for an interim period of six months. I brought my leadership skills to this administrative team at the critical juncture when we were finalizing plans for the new hospital. It was a challenging experience, and I worked both roles seven days a week. I believe that I provided an opportunity for the corporate team to see a nurse administrator functioning effectively in a classic hospital administrative role, and I was successful in it. As recruitment began to fill this position, I was encouraged to apply for it on a permanent basis from no other than members of the medical staff. Again, I analyzed my choices and determined that I wanted to continue to provide leadership for the nursing community.

In my seven years at the University of Michigan, I learned to establish networks of influence from a staff position that motivated the nursing leadership and supported the nursing staff to strive for excellence in the provision of care in a unionized environment. As assistant dean, I participated with the faculty in enhancing collaborative projects with clinical specialists. This was the first organization in which I could justify a nurse researcher in the nursing department, who provided me and the nursing staff with the skills of scholarly thinking and inquiry into practice issues. The catalyst that was useful in providing the momentum, and the funding for selective initiatives, was the move into the new medical center that would completely replace all facilities. This was a time and an opportunity not to be missed, and I utilized my leadership role to the maximum to facilitate positive change. The current buildings were 1910 vintage, many wards inefficient but beloved by all who had trained there. To move into the new facilities required envisioning the best designs for patient care and patient flow; however, to work in the new facilities required new models of practice assignments and patterns of teamwork. As the new structure had all semi-private or private accommodations, the ability to help other nurses by being visible in the common wards was gone. It required flexibility and adaptability to change old habit patterns but in a relatively short time the new facilities became comfortable to both patients and nursing staff. Turnover rates came down, recruitment was enhanced, master's-prepared nurse managers assumed responsibility for the clinical units, and professional nursing concepts became integrated into the provision of patient care services.

Every three years the nurses' contract was renegotiated, and I experienced my first strike on my own campus for the first time. The time and energy that was expended in this process was phenomenal as we brought the hospital census from 800 to less than fifty percent occupancy in order to provide safe patient care. At the next contract negotiation, the administration took the nurses' union to court to argue that it was denying access to patients in the state who required specialty care. This argument was upheld, and the nurses returned immediately to work with no adverse attitudes. In spite of these difficult negotiations, it was possible to develop a professional practice model and a spirit of collaboration with University Hospitals that allowed it to become one of the early leaders in quality improvement efforts.

With the nursing environment stabilized and leadership within the diverse components matured and professional nursing recognized, another opportunity presented itself for me to choose to stay and conclude my career at University Hospitals, or return to Vermont in a joint-appointment position with The University of Vermont School of Nursing and the Medical Center Hospital of Vermont. I believed that it was timely to leave and to seize the opportunity to develop new skills in the teaching of graduate courses in management and leadership at the school, and to develop a new role with the medical center to enhance nursing practice. This opportunity was the embodiment of all my visions of collaboration between nursing service and nursing education and many degrees of freedom to do what I wanted to do.

Working with the graduate students was a great challenge and the most rewarding experience. I was so impressed with these mid-career nurses working in Vermont as they traveled miles to participate in this educational effort. They were bright, enthusiastic, and motivated students, and I learned as much from them as I hope they did from me.

At the Medical Center, I established a Center for Nursing, designing it to be a collaborative effort between the school and nursing service. Within the Center were the staff development, research, and quality programs and opportunities for consultation in practice. One of my significant accomplishments was to convene a nursing strategic planning committee that worked and learned together to articulate the future vision for the Medical Center in a document entitled "The Nursing Quality Initiative." Concurrently, the Vermont Organization of Nurse Executives were successful in receiving a Robert Wood Johnson/Pew Charitable Trust grant to "improve hospital nursing services in the delivery of patient care." The collaboration of all the nurse executives in the state on this project is one of the major reasons for receiving the award: out of over 700 applications, only twenty projects were awarded one million dollars over a five-year term to plan, implement, and evaluate their project titled the Vermont Nursing Initiative (VNI). The nursing leaders who were responsible for obtaining the Robert Wood Johnson "Pew" Charitable Trust grant were Carolyn Roberts, CEO at Copley, and the nursing administrators in the state. Toni Kaeding was the project director, Ellen Ceppetilli was the associate director. This grant was a tremendous stimulus for the state and has written reports documenting its initiatives and outcomes.

I became involved with VNI and negotiated with them to take responsibility for one of their initiatives, i.e., to establish a state-wide educational network. For five years, I planned and implemented educational programming to meet the needs of the grant project, including an annual retreat in the mountains where I utilized my network to bring in colleagues who had achieved national recognition for their leadership efforts. Some of the national nursing leaders that came to Vermont as a part of the VNI educational programs were Mary Ann Fralic, DrPH, RN, FAAN, Senior Vice President for Nursing at the Robert Wood Johnson Medical Center in New Jersey, who had published some excellent work on redesign of nursing; Marjorie Beyers, PhD, RN, FAAN, Executive Director for American Organization of Nurse Executives; Roy Simpson,

RN, FAAN, Executive Director for Nursing Affairs, HBO and Co., a major computer systems company; and other nonnurse leaders, including Dr. Larry Weed for his work on knowledge couplers. It was a time to learn and to applaud the work being done in the state to improve nursing practice and to have fun. Our motto was "Virtually Nothing Is Impossible."

The year 1993 was a banner year for me. I was privileged to receive the Vermont State Nurses' Association Nurse of the Year award. I was inducted as a Fellow into the American Academy of Nursing, the only nurse in Vermont with that distinction. I was thrilled to receive an honorary doctorate in nursing from Norwich University. And I successfully influenced my network to recommend me for the first nurse-at-large position on the Joint Commission on Accreditation of Healthcare Organizations (JCAHO). I had served as the American Nurses' Association representative to the JCAHO Hospital Accreditation program for seven years, and been part of nursing's twenty-five year struggle to get a seat on the Board, so it was very meaningful to me to be appointed to this position. I am now in my second term and am on the Executive Committee (a first for nursing) and chair the Accreditation Committee. I am on the JCAHO Board of Governors of the new Institute for Healthcare Quality and on the oversight committee for Joint Commission International. It has been a very stimulating experience to participate within this twenty-eight member board, composed primarily of physicians and administrators plus six public members to strategize on the issues of quality care and quality outcomes.

After forty years in nursing, I moved into consultation in 1995, working with The University of Vermont Continuing Education programs. I enjoyed the opportunity to develop educational programs for nurses and other health care workers which utilized distance learning technology. I continue to participate on a much more limited basis, sharing my network of colleagues and their expertise.

My current activities include additional board responsibilities. I am in my third year on the Board of Trustees of Fletcher Allen Health Care in Burlington, Vermont, the result of the merger of the Fanny Allen and Mary Fletcher hospitals. To bring together these diverse constituencies with their unique values, budgets, and goals has indeed been a challenge. As a Board, we have had to work through key leadership changes, critical budgetary issues, low morale, and quality concerns, as we try to position Fletcher Allen in the managed care environment that is driving health care decisions and outcomes. I was fortunate to have had previous Board experience in order to function effectively on Fletcher Allen's Board. I currently chair the Planning Committee, which is bringing forward the $100 million dollar capital plan to build a new Ambulatory care facility and parking garage as well as other critical renovations to provide better facilities for coordinated health care services. I also serve on its Executive Committee and the Committee for Quality and Patient Care systems which recently met with members of the nursing staff for two full days of hearings to hear their concerns for quality of care. This was a difficult assignment for me as I related so closely to their concerns, and yet I had to maintain a relative objectivity in terms of their perceptions and the realities that we are facing in managing this health care system. I also serve as the Board's liaison to the Visiting Nurse Association and to the Champlain Initiative, which seeks to develop insights and strategies to improve our community quality of life.

A new organization, the Florence Nightingale Institute for Health Care and the Environment, has captured my interest and I serve as its chairperson. Its mission is to raise awareness of the role that nursing has in minimizing the negative impact on the environment generated by hospitals in managing their waste products or in their use of such toxic agents as mercury. I also serve on a newly formed for-profit organization which is planning to launch a distance learning network to provide timely education and information to three targeted audiences: higher education, health care, and public administration. Currently we are conducting market research in these areas, and my network of colleagues becomes essential in seeking wise counsel and advice. I also serve on The University of Vermont's School of Nursing Advisory committee.

Choices and Challenges for the Future

The health care industry will continue to experience overlapping waves of change within its organizations. The delivery systems will be extensive and complex, requiring the ability to envision that totality of health care needs require multidisciplinary strategic initiatives. It is essential for professional nursing to have a clear vision of where it can make a difference in the health care of the communities it services.

Professional nursing leadership is necessary at points of care, at the corporate table, and in the political arena. It is speculated that another nursing shortage will be occurring in the next ten years. Sound data must be gathered to affirm or deny this speculation, so that an adequate supply of nurses continues to be available to provide care to the sick and the well of the community.

The economic and political forces will continue to influence access to care. Every effort must be made to keep nurses informed and prepared to address the numerous issues surrounding access and quality care. This is especially true of rural areas in Vermont, where attention to national and global issues might not seem to have as great an impact on our environment. Nurses must be attentive to the environment in which they practice and work collaboratively to assure quality nursing care.

Collaborative models with schools of nursing will assist in providing students with an appreciation of the reality of the healthcare environment. Vermont has a unique opportunity to seek out models and test them for the most effective methods of nursing practice. In our small state, faculties and staff know one another and can more easily collaborate on issues of mutual concern.

Issues facing the nursing profession into the millennium will be more complex, such as anticipated ethical dilemmas, issues of social justice, supportive care for the dying, and the continuing advances in medical technology, gene therapies, and pharmaceuticals. None of these issues should be faced alone; rather, there is opportunity for collaborative dialogue and research with our colleagues in medicine and other fields of science.

As we await the twenty-first century, the health care system will continue to evolve at a fearsome pace. How the future will unfold is best described by one of our historic leaders. Florence Nightingale, in her 1860 *Notes on Nursing*, said, "No system can endure that does not march. Are we walking to the future or to the past? Are we progressing or are we stereotyping: We must remember that we have scarcely crossed the threshold of uncivilized civilization in nursing, there is so much to do. Don't let us stereotype mediocrity. We are still on the threshold of Nursing."

I hope that nurses in Vermont will march with vigor, with creativity, with a passionate commitment to quality patient care, remembering the slogan, Virtually Nothing is Impossible.

—Sally A. Sample, RN, MN, FAAN

When The Patient Is Vermont: Public Health Nursing

PUBLIC HEALTH NURSING as a nursing specialty in the United States celebrated its 100th birthday in 1994. In 1894, Lillian Wald and Mary Brewster began home visits to the immigrants living on the lower East Side of New York City. Their work was the beginning of the Henry Street Visiting Nurses and the forerunner of public health nursing in the United States. In the early part of the twentieth century, the first visiting nurses—providing bedside care at home and school nursing—were hired in Brattleboro and Burlington, and several other Vermont communities soon followed suit.

The passing by Congress of the Sheppard-Towner Act in 1921 gave further impetus to the development of pubic health nursing, strengthening and expanding the functions of the Children's Bureau by providing federal grants to the states to encourage the development of programs to reduce maternal and infant mortality. Child health conferences (originally known as Well Baby Clinics) were established, providing medical examinations and immunizations. Families were taught health promotion practices by the nurses.

In 1925, the Vermont State Department of Public Health received $5,000 as a result of the federal Sheppard-Towner legislation, and employed its first nurse. In 1934, the Division of Public Health Nursing was created by changing the name of what had been the Division of Maternity and Infancy. In addition to state-employed public health nurses, there were community nurses employed in schools, towns, and visiting nurses agencies.

The following history begins with the war years; the early years of public health nursing are addressed in *We Who Serve.*[1]

In 1941, a generalized public health nursing program was in operation in sixty-eight towns served by twenty-one public health nurses, four nursing supervisors, and one director of nursing, Nellie Jones. Jones had

---

This chapter on public health nursing history is dedicated to Esther Martinson, who was Director of Public Health Nursing for the Vermont Department of Health from 1948 to 1967. Esther was a nursing leader in Vermont during that time, and is acknowledged as an outstanding contributor to the development of public health nursing in Vermont.

joined the State Health Department as a Sheppard-Towner Act nurse in 1926. This program later became the Maternal and Child Health Division. In 1936, Jones was named the first director of the newly formed Division of Public Health Nursing.

The main office of the Health Department was located at 2 Colchester Avenue in Burlington, and Dr. Charles Dalton was the State Health Officer. Nurses were also employed in two specialized public health areas:

1. Tuberculosis: Six staff nurses, paid by the Vermont Tuberculosis and Health Association, were supervised by Evangeline Galaise, RN, and followed tuberculosis patients statewide.
2. Crippled Children's Programs: Lillian Kron, RN, oversaw the program with six nurses who worked out of their own homes. These nurses staffed clinics statewide to follow up on child polio patients.

In 1940, Esther Martinson was hired as a nursing supervisor by the Vermont Department of Health. At the time, the Public Health Nursing (PHN) office was located in Burlington in an old school building at 348 College Street. Hortense Harwood, a nursing supervisor, oriented Esther, and she was assigned to the northeastern section of Vermont with staff nurses in Concord, Lyndonville, Wells River, Morrisville, Stowe, Hyde Park, Johnson, and later the Enosburg and Highgate area. As Esther recalled, "To reach Miss Jones, one entered a large room on the second floor of 348 College Street. Dr. Viola Russell, Director of Maternal Child Health, occupied separate office space reached by going through Miss Jones' office."[2] This close proximity between public health nursing and Maternal Child Health was based historically in the roots of Maternal Child Health (MCH). Through federal funding, public health nurses at the local level provided home visits to families with newborns and staffed Child Health Conferences. These nurses also served in the public schools and occasionally attended home deliveries.

In addition to federal funding to promote and improve MCH in rural areas, both John Hancock and Metropolitan Life insurance companies sold policies to families that provided coverage for nurse visits to pregnant women and newborn babies. These visits were viewed as a means of preventing illnesses and complications, thus saving money for the insurance companies.

War Years, 1941–1945

Many Vermont nurses were called upon to serve in the military. Esther Martinson shared with this author a copy of her military paper, a notice of classification from the State Committee for Nurses for the Division of Procurement and Assignment of the War Manpower Commission. Those classified as essential for civilian nursing were encouraged to continue working in Vermont. For example, a Public Health Nursing Supervisor or a Visiting Nurse Association (VNA) Director were classified as essential, because chances of finding a satisfactory replacement were small. Staff nurses in public health were classified as available for military service. They were encouraged to contact the Red Cross Recruitment Committee and apply to enlist in the Army or Navy Nurse Corps. A number of public health nurses were recruited for service.

Ruby McKewen, a public health nurse working in Grand Isle County during the war years, recalls continuing the traditional nursing activities including infant and preschool clinics, school health inspections, and home visits.[3] In addition, public health nurses organized classes in first aid and home nursing, and enlisted volunteers to stock closets with first aid supplies for emergency use. They encouraged the planting of gardens to supplement limited food items, because food rationing was in place. The nurses taught women with infants how to use additional ration books available to them to provide the necessary nutrition essential for growing babies.

During 1942–43, Esther Martinson, as a public health nursing supervisor, was asked to visit industries in Vermont, which at that time employed about thirty occupational health nurses. As a result of the war effort, many men who had worked in industry had been drafted, so a high number of women entered the work force and were employed in factories. The Health Department reported the need "to encourage adequate rest periods" and sufficient bathrooms for these women. According to Esther, "a review of the nurse program and safety provisions were made because many more employees were necessary to meet the war needs. As a result of these contacts, we ultimately formed an industrial nurses group in the Vermont State Nurses' Association."[4] The first meeting was held in Rutland, near the site of the Proctor Marble Company, the company which employed Ada Stewart as the first industrial nurse in the United States.

In 1948, Nellie Jones retired as Director of Public Health Nursing after eleven years in that post, and was succeeded by Esther Martinson. In 1949, major public health legislation led to the reorganization of the Vermont Department of Health with the first Commissioner of Health, Dr. Robert Aiken. Under Aiken's and Martinson's leadership, public health nursing was poised to enter a significant era when the program would become statewide.

1950s

In 1951, the Public Health Nursing office was moved to an old building at the airport, continuing a long practice of having health department units located in various places throughout Burlington and the state of Vermont.* The Industrial Hygiene Division was located in Barre to better serve the needs of granite workers. Chest Clinics were also located in Barre and Rutland to assure adequate follow-up for the many tuberculosis patients who were employed in the granite and marble industries. These patients also included those who developed silicosis, a consequence of long exposure to silicon dust from working in quarries.

Prior to 1951, the twenty to twenty-five nurses employed by the Health Department provided generalized services to a limited number of Vermont towns. These nurses were funded by town money supplemented by state and federal funds. Public health nurses who worked in these towns encouraged members of the health committee to go each year to the town meetings, to secure a sum equal to 1% of the Grand List taxes to support the services provided by the nurses for the following year. These funds were sent directly to the state treasurer.

At about this time, the fact that a number of towns in Vermont were not receiving public health nursing services was identified. This disparity indicated that the Health Department's mandate by legislation and mission—to serve all citizens of Vermont—was not being implemented, and that state and federal funding was not being equitably distributed. Martinson, in response to this disparity, expanded the public health nursing program to cover the entire state.† Core services were provided to all towns, and included:

- Well Child Conferences
- School nursing: consultation with schoolteachers regarding health of students, home visits to follow up on concerns identified, hearing and vision screening, patch tests for tuberculosis, dental education
- Prenatal and postnatal education and services and home visits
- Communicable disease investigation: locating contacts for venereal diseases, follow-up of cases of scarlet fever, measles, diphtheria, including quarantine

* During this move, many books and papers of historical significance to the Division of Public Health Nursing were lost. In 1978, when the Division was disbanded, more materials were lost, making this history difficult to reconstruct.

† This was accomplished with no additional staff and with no additional funding.

- Limited home visits for care of the sick, including teaching of family members
- Tuberculosis follow-up, including clinics
- Crippled Children's Clinics

Overcrowding and lack of adequate space plagued the Health Department, making it difficult to coordinate the work of the many divisions. Since Public Health Nursing was a program for the implementation of many of the department's programs, close communication with division and program heads was essential.

At last, in 1952, the Health Department moved to a new building at 115 Colchester Avenue. At the time, there was a plaque in the main entrance with the motto, "An Ounce of Prevention." In later years, Commissioner of Health Aiken, humorously changed it to "a ½-ounce of prevention," in response to severe legislative cuts in the Health Department budget.

There were now nine divisions in the Health Department: Sanitation, Communicable Disease, Laboratory, Statistics, Maternal Child Health (including Crippled Children's Program), Dental Health, Industrial Hygiene, Public Health Nursing, and Administration. Much of the work of these divisions, most often Maternal Child Health and Communicable Diseases, was implemented by the public health nurses.

During the decade of the fifties, the Public Health Nursing Division provided strong leadership and guidance to the local supervisors and staff. Offices were eventually located in eleven communities: Barre, Burlington (Essex Junction), St. Albans, Newport, St. Johnsbury, Rutland, Brattleboro, Middlebury, Bradford, Chester, and Bethel. The location often depended upon the availability of space. It was the responsibility of the supervisor to find adequate space and then suggest the location to the State Buildings Division, which would negotiate the lease for the space. In addition to supervising two offices, the supervisor also was required to transport necessary office and medical supplies from the monthly supervisors' meeting at the Central Office to the local office. The supervisor also assisted in hiring nurses and the one secretary who staffed the office—answering the phone, typing medical records, and doing general clerical work.

All nurses were hired by the nursing director. Many nurses recalled the trip to Burlington for the interview with Miss Martinson, who set a very high standard for the nurse to follow as a representative of the Health Department in the community. All nurses were also expected to be members of their professional association, the Vermont State Nurses' Association (VSNA).

One thread that runs through public health nursing history is the relationship between the local offices and the Central Office. During the

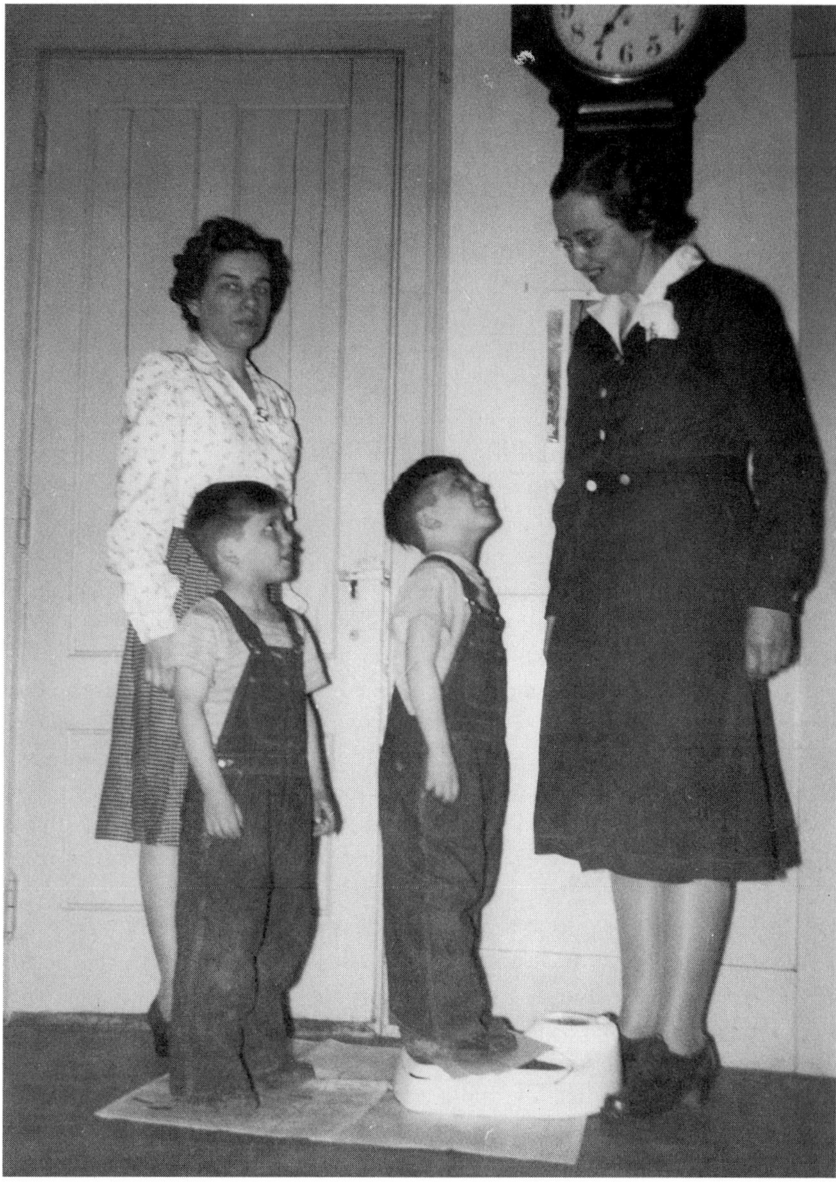

Courtesy Vermont Department of Health

Public health nurse and teacher perform screening at a school in the 1950s.

1950s, the Divisions and the Department provided the theme, program guidance, and written guidelines for public health nursing actions. Nurses then took this to their local towns and adapted the program/activity to the local community. There were thirty-four nurses, who each had five to seven—or more—towns grouped geographically for economical travel and according to population density. Each nurse was encouraged to form a local health committee for each town (a continuation of the local health councils of the 1930s and 1940s). These groups served in an advisory capacity to the nurses and provided for the recruitment of volunteers to help staff Well Child Conferences and perform vision and hearing screening in the schools. Under the nurse's guidance, these committees also worked to raise funds to help needy families who required specific assistance with medical needs such as eyeglasses, hearing aids, or medical equipment.

Although public health nursing services were statewide, some towns continued to hire local nurses. Veronica Williams was hired by the town of Poultney and paid by the Women's Club and the town.[5] She worked as the town nurse from 1948 to 1955. She had three responsibilities: school nursing, home nursing, and follow-up of welfare needs. For home visits, she collected $1.00 from those who could pay. She organized school clinics, and was taught to do hearing and vision screening by Rutland public health nurse Agnes McElroy. In 1955, she was hired as a public health nurse in Rutland.

Public health nurses continued to follow up on individuals who had communicable diseases such as diphtheria, measles, and scarlet fever. Vaccines were available for smallpox, diphtheria, whooping cough, and tetanus. On January 11, 1952, the *Rutland Daily Herald* headlined, "Health Department Reports Shocking Situation." Vermont children were not being adequately immunized for smallpox or diphtheria. In one town, 73% of the children surveyed were without protection against smallpox, diphtheria, or tetanus. Local public health nurses intensified immunization efforts to address these needs.

In 1955, a major public health event was the introduction of the long-awaited polio (Salk) vaccine. Public health nurses and school nurses mobilized statewide to organize mass clinics to immunize children against the disease that caused so much death and disability in Vermont. Veronica Williams recalls spending many hours sterilizing needles and syringes with ammonia, experiencing many a tearful moment! The polio immunization campaign was the start of a long and successful public health effort to immunize the entire population, especially children, against commonly occurring childhood diseases.

Public health nurses were expected to provide confidential case and contact follow-up for venereal diseases such as syphilis or gonorrhea. This proved to be a major challenge, as most public health nurses were well-known in the local area. Occasionally a nurse was assigned a case in another town in order to avoid placing the local nurse in an uncomfortable role with a relative, friend, or neighbor. To enhance their investigative techniques, the nurses attended an educational program in Brooklyn, New York, to perfect interview skills and elicit essential contact information.

During this decade, the Health Department, under the leadership of Martinson and Don Bergstrom, head of statistics, developed a system to accurately record nursing activities (home visits, clinic attendance, etc.) by age, town, and other demographic characteristics. The data were sent from the local PHN office to the Central Office for data entry and processing, with summaries sent to each town for inclusion in the town's annual report.

Esther Martinson was acknowledged as a significant force in public health nursing on the state and national level. She served with distinction as an officer in the Vermont State Nurses' Association (President, 1949–51) and also as an officer in the Association of State and Territorial Directors of Nursing (ASTDN). In this national role, she had tea at the White House with Mrs. Eisenhower in 1959. She was president of ASTDN when the association honored Pearl McIver, a nursing pioneer, upon her retirement as the first nurse director in the Public Health Service.

In the 1950s, the Health Department began an arrangement with The University of Vermont (UVM), in cooperation with Laura Dustan and then Faith Emerson of the School of Nursing faculty. Nursing students met and traveled with public health nurses, providing a rich introduction to the daily health promotion and disease prevention activities in official agency settings. Some of the student placements were in District Offices which were too many miles distant for the students to commute to and from the University, so they rented rooms for the eight weeks for this valued experience. The Vermont Association for Tuberculosis and Health helped finance travel for some of these students. The staff nurses were most helpful in providing meaningful learning experiences for the students, and took an interest in their personal as well as professional welfare while they were away from UVM. The students also had some interesting living experiences. Two of the students one night went to the St. Johnsbury House for dinner and decided they'd try tripe. They were not enthused with the flavor, but ate it. The next morning, they told the staff about their meal and were told what tripe was. They were disillusioned, to say the least! Eventually, time constraints for the public health nurses, and the difficulty for the UVM instructor to closely supervise, ended this cooperative agreement during the 1960s. It was re-introduced in the 1980s using District Offices in closer proximity to UVM.[6]

Although the salary was low, many Vermont nurses felt that employment as a public health nurse was a desirable job. It allowed the nurse to practice a variety of functions with independent responsibilities, and provided leeway for more one-to-one instruction with families. Another benefit was the chance to work regular daytime hours with little weekend or holiday duty.

Transportation for nurses in Vermont communities has been a major concern in providing public health nursing services. Nurses were known to ride through rural areas on horseback as late as the 1920s. In 1951, Dr. Aiken noted that the low salaries offered to the nurse prohibited many nurses from accepting the position because of the high cost of maintaining a vehicle which would permit travel in the remote areas of Vermont.[7]

Edith French, a public health nurse in the Morrisville-Stowe area in the 1940s, recalled:

> When I arrived to begin work, I had a 1936 Plymouth Coupe and was feeling pretty important. Little did I know the weather ahead. There were no special tires—it was chains and courage. Whenever I headed for the hills, where many of the one-room school houses were, the kind farmers would watch for me to come back down the hills and if it seemed a long time, they'd come looking for me. More than once they'd find me off the road or in a snow bank! There was one incident in mud season. As I was driving down from West Hill School, the road just separated and there I sat with the front end of the Plymouth nosed into the separation. It was a nearby farmer who came with his team to the rescue![8]

Public health nurses during the 1950s assumed leadership roles in Vermont nursing organizations. The Public Health Nursing Section of the Vermont State Nurses' Association was formed in 1935 and consisted of fifty-two nurses; thirty were members of the VSNA. In 1940, the rules of the PHN section were adopted with the purposes to, "promote the interests of public health nurses and to provide an opportunity for the consideration of problems of special interest to public health nurses."[9] Membership was limited to those engaged in public health nursing and to VSNA members interested in public health nursing. The members included state-employed public health nurses, visiting nurses, some town nurses, and school nurses.

Interesting insights into public health nursing's past can be gained from a perusal of the minutes of its professional organization.[10]

- In 1943, the meetings addressed such war-related topics as nursing in defense, family nutritional needs, and the constraints of food rationing. From the June 24, 1943, Section Report: "Meeting new situations and learning to cope with all sorts of problems as a result of the war effort has taxed the ingenuity of the public health nurse and made her realize more strongly than ever that a public health program must be elastic in order to serve the needs of the community."

- In November 1944, the group planned a spring meeting in Bennington and decided to invite the occupational health nurses. "It would be best to have them take part in the public health program. There being so many industrial nurses in Bennington, it would be an opportune time to invite them." (Agnes McElroy, Chairman)
- At the June 7, 1945, meeting, Dorothy Allen, Public Health Nursing Supervisor, reported on a new antibiotic—penicillin—its history, method of production, uses, distribution, dosage, and characteristics.
- At the October 1952 program, the topics addressed included: "Dental Health and Use of a Dental Hygienist in a School Dental Program," and "Future Plans—Lay People as Members of the Public Health Nursing Section."
- At a Community Health Institute sponsored by the Section on May 21, 1954, the topic was "Health is Everybody's Business," with Dr. Carlton Haines of the Division of Cancer Control of the Health Department. The registration fee was $.50 and dinner was $2.00. The Section reported expenditures of $2.55, including the purchase of 50 three-cent stamps.
- The last reported meeting of the Public Health Nursing Section was on September 26, 1955. Emily Smith from the United States Public Health Service was the speaker. The topic was "Opportunities In Nursing" in the newly organized noncommissioned reserve corps for civilian defense and disaster duty.

In addition to the educational programs provided by the PHN section of the VSNA, educational assistance was provided by the Health Department. Nurses who initially were hired as public health nurses were often lacking the formal preparation for public health nursing, which included health promotion teaching, communicable disease content, community organization, etc., as offered in a baccalaureate degree program. After one year of employment, they were sent to out-of-state colleges for a one-year course in public health nursing. This was paid for through maternal child health funds in the budget.

This commitment sometimes caused considerable upheaval in the lives of individual nurses. Veronica Williams attended Simmons College in Massachusetts for one year in 1957–58. She had two teenagers who went with her and went to school while she did. They lived in the family motor home. Another nurse, Jean Shepard of the St. Albans office, left her three daughters at home with her husband while she attended St. Anselm's College in New Hampshire for one year. One nurse from the Barre area was a single parent who arranged to have her three children board at St. Joseph's in Burlington while she completed her year of education. These nurses demonstrated incredible dedication to their positions to complete the essential course work.

In 1952, a report of the Vermont Survey of Nursing Needs and Resources[11] gave a a national guide for public health nurse staffing: a ratio of 1 PHN to 5,000 population, with a long-range goal of 1 PHN to 2,000 population. The Health Department reported six nursing supervisors and thirty-one staff nurses. The report noted that it would take twelve additional nurses to bring the ratio to the 1:5,000 guideline. Vermont's Public Health Nursing Division was woefully understaffed.

1960s

The public health nursing role in the early 1960s continued as it had through the 1950s, with an increase in the need for maternal child health services. Public health nurses had also assumed the follow-up for tuberculosis patients, as the Vermont Tuberculosis and Health Association discontinued providing nurses for this purpose. The introduction of the measles vaccine again brought mass immunization clinics, though this time the effort was helped by the use of disposable syringes and needles. Another responsibility assigned to the public health nurses was to assist with orthopedic clinics conducted in local communities, as the emphasis shifted from the specific polio focus of earlier years to the more general common orthopedic problems of children.

For public health nurses in Rutland, St. Johnsbury, and Brattleboro, another Handicapped Children's Program that required nursing service was the Hearing Program. Clinics were held in these locations, and nurses from the local office assisted the staff from Central Office and local physicians who provided care for the children referred to the clinic. In coordination with the Chronic Illness Division, the public health nurses from the Rutland office assisted the local physician at the monthly tumor clinic held at the Rutland Hospital. The office also housed the clerical support for the Tumor Registry.[12]

Public health nursing practice continued to reflect the Health Department's mission and goals. An increase in MCH funding resulted in the development of programs to educate nurses in evaluating the health status of preschool children. The Department hired a maternal child health nurse consultant, Claire LeFrancois, a former public health nurse and supervisor, who had completed her master's program in maternal child health nursing and returned to the Health Department. Claire provided extensive educational support, encouragement, and assistance to the nurses in improving nursing practice in newborn assessment and preschool evaluation. Additional administrative assistance was made available when Joyce Stickney, who had been a nursing supervisor in Rutland, joined the Central Office as assistant director under Esther Martinson.

In 1964, President Lyndon Johnson proposed major legislative changes in social and health areas that were passed by the Congress. These changes impacted Vermont and the Health Department in a profound way. The Department began to rely more heavily on federal funding in its budget, particularly in maternal child health. Although there was no increase in the number of nurses and supervisors (the number of staff nurses remained at thirty-five and the number of nursing supervisors remained at six from the 1950s to the 1970s) there was more money available to enhance maternal child health activities on the local level.

Two of the most significant pieces of national legislation to impact public health nursing practice occurred in 1965. The first was Public Law 89-97, the Medicare Program. Until the introduction of this health insurance program for those aged sixty-five and over, there was often a patchwork set of services at the local level, especially in home health coverage. Although there were visiting nurse agencies located in larger communities, many rural areas lacked services that could deliver the skilled home nursing care that Medicare would reimburse.

Commissioner Aiken knew the Health Department was at a crossroads. There was little prospect that the state legislature would vote for additional nursing positions, and with only thirty-five public health nurses statewide, the Department was unable to consider offering extensive home health services. The limited resources of the Department needed to remain focused on disease prevention activities, which had always been a major responsibility of an official agency. Aiken determined it would be in the best interests of Vermont to use the flow of federal funding to develop new home health agencies and to assist the existing visiting nurse agencies with the process of certification to deliver home health services under Medicare. The goal was to assure that every Vermonter sixty-five years of age and over would have access when needed to a local home health care provider.

Thus began a tremendous effort by the Health Department Central Office to meet with local communities to encourage them to develop the necessary structures—including boards of directors, professional staff, and administrative support—to become certified home health agencies. Much of the effort to motivate the local communities fell to the assistant public health nursing director, Joyce Stickney. She traveled the state focusing on potential interested communities, meeting with local medical providers, influential community members, and citizens. She spent countless hours on the road at evening meetings helping the communities to understand the Medicare requirements for certification. Local public health nursing supervisors often helped by serving as initial board members of these agencies. Several new agencies, including Caledonia Home Health, Franklin County Home Health, and Addison County Home Health were established during this time.

In 1967, Esther Martinson retired as director of the Division of Public Health Nursing. Joyce Stickney became director and Priscilla (Pat) Allen was hired as assistant director. Allen assumed the vigorous role established by Stickney in working with the home health agencies, and was also responsible for inservice education.

As the number of home health agencies grew and flourished, the previous very clear boundaries between public health nursing and home health practice began to blur. Several home health agencies began to develop or enhance existing maternal child health programs with visits to pregnant women and newborns. Some began community health education efforts in the areas of chronic diseases and childbirth education. To the community and to the legislature, the services provided by home health nurses and public health nurses started to look the same.

By 1969, there was increasing pressure to consolidate what appeared to be very similar nursing services at the local level. The state legislature began to question Commissioner Aiken about the duplication of nursing services and how better to spend the funding for health care. This challenge affected the morale of the public health nursing staff, who for several years had felt threatened with the loss of jobs. They also sensed a decline in the Health Department's appreciation for the value of their work. For these nurses, there was the long tradition of the familiar public health nurse making the rounds in her crisp navy blue uniform, carrying the traditional black bag containing basic supplies for home visits. These were nurses who lived in the community and were known to generations of Vermonters through their school, clinic, home, and community services.

At this time, also, a second major piece of legislation, the Elementary and Secondary Education Act, was passed in 1965. This act provided federal funds to encourage schools to hire their own school nurses. School nursing was a major component of the public health nurse's daily work, representing, in some cases, more than 25% of the total time. An individual nurse was often expected to cover ten or more schools. It was almost unrealistic to expect that basic screenings such as vision and hearing and the subsequent follow-up was performed in a timely manner. Contacts with local schools often resulted in requests for home visits to meet with a parent about a health concern noted by the classroom teacher. Sometimes nurses became involved in health education with individuals and groups on topics related to health such as nutrition and positive behaviors that promote health.

The need was great, and many schools acknowledged the essential role of the nurse as modeled by the public health nursing staff. Said one superintendent:

> The nurse that has come to the communities of Morrisville and Stowe has sold herself with her work. As I have visited conferences held in my rural school areas, the thing that impressed me is the fact that young married women from our poor families show on their faces the love and devotion toward the bringing up their children and this look is one that I have not seen before. It is there because they know the nurse is there to help them and they have a reasonable hope of success in being a parent.[13]

Beginning in 1965, most schools in Vermont took advantage of the federal funds and hired their own nurses. Public health nurses then became teachers, passing on to these new nurses the philosophy of viewing the child as part of the family, and serving as a resource to the school's teachers on matters relating to the health of the children in their classrooms. Public health nurses shared the importance of health education with the new school nurses and helped pave the way for their acceptance. This partnership continued over the years as the nurses worked together on disease outbreaks and mass immunization clinics.

As the public health nurses were phased out of their school nursing responsibilities, they increased the time spent with families teaching health prevention and care of newborns, infants, and preschoolers. By late 1969 to 1970, more emphasis was placed on preschool screenings to determine if these children had any health problems which might affect their ability to learn—again done in partnership with school nurses in many areas.

The Health Department continued to upgrade programs as federal funds increased. A new Division of Chronic Illness was created that developed programs for early diagnosis of chronic conditions like glaucoma and amblyopia. Public health nurses were taught to do amblyopia screening as part of the preschool clinics.

After the introduction of Medicare and Medicaid, the Health Department also created the Division of Medical Care, which was responsible for certification of home health agencies and monitoring nursing homes for compliance with federal regulations. Margery Kemon, became the nurse surveyor for home health agencies in this Division. Public Health Nurse surveyors were hired to travel statewide to visit nursing homes and

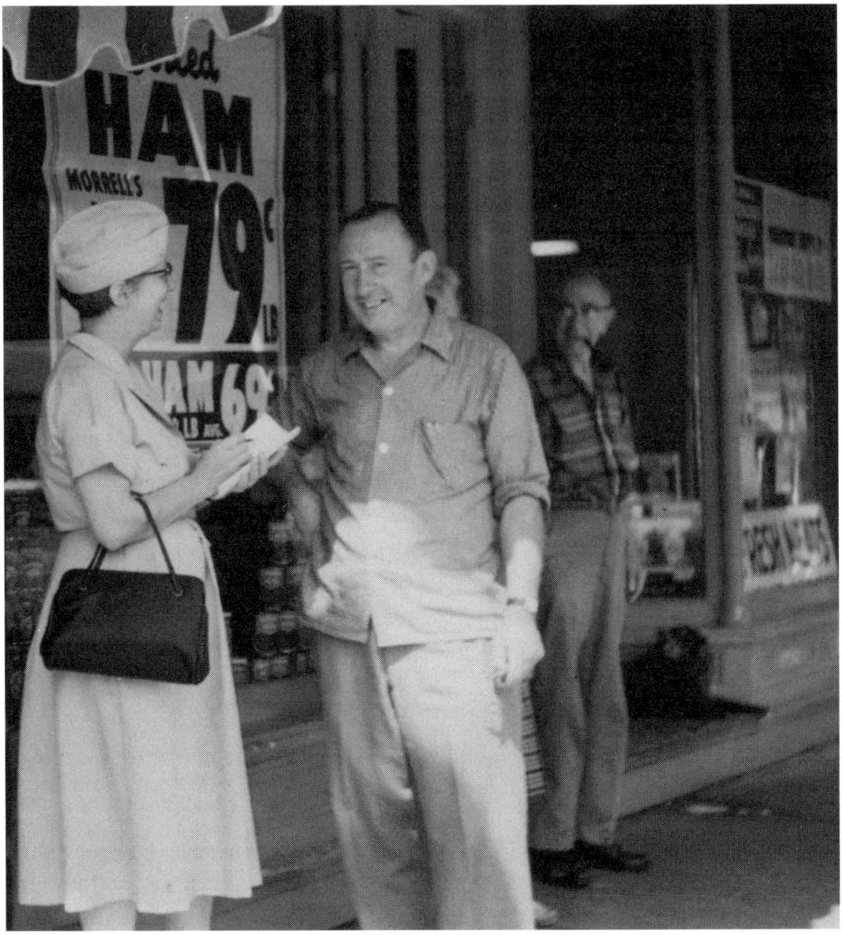

Courtesy Vermont Department of Health

Public health nurse visits with a client, 1960s.

home health agencies. Prior to the hiring of these surveyors, public health nurses had sometimes been asked to visit nursing homes to critique the care provided.

New vaccines were introduced, and there were changes in the treatment of communicable and chronic diseases. Frequent outbreaks of communicable diseases often strained the resources of the thirty-four staff nurses and six supervisors.

In 1969, an internal event united nurses as employees of a government agency. The entire state employee job grading system was re-evaluated. One of the results was the discovery by public health nurses that their pay grade was several pay grades lower than that assigned to social workers employed in social services and welfare. The nurses rallied and petitioned the Department of Personnel through the appeals process. They gathered documentation of the professional skills, independent judgment, and specialized knowledge required to practice public health nursing in rural Vermont. Public health nurses felt their practice was closely related to that of the social workers, who also made home visits and carried challenging caseloads. The nurse and social worker often visited the homes of some of the same families for different purposes. In addition, public health nurses established and ran clinics in less-than-ideal facilities such as schools and church basements. They acted independently, and made professional decisions in assessing the health status of individuals on home visits, such as performing physical assessments on newborns to determine if growth and development were within normal limits. Their arguments were heard and the appeal was successful. Two different pay grades were established for public health nurses: one for those without public health nursing experience, and another for those with experience or equivalent education such as the BS degree in nursing.

Ahead lay yet the greatest challenge to the core philosophy of public health nursing practice by state employees. By 1970, there was considerable legislative and community pressure to contract with local home agencies to provide the services being provided by the Health Department nursing staff. For the Vermont public health nurses and nursing supervisors, the long tradition of state public health nurses in the local community—started in the 1930s under Nellie Jones—was coming to an end. This practice of State Health Department employees providing direct services to families was unique to Vermont. Because of its population and size, Vermont's state health department functions as would a county health department in most other states; large cities like New York have city health departments which provide direct services.

1970s

The 1970s dawned with the prospect of contractual nursing services clouding the future of public health nurses as state employees. The first community agency chosen for such a contract was the Burlington VNA, which had a long history of providing services in maternal child health as well as home care. They had established Well Child Conferences in Burlington, and provided maternal child health visits in certain Chittenden County towns. They also developed one of the first childbirth education programs in Vermont. Health Department nurses provided maternal child health visits and well child clinics in rural Chittenden County and parts of Grand Isle County, venereal disease and tuberculosis follow-up, and staffed handicapped children's clinic.

This author was seeking employment at this time. When I was hired as a staff nurse in the Burlington office in November, 1971, Joyce Stickney interviewed me at the Central Office along with a representative of the Burlington VNA. She made it clear that if I was interested in a long career as a state employee, this was not the position for me.

The three public health nursing positions in the Burlington office were to be contracted with the Burlington VNA within a year. The public health nurses in the Burlington office resigned or transferred to another District Office of the Health Department. The public health nursing staff took their concerns about the impact of this contracting with local communities to the Vermont State Employees' Association (VSEA), the bargaining agent for state employees. The VSEA requested an opinion from the Attorney General's office regarding the existing state employees' contract and the Health Department's intent to contract for services. The Attorney General's office issued an opinion in 1972 indicating it was a violation of the VSEA contract to initiate a contract for any services being provided by existing state employees that would result in the loss of positions. This temporarily postponed any contracting for public health nursing services, although other alternatives in public health nursing service delivery were initiated during this decade.

The Health Department turned its focus to strengthening Health Department programs. Dr. Joan Babbott, the director of the Division of Child Health Services, hired several nurse consultants to supplement the services of Claire LeFrancois. Carolyn Harris was hired in 1971 as School Nurse Consultant and Elizabeth Miekle came on board as a Rehabilitation Nurse Consultant in the Central Office. There was a complete reorganization of Well Child Conferences, beginning with a regionalization process in many communities. In small Vermont towns, Well Child Conferences were held once a year, often in the spring, for preschool screening. As the immunization schedule became more complex and the standards for well child care of the American Academy of Pediatrics were adopted, the infants and preschoolers were seen more frequently for physical examinations including screenings and immunizations.

The nurses attended educational programs which would improve their Well Child Conference skills in clinic organization, nurse interviews, parent education, screenings, immunizations, and volunteer recruitment. The nurses then returned to the local areas and developed monthly regional clinics that would accommodate families from a group of towns. An extensive Well Child Clinic manual was also developed. In some areas of Vermont, there was insufficient physician coverage for well child services.

In 1973, the new director of Maternal and Child Health, Dr. Roberta Coffin, visited local physicians throughout Vermont, accompanied by Assistant Director of Public Health Nursing Audrey Swarkowski, and Maternal Child Health Nurse Consultant Claire LeFrancois, to enlist their support. Coffin also arranged with Dr. James McKay, chairman of pediatrics at the UVM Medical School, to use medical students to assist with staffing (with local pediatrician supervision) at Well Child Clinics in Newport, St. Albans, and Pittsford. This allowed medical students the opportunity to have an additional learning experience in child health care.

There were still not enough physicians available to meet the demand. In 1974, under the leadership of Roberta Coffin, Claire LeFrancois, and Joyce Stickney, the Health Department developed an internal Pediatric Nurse Practitioner Program. There were six public health nurses selected for the program: Donna Mason Reed, Barre; Mary Lou Waite, Chester; Sr. Marie Clory, Burlington; Virginia Blackwood, St. Johnsbury; Alice Howes, Brattleboro; and Glenna Smith, St. Albans. The nurses worked with local pediatric preceptors to learn physical assessment skills, and later worked at local Well Child Clinics. In other areas, local physicians continued to provide services on contract with the Health Department.

The 1970s also brought experiments in the combination of services with home health agencies. Although services could not be formally contracted out, there was still considerable interest in trying to combine home health and public health nursing staff in several areas. Two areas of Vermont lacked home health agency coverage despite much energy from the Health Department in promoting agency development. These areas were Randolph and rural Windham County. New or long-established home health agencies were present in most other Vermont communities. When no community group stepped forward to organize an agency in the Windham County area, the Health Department decided to offer the services. The State Health Department staff in the Brattleboro office learned home health care skills, a billing system was developed, and under the leadership of Public Health Nursing Supervisor Frances deFlorio, a small home health unit was established. The staff in the Brattleboro office provided both home health and public health nursing services in towns which had lacked home health care coverage.

In Randolph, the Gifford Hospital and state Health Department joined forces to establish a combined agency, employing staff who would also provide both home health and public health services.

In 1972 in Burlington, the public health nursing staff was co-located to the offices of the Burlington VNA. As new public health nurses and VNA nurses were hired, they were prepared in both Health Department and home health care programs, and it soon became impossible to tell which nurse was employed by which agency. Only a statistical and fiscal system kept track of program services.

On the communicable disease front, there was a major change in the way the Health Department would approach treatment and follow-up for reported cases of tuberculosis. With the assistance of the Centers for Disease Control, the Health Department developed a new tuberculosis program. There was a marked decline in the number of patients diagnosed with tuberculosis. It was felt that Vermont could be one of the first states to eliminate tuberculosis. No longer were tuberculosis patients sent out of the community to a sanitorium for in-patient care. With the advent of powerful new drugs, individuals could be treated at home in the local community. For those with more debilitating forms of tuberculosis or other co-existing conditions, the State contracted with the Truax Nursing Home in Richmond for a number of beds for longer-term in-patient care. The major focus in the elimination of tuberculosis was skin testing of contacts, and providing Isoniazid (INH) chemoprophylaxis to contacts of active cases to avoid future cases among those contacts. Public health nurses would regularly monitor the individual on INH to assure that those on INH would complete one year of treatment. Chest Clinics in Rutland and Barre continued with tuberculosis follow-up with a PHN from the local office assigned as staff. The Rutland Chest Clinic closed in 1985.

Responsibility for venereal disease follow-up, a public health nursing responsibility since the 1930s, was transferred to specialists in the Central Office in 1973. Also in the 1970s, there were major measles outbreaks on college campuses thought to be the result of this age group receiving less potent measles vaccine as youngsters. Many of the public health nursing staff were sent to The University of Vermont, Middlebury College, Castleton College, Norwich University, and Vermont College for mass immunization clinics and case follow-up.

In 1976, Vermont as well as the rest of the country undertook the Swine Flu Program, immunizing thousands of Vermonters in mass clinics statewide. Both public health and home health nurses were called upon to immunize many individuals in local clinics. Recalls Anne Logsdon, a nursing team leader at the Burlington VNA:

> We were setting up the very first clinic in Alburg. There were many elderly people all lined up and ready. We were preparing the vaccine and there were reporters, cameras, and media present from the major networks. Suddenly, Dr. Marshall McBean, the Commissioner of Health, stood up on a table and called a halt to the clinic. It seems there was a report of a vaccine reaction from a clinic in Philadelphia so it seemed

prudent to stop everything. It was quite a disappointment to all who had gathered![14]

The clinics resumed shortly after, and thousands of Vermonters were successfully immunized.

The anticipated outbreak of Swine Flu was another test of the public health response system to actual or potential communicable disease threats which are public health emergencies, and the Public Health Nursing Division was exceptionally well prepared, organized, and efficient in providing these clinics. Mass immunizations and immediate response to communicable disease threats became a major focus for the Vermont State Health Department. The Communicable Disease Division recognized the contribution of public health nurses as vital to the Health Department's prompt follow-up of communicable disease outbreaks. The Health Department developed a specialized role for selected public health nurses in each district office. It was difficult for forty-five nurses to remain current in all aspects of the increasing number of reportable diseases including tuberculosis, salmonella, shigella, meningitis, and measles. In each office, one public health nurse was trained for epidemiological follow-up, assuring that each case reported to the local office was followed according to established protocol. Jean Stevenson, of the Burlington office, one of the early epi-designees, made a significant contribution to the initial development of this specialized role.

With increased MCH funding the Health Department, under the leadership of Dr. Coffin, was able to expand its maternal-child health services that depended on the participation of the public health nurses. A vigorous new program for newborn follow-up was introduced. The previous method of using birth certificate information as the referral for home visits was inadequate, as the infant was often three months old before the information was received in the local office. In close coordination with hospital maternity units, a newborn referral process was developed including use of a referral form. Public health nurses began visiting infants shortly after hospital discharge. The number of visits increased substantially, and more timely intervention for newborns and their families meant better follow-up with pediatricians and obstetricians, improved breast feeding, and opportunities for teaching new parents about normal growth and development, nutrition, and preventive health practices including immunizations.

In 1974, a Leadership Training Program was instituted for nurses who would learn group techniques for expectant parent classes. For many nurses interested in teaching these classes, there had been no option except to go out of state for formal classes in childbirth education. Nurses, including public health nurses and maternity nurses from local communities, attended the first session in Burlington. Several more sessions were held in Vermont in the 1970s, where nurses and nonnurses learned about group methods. Classes in local areas proliferated as hospitals began changing their philosophy of obstetrical care by adding rooming-in and including fathers in the labor and delivery experience.

In 1974, once again the federal government provided major change in the daily life of the local public health nurse. Congress enacted the Supplemental Food Program for Women, Infants, and Children (WIC), through the Department of Agriculture. With the assistance of Senator George Aiken, Vermont was selected for one of the first pilot programs. Vermont, as always, was unique in its response to establishing the WIC Program. In acknowledgment of the rural nature of the state, the program was implemented statewide using the network of thirteen PHN district offices as a base. Thirteen public health nurses, the largest increase since the Division was established in 1934, were added. Clinics were provided in many rural areas, and more than three thousand individuals were enrolled. Families received their foods through a home delivery system, with local dairy delivery drivers bringing food directly to the family's door. Nurses were key individuals for nutritional assessment and education, working closely with nutritionists as part of the WIC program. It was a natural addition to the PHN program because many of the young families were already seen by the public health nurses in well child clinics and on home visits.

Services in maternal and child health continued to expand. Another program, Early Periodic Screening, Diagnosis, and Treatment (EPSDT), a Medicaid outreach program for children, was added to the Health Department through an agreement with the Department of Social Welfare. Ten outreach workers were added to the staff of the local offices. These new staff members worked closely with the public health nurses, helping families with children under age twenty-two on Medicaid to make and keep medical and dental appointments and to provide transportation to appointments as needed.

The 1970s led to increased pressure for specialization in the PHN role. It seemed ineffective to prepare all nurses to be generalists (i.e., able to carry out all of the public health nursing responsibilities), as had been the expectation since the 1930s. A new model for PHN practice was needed to adapt to the growing number of specialized programs which had been added.

One need for a specialized role came from the maternal-child health constituency. On the national level, there was an increasing need for support for parents who lost infants to the tragedy of Sudden Infant Death

Syndrome (SIDS). In coordination with the Chief Medical Examiner, Dr. Lawrence Harris (and later Dr. Eleanor McQuillen), the Health Department established the Vermont SIDS Program. In each local office, one nurse received intensive education to work with families who experienced a sudden infant death, which averaged about ten to twelve infants each year.

For the local district office, this meant still another nurse was selected from the generalized staff to once again focus on a select population and receive specialized preparation. The specialists now included epidemiology designees, pediatric nurse practitioners, SIDS nurses, home health nurses, and those teaching prenatal classes. This generalist versus specialist trend continued into the 1980s and 1990s, presenting a supervisory and administrative challenge.

By 1976, another program using nurses and outreach staff was added to the local office. The Cervical Cancer Screening Program, which was federally funded, hired nurses and outreach staff to encourage low-income women to have Pap screening to test for cervical cancer, and to learn breast self-examination. These staff members were also housed in the district office, making space and communication a challenge for the public health nursing supervisor and Central Office staff. The supervisors traveled between two offices, and the additional program responsibilities were stretching nursing staff to the limit. Throughout most of the 1970s, Joyce Stickney was the Director, and the nursing supervisors were: Frances deFlorio, Brattleboro/Chester; Veronica Williams, Middlebury/Rutland; Audrey Swarkowski, Burlington/St. Albans; Carol Fielders, Newport/St. Johnsbury; Doris Fish, Barre; Ann Ruotsala, Bradford/Bethel.

During this time, the nurses who were working closely with home health agencies requested that the Division consider eliminating the requirement for uniforms. The dark blue uniform and cap along with the black leather bag were all a part of a tradition dating back to the origins of public health nursing in the 1890s. Most home health staff had no uniform requirement. The issue seemed to split the staff, with much discussion of the pros and cons. The existing "uniform" was not as formal as most—dark blue skirt or slacks, white blouse, and navy blue cap. The requirement for uniforms was abolished by 1975, and informal attire became the standard.

Internally, the Health Department was preparing for a major reorganization. When Dr. Aiken retired in 1973, Dr. Anthony Robbins became Commissioner and was followed by Dr. Marshall McBean for a short time in 1976. Dr. Lloyd Novick succeeded McBean as Commissioner. On the local level, Health Department staff located in the same office were reporting to four or more different supervisors for the following programs: public health nursing, WIC, EPSDT, Environmental Health, and

Cervical Cancer Screening. In 1978, after much internal discussion and deliberation, the Medical Services Division was formed, bringing together related programs providing direct services on the local level—maternal child health, WIC, EPSDT, Handicapped Children's Clinics, Child Development Clinic, Cervical Cancer Screening, Immunizations, and the Tuberculosis Program—all under the direction of Dr. Roberta Coffin. There were thirteen local offices including Randolph and Morrisville. The Division of Public Health Nursing, after more than forty years of existence, was eliminated. The existing group of nursing supervisors—Frances deFlorio, Brattleboro/Bennington; Barbara Herrmann, Barre; Audrey (Swarkowski) Larrow, Burlington; Carol Fielders, Newport/St. Johnsbury; Patricia (Pearson) Berry, Morrisville/St. Albans; Sylvia LeBourveau, Randolph; Veronica Williams, Middlebury/Rutland; and Catherine Foster, Bradford/Chester—were promoted to district managers with the responsibility of supervising local staff from all programs, not just nursing. This was a challenging yet stressful time, and the nursing supervisors and staff were saddened by the loss of the Public Health Nursing Division. Joyce Stickney resigned at this time, leaving a void in public health nursing leadership in the Central Office. Nurses, however, continued to provide the skills and leadership in the role of local district managers and provided a public health nursing presence until each district could add a nursing supervisor to replace the manager in the nursing role.

Environmental issues in the 1970s that involved local nursing staff included mercury poisoning at a thermometer plant in Poultney, severe flooding in many Vermont towns in 1973, and preparing for a nuclear incident at the Vermont Yankee Nuclear Power Plant in Vernon (Brattleboro staff).

By the late 1970s, the combination experiments with home health began to unravel. The Health Department's focus on preventive health and the broadened Medical Services Division teams at the local level, redirected the PHN priorities away from home health activities. The Burlington office separated from the Burlington VNA by 1980. The Randolph office became a separate home health agency, with the Barre Health Department office resuming responsibility for Health Department services in Randolph. The Brattleboro office continued to provide home health services until a local agency was formed in the mid 1980s.

1980s

This decade was marked by more change within the Health Department. Lloyd Novick left to become Secretary of the Agency of Human

Services, the parent organization for the Health Department. Roberta Coffin became Health Commissioner. There continued to be a vacuum in public health nursing leadership at the Central Office. The Department was facing some major program cutbacks: The Reagan administration was imposing major cuts in federal funds, which made up the major portion of the Department's budget. Positions were being cut, the Morrisville office was closed, the WIC Program had to put families on waiting lists to receive food, and the Cervical Cancer Screening Program was eliminated. At the same time, the district managers were facing the challenge of taking separate program units and forming a united team to provide direct services.

The Agency of Human Services (AHS) began to exert a significant impact on the functioning of the local offices. Co-location with other departments in the Agency (such as Social and Rehabilitation Services, Corrections, and Social Welfare) became a priority, and many offices moved to new space shared with these departments.

Despite these new initiatives, there remained some unfinished activity with the home health agencies. A renewed effort to contract for services began in 1982. The Vermont State Employees' contract was changed to allow contracting for state employee services under certain conditions—for example, if the state work force lacked the required expertise, or if it was financially advantageous to contract for services. Requests for proposals were sent to the local home health agencies in the Agency of Human Services administrative districts, inviting them to submit plans and budgets that would allow for contracting of existing health department services, including the programs in public health nursing, WIC, and EPSDT. Several agencies expressed interest. The proposal, however, was to include the area within the AHS administrative districts, and the Burlington VNA, one of the interested parties, was aligned with Addison County. A public hearing was held in Addison County and later Dr. Novick, AHS Secretary, ruled that such contracting would not be feasible or cost effective.

Leadership in the Medical Services Division changed in 1984. A vacancy in the position of Chief of Field Operations, which oversaw the twelve local offices, was filled by Patricia Berry, a former public health nurse, supervisor, and district manager. Under Berry's leadership, there were several new initiatives including the development of programs for prenatal care and teen pregnancy prevention that relied heavily on the public health nurses for implementation. In addition, new district managers and new nursing supervisors were hired for each local office so that it was no longer necessary to cover two offices. In 1988, the local offices were reorganized under the direction of Berry into a new Division of Local

Health. There was renewed emphasis on community involvement with increased participation in preventive health activities in local communities.

By the late 1980s, several new programs were introduced. In response to the concern about a new disease called AIDS, the federal government provided funds for AIDS education to each state. Vermont established a program for AIDS education within the Health Department. The focus was on education of the community and professionals about the disease. Public health nurses were selected in local areas to receive preparation in AIDS education, and each nurse in turn spoke to thousands of Vermont citizens in numerous AIDS education sessions held in local communities.

The Epidemiology Division continued to work in partnership with the nurses at the local level strengthening and enhancing the role of the epidemiology nurse-designees created in the 1970s. The Prenatal Program was initiated in 1988. Public health nurses began to focus efforts on identifying and counseling high-risk pregnant women, including teens. Extensive educational preparation allowed the nurses to improve their assessment skills and teaching strategies with this population. A prenatal risk screening tool was used to assess each pregnant woman's risk factors, and risk-specific interventions by the public health nurse and nutritionist were planned. The prenatal and pregnant teen intervention programs became an increasingly important part of the public health nursing caseload.

In the early 1980s, an influx of refugees from Vietnam relocated in Vermont. The Vermont Refugee Resettlement Program and the Health Department developed a system of screenings and follow-up for certain communicable diseases. The public health nurses, particularly in the Burlington office, worked with the individual refugees to assure that they were free from active communicable diseases such as tuberculosis, hepatitis, and/or parasites. As world conditions changed, refugees from Eastern European countries and Russia also came to Vermont requiring similar follow-up.

Another role developed by public health nurses involved the International Travel Clinic. The Epidemiology Division was searching for a unit in Vermont to offer the immunization for yellow fever. Since a clinic needed to be licensed to administer this vaccine, the Burlington local office took on the responsibility in the early 1980s and developed a nurse-run clinic with physician back-up that offered extensive teaching about international travel, as well as many vaccines in addition to yellow fever. The International Travel Clinic was different from the other Health Department clinics in several ways. A fee for service system had to be developed because the clinic needed to pay for itself, and charging for a service was not a familiar practice for the public health nurse. The clinic attracted people from many areas of Vermont.

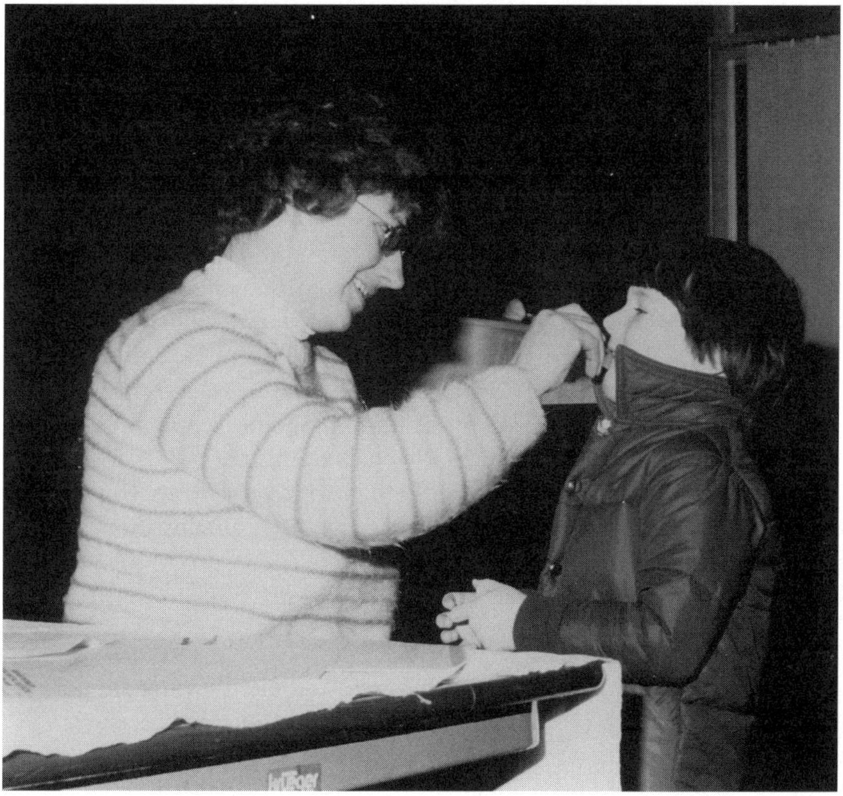

Courtesy Vermont Department of Health

Georgianna Spooner, RN, administers oral polio vaccine at a local clinic, 1980s.

During this time, the public health nursing staff began to provide services to other Vermont state employees. The Department of Fish and Wildlife and the Health Department worked together to see that game wardens received rabies vaccine. Public health nurses administered the vaccine to the game wardens and later drew titers to assure adequate protection as rabies was spreading in the fox, raccoon, and skunk populations in the state. Later, the nurses worked with the Vermont State Police to administer Hepatitis B vaccine—protection from a disease for which officers were at risk of exposure (from injured accident victims or individuals in custody).

As part of the State Employees' Contract, the Health Department was asked to develop a health program for state employees. Public health nurses went to work sites to offer blood pressure and cholesterol screenings, and health education about nutrition, exercise, weight loss, smoking cessation, and other health promotion practices. This program proved very popular with state employees, who welcomed the nurses who came to their workplace—whether it was at the local transportation garage, airport, or office setting.

As the 1980s were drawing to a close, the public health nursing staff noted an increase in the number of clients served by the various programs. These programs now included: home visits to pregnant women and newborns, WIC and Well Child Clinics, EPSDT home visits, epidemiology investigations, state employee health promotion and screenings, administration of rabies and hepatitis B vaccine to special populations, routine immunization clinics, refugee health, international travel clinic, mass immunization clinics for disease outbreaks and prevention, SIDS follow-up and community education, and a variety of other public education programs including AIDS education. Many of these programs required the nurses to have specialized preparation, so the challenge as the 1990s arrived was to once again balance the growing demand for services to groups with special needs with the need to cover the generalized nursing programs.

1990s

The complexity of the nursing programs required greater support for the local supervisors and nurses. A public health nursing specialist, Cynthia Ingham, was hired for the Central Office. She offered technical and professional support to the nursing supervisors, helping to develop educational programs and providing much-needed program guidance.

In 1990, Patricia Berry employed Audrey Larrow as Public Health Nursing Chief. Public health nursing administration returned to the Central Office after a twelve-year absence. The new nursing unit began to work on organizing the multiple programs requiring nursing expertise, and began responding to a variety of requests for nursing from many sources.

One of the requests was to expand the immunization program. Public health nurses were always active in offering immunizations to Vermont children, whether individually in Well Child Clinics or through mass immunization clinics when new vaccines were introduced. Federal funds increased, and new nurses were hired to offer immunizations to preschool children and to review the immunization status of children enrolled in local daycare centers. Unlike the schools, daycare facilities did not have any regular supervision by nurses. In cooperation with the Day Care Licensing Unit, public health nurses visited local daycare centers to review immunization records and to offer assistance to families in obtaining the age-appropriate vaccines. Families received help with making appointments at the pediatrician's office or at the local immunization clinic, and help with arranging transportation for the immunization appointment.

During the 1980s, there had been an increased awareness regarding the incidence of lead poisoning. With increased federal funding, the Health Department's Environmental Health Division developed a lead screening program, and the Division of Local Health hired additional public health nurses to offer lead screening clinics in communities. The nurses also continued to follow up on children identified with elevated lead levels to assure appropriate medical and environmental follow-up. In addition, there was an agreement with the Vermont Housing and Conservation Board for the nurses to participate in a study to identify housing that contained lead paint. Young children in these homes would have blood tested for lead levels, and environmental testing would also be done. Funds were available to the homeowner to eliminate the lead-based paint.

Another major program, which added a number of nursing positions, was the Healthy Babies Program. This program was a natural continuation of the prenatal program of the 1980s, and was one facet of Vermont's efforts to improve the health of pregnant women, infants, and preschool children on Medicaid. Coordinated efforts by obstetricians and pediatricians were a major element of the program. The physician's office would complete a risk assessment for each pregnant woman or infant and coordinate follow-up with the Healthy Babies Nurse. Each pregnant woman on Medicaid was offered these enhanced services including childbirth and parenting education and home visits by a public health or home health nurse. After the baby was born, nursing visits would continue and visits by a family support worker from the local parent–child center would be offered.

The Healthy Babies Program was one component of the Success By Six Program in local communities, where concerned citizens, health and education professionals, and parent–child center representatives would coordinate efforts to offer every child the opportunity to enter school ready to learn. The Healthy Babies Program once again combined the efforts of home health and public health nurses at the local level to provide home visits to pregnant women and newborns on Medicaid.

Dr. Jan Carney had assumed the position of Commissioner of Health on October 11, 1989. In 1992, the Health Department moved to new quarters at Cherry Street in downtown Burlington. The Chief Medical Examiner's Office was located elsewhere in Burlington; only the laboratory remained at the building at Colchester Avenue. Even the Occupational Health Division, which had been in Barre/Montpelier since its beginning as the Industrial Hygiene Division, moved to Cherry Street. It was an exciting time for the Department; at last, after years of being separated in five or more locations in Chittenden County, the many divisions and programs could better achieve the goal of close coordination and communication.

In 1993, the Division of Local Health, reaching back to its roots in the schools, began an arrangement with many local schools to help them maximize funding available in EPSDT. Using a complex formula, each school district was able to use existing services for Medicaid-eligible children to gain additional funding for support services for children. Some schools hired more nurses, others chose to hire social workers or contract with the local mental health agency to better address the physical and mental health needs of the students. The Health Department hired additional public health nursing staff to work on the EPSDT arrangements with the schools.

Sadly, one long-standing program, Well Child Clinics, was eliminated in 1993. This was due to a variety of factors, including declining attendance, improved accessibility to private physicians in Vermont, and funding through the state's Dr. Dynasaur Program for routine visits to pediatricians, family practice physicians, or nurse practitioners. Many preschoolers were also attending preschool screenings in their local community, which often duplicated many of the services of the Well Child Clinics. These clinics had existed from the early 1900s and demonstrated to communities and government the importance of preventive and health promotional care for infants and children.

By 1995, the public health nursing staff had expanded to thirteen nursing supervisors and sixty-five full- and part-time nursing staff working in a variety of programs. In the evolution of public health nursing practice, the basic components of the nursing role have remained: blending together the theory, principles, and practice of nursing and public health. Central to the nursing role over the years had been maintaining a focus on the community while providing nursing intervention with individuals, families, and groups. Changes in public health nursing practice can be traced to changes in technology and advances in knowledge of health risks and disease prevention. The role of public health nursing today reflects the current health issues in the community and the population.

Sharon Moffatt, the current State Director of Public Health Nursing at the Vermont Department of Health, shared her thoughts on the future:

> The role of public health nursing for the future will continue to emphasize skills of assessment, community collaboration, problem solving, and evaluation. Public health nurses are already expanding their role as they provide the essential services of public health in their partnership with other disciplines in public health. For example, a critical role is in envi-

ronmental health, working with individuals and communities to identify health problems and health hazards in the community. Public health nurses will also play a key role in planning for and responding to disasters and threats of bioterrorism. Their current knowledge of epidemiology and skill of community mobilization will be invaluable. Another area on which public health nurses will focus is the health promotion and disease prevention needs of our aging population. Although long involved in focusing on the health needs of the maternal child health population, these same skills of assessment, policy development, and evaluation will be the bases as we shift more of our attention to a maturing population.[15]

—AUDREY LARROW, RN, BS, MA*

NOTES

1. Vermont State Nurses' Association, *We Who Serve: A Story of Nursing in Vermont* (Winooski, Vt.: Vermont State Nurses' Association, 1941).
2. Esther Martinson, written communication with the author, 1995.
3. Ruby McKewen, written communication with the author, 6 November 1995.
4. Martinson, written communication.
5. Veronica Williams, conversatio with the author, Poultney, Vermont, July 1998.
6. Faith Emerson, written communication with the author regarding The University of Vermont student affiliation with Vermont Department of Health, April 2000.
7. Vermont Department of Health, *Annual Report*, 1951.
8. Edith Bengston French, "Memories of the First Morristown/Stowe Public Health Nurse," *The Transcript* (Morrisville, Vermont) 16, no. 30, 26 September 1988, 2.
9. Vermont State Nurses' Association, Minutes of the Public Health Nursing Section, 1940. Vermont State Nurses' Association Special Collection, Library Research Annex, The University of Vermont, Burlington, box 5. (Hereafter cited as VSNA Archives.)
10. Vermont State Nurses' Association, Minutes of the Public Health Nursing Section. VSNA Archives, box 5.

---

*A very large thanks go to the following: Esther Martinson, who shared her thoughts in writing, along with some important public health nursing memorabilia; Veronica Williams, who shared so much of her experiences during a personal interview; Marian Segale and Priscilla (Pat) Allen, who reviewed the original manuscript and added much from their personal experiences; Frances deFlorio, who provided validation of some content; Sharon Moffat, who shared her thoughts and provided the practical support in obtaining the photographs; the Vermont Department of Health for the photographs, and for being one of the best employers a nurse in Vermont could have; the many nurses and staff of the Vermont Department of Health whose experiences are represented in this history; Faith Emerson, whose excellent critique and editing of this manuscript greatly enhanced its representation of public health nursing in Vermont; and Jo-An Tudhope, whose technical support got this material from the typewriter to the computer.

11. Edyth Barnes, ed., "Report of the Vermont Survey of Nursing Needs and Resources," U.S. Public Health Service, 1952.
12. Marian Segale, conversation with the author, Middlebury, Vermont, August, 1999.
13. Milton Moore, Superintendant of Schools, Morrisville and Stowe, in a report to the Vermont Department of Health, 1940. Reported in "Memories of the First Morristown/Stowe Public Health Nurse," 3.
14. Anne Logsdon, conversation with the author, South Hero, Vermont, July 1999.
15. Sharon Moffatt, written communication with the author, September 1999.

Voices of Community Nursing

In September 1940, Lillian Wald, "one of the great urban pioneers,"[1] died. She was the founder of the Henry Street Settlement in New York City, from which evolved the Visiting Nurse Service of New York. Her work in the poverty sections of New York City formed the concepts of public health nursing and home nursing care that endure today. She saw "the whole movement . . . full of promise for homes, schools, and communities."[2] Nurses provided nursing care for the ill, checked on epidemic disease, conducted milk inspections, and assessed the health of new infants. She fought constantly to build provisions for justice and human welfare into the social structure of the country, recognizing the social, as well as the disease, determinants of health. That vision remains viable today and, hopefully, will be the base for home health and community nursing in the new millennium.

The history of the Central Vermont Home Health Agency is typical of the origins of home care in Vermont:

> 1911 – Nursing care at home began. The Montpelier Women's Club hired Miss Eleanor Black as the first District Nurse. During those first years the citizens of Montpelier were of great assistance in this work, helping financially and furnishing carriages and automobiles to help the nurse reach her many patients.
>
> 1912 – The Barre Visiting Nurse Association was founded. It was a voluntary not-for-profit agency originated by the Barre chapter of the American Red Cross. Miss Elizabeth Noonon served as Director for forty years!
>
> The Communities' nurses taught sanitation and cared for the sick with great dedication. The fee for a house call was 75 cents, or what people could pay. World War I, no health insurance, very little money and travel by trolley or horse and buggy made care for the sick difficult. The trolley ran through Barre and up Washington Street. Doctors made house calls, many babies were born at home and silicosis and TB were common illnesses with which Barre's granite workers had to cope. For many years, to

The author thanks Nancy Serrell Coonley for allowing reprint of many of the stories in this article.

> raise funds, the Montpelier Women's Club published cookbooks and sponsored popular gala charity balls. At the end of World War I cars became more plentiful and a greater area could be covered.[3]

The period between 1940 and 1945, of course, was dominated by World War II and the devastating effects of the holocaust. During that period, many Vermont nurses joined their husbands at different training sites, and the push was for schools of education to recruit and graduate more nurses for both the war and civilian work. Through the 1940s and until the early 1960s, home health agencies and visiting nurse associations in Vermont continued to focus primarily in the more densely populated areas, with town nurses and public health nurses filling the gaps in certain regions of the state. Several agencies were started by women's church groups, such as the Kings Daughters in Springfield and Woodstock. The focus was on prenatal, postnatal, and infant care, running Well Child Clinics, conducting educational programs, and offering limited services for the ill and disabled.

> LUCILLE WALDO: Back in '38, when I was the district nurse for Woodstock, Bridgewater and Pomfret, Vermont, I boarded and roomed in a home in Woodstock. Wherever I was, everybody had a big kitchen. Of course, the mother didn't work out of the house in those days so she was always home. There would be a rocking chair, padded with quilts, near the stove and half the time a cot, too. That's where the aunt or uncle would be, or the grandmother or grandfather.
>
> Every year we had a tonsil clinic in the town hall, when we'd take out tonsils and adenoids—now they don't even believe in it. Sometimes there were four or five children from one home. They had them on low cots; I went around and gave them the cone ether; and one of the doctors came along behind me, took a scalpel, and yanked their tonsils out. The next morning I had to visit every home. It scares the heck out of me to think about it—now everything is done under sterile procedures—but we never had any casualties, never had to send anyone to the hospital.
>
> There was one Christmas day when I was home with my three kids and husband and they called me from the hospital in Hanover and said they had a mother who was terminally ill with cancer. She could come home for the day to be with her five-year old daughter if I would come down there at 10, 2, 6 and 10 at night to give her shots, Demerol I think. That's how I spent that Christmas.
>
> Another time, in the spring, I got a telephone call from a doctor in Bridgewater about a woman who didn't have a telephone or any electricity. When the kids came to school they brought the news their mother was going to have another baby. The doctor said he couldn't come, would I go. So, I parked my car at the foot of the hill near a big field. I was strolling along with my bag, picking May flowers, and this robust man

with reddish hair came down in a horse-drawn wagon, with a seat over the flatbed, and told me it was his wife in labor, come on up. Up I went and sat with her. They had kept their 10-year old girl at home, to get the noon meal, I guess. She'd made a cake and put a lot of chocolate junk over the top—the flies were abundant—and she made boiled potatoes and salt pork that had hardly touched the stove. I couldn't say I had already eaten, since I was there a long time, but I don't think I've touched a boiled potato since. The doctor said he'd stop by, but I didn't think he would, and he didn't. The baby came out fine.[4]

Martha Lussier: I've taken care of somebody in almost every house in this town. I'm a Woodstock person; I was born here. It was 1937 when I graduated from nurse's training at Mary Hitchcock Hospital. They were pretty hard on us. In the morning they would teach us to do something (rub a back or give a bed bath), and then in the afternoon we went right on the floor to do it.

For several years, I did private duty nursing in Woodstock. I left private duty after a town meeting, when some people asked me to prove we needed a nurse for the town. I knew Woodstock had a very bad record of immunizations for the children. It was a black eye for the town. I took on the job part-time and went to work for the Visiting Nurse and Public Health Society making a lot less money. I think I did 11 immunization clinics that first year. I loved doing those clinics. Later, when it came time for flu shots, I set up right on the street in front of one of the drug stores, stood there in my uniform, and gave shots to people walking by.

I worked out of our home, so there were always syringes boiling on the stove and rubber tubing soaking in Lysol in the bathroom. My children knew not to touch them. My mother lived with us for 10 years and took the calls when doctors wanted me to come take care of a patient. Everything was an emergency, you know; I had to laugh. The funeral parlor had the ambulance—there were no EMT's back then—and when they were transferring someone to the hospital and needed a nurse to ride along they would call and say, "We'll be right along, can you meet us?" I'd run down to the foot of Hartland Hill. I loved it! I knew them all, of course, the drivers and the patients. That ambulance could be pretty cold, freezing cold.

I worked for four years on my own, no help, and it got so I was making five or six calls a day. Sometimes, if you believe in a thing you have to sell it. I went to a meeting in town and said, "I don't like what's happening. I need more backing or I'm going to leave." But, they didn't want to spend the money. Towns never felt they needed anything like that. Years ago, people lived on farms with three/four generations, and people took care of their own.

But at the next meeting all the ladies from the Congregational Church came. We got an office down near the health center, and I started hiring nurses.[5]

Research of the visiting nurses in Bennington revealed that the Red Cross was the first organized unit of such nurses, and since Bennington was a small town, the Red Cross provided school nurses who extended their school nursing into the homes by following up on communicable disease trying to meet the needs of whole families.

> In 1947 the Town of Bennington hired Mrs. Elizabeth Burke, RN, to care for the sick in their homes. She worked from her home, using a calendar as her only record of care given, charging the patients what they could afford, usually 25 cents to a dollar per visit. Receipts for these calls were given to the Town Treasurer once a week. Mrs. Burke was on salary and was provided with a vehicle.[6]

In the early 1960s, the needs of people coming home from the hospital began to change. With the reduction of infectious illness and communicable disease, with people living longer, and with the increasing prevalence of chronic conditions, it became apparent that more comprehensive home care services were needed. Those of us practicing nursing at that time were providing not only the treatments and procedures necessary for sick persons, but attempting to fill the gap in other services needed, such as in meal preparation; sometimes even chopping wood and filling the stoves for persons isolated at home and unable to manage independently. It became a challenge for nurses and others in the community to support these patients determined to keep their independence and to remain in their own homes. Home care nurses speak of this:

> ANGELA JOHNSON: You never really know what you're going to get, even in (maybe I should say especially in) the rural parts of Vermont. People here are very independent and expect to live their lives the way they want to, which I respect and enjoy. I know what that is. My family has lived in this area for many, many generations.
>
> There are situations where there's no running water, sometimes no indoor toilet, just shacks that people live in. They won't have it any other way, because that's what they're used to—whether or not it's the standard other people consider to be correct.[7]

> SHEILA AUBIN: Maybe it's just New England. There's a belief that you should take care of your own, that it's a responsibility to take care of our own, to be self sufficient, that if you have to rely on outsiders then maybe you're not as worthy as somebody who doesn't have to.[8]

> ANGELA JOHNSON: I'm thinking of one man who didn't want a nurse to visit him at all. He wanted to die. He knew he had something wrong with him—he'd gained a large amount of weight, fluid weight. So I said to him, "I don't have to do anything you don't want me to do. If you

don't want to go to the hospital that's fine. But, it's hard to you to breathe, you can't walk around very well, you can't even cook your own meals. I want to see if there is something I can do to make you more comfortable. And, if you choose to die, then that's your choice, and I will help you get through this stage of your life." I couldn't push, because when I pushed too hard he shut off, he'd close down, and so I would pull back.[9]

President Lyndon Johnson brought the vision of a Great Society with numerous health and welfare initiatives, among them the Medicare Act of 1965. Fortunately, the leaders in nursing on a national level were able to press for inclusion of a home health benefit, recognizing that there were needs of persons coping with chronic illness or needing support and rehabilitation after hospitalization. The Visiting Nurse Association in Burlington recognized the importance of continuity of care, and convinced the two hospitals in Burlington to allow a nurse to participate within the hospital in helping to plan and coordinate care post-hospital. Liz Stouch filled one of the first hospital liaison positions created in Vermont and in the Northeast.

The advent of Medicare brought both opportunities and challenges. Fortunately, there were Federal grants to help agencies gear up for what was anticipated to be a major role for and growth in home care services. There were mixed reactions to the Medicare program, expressed by community nurses:

Frances Field: When I began nursing in the 40s, health care was pretty much divided between the well-to-do people with their private doctors, private nurses, and private rooms in the hospital and people who couldn't afford that. Those were the people on hospital wards, the people seen in the community clinics or in their homes by visiting nurses, without charge. Once Medicare was passed health care could be available to almost everybody; it didn't have to be charity. Each state department of health was given the right to license the health care agencies in their state, meaning they had to assume certain standards to be reimbursable for Medicare and Medicaid. There was quite a challenge here, and this tremendous potential.[10]

Sally Munro: Everybody was listening to the radio to see how the vote went. Physicians just thought that was the end of the road, "Well now they've done it, now they've really done it." Because now they were going to have to provide services for certain fees, and they didn't like that. I think they were afraid they were going to lose business, or they were going to lose money. Some people were saying it was a step toward socialized medicine. I think nurses saw it in a very different light. Finally, there were going to be some services provided for people in need. The government was finally going to pick up the tab.[11]

> Pat Harford: When I started nursing in Windsor, Vermont, the town gave us money to be their town nurse, and patients paid if they could—two to three to six dollars, I think it was, but we weren't set up to get Medicare or insurance reimbursement. Going through that change to get certified entailed a whole lot of paperwork. We found it hard; it took a long time.[12]

> Martha Lussier: The morning after our agency signed up, the Rutland Herald ran a story about Medicare that had a black border all around it. It scared the life out of us. They said it would never work.[13]

It was an exciting time, as several of us around the state planned for developing physical therapy, occupational therapy, and home health aide services. Interestingly, the major concern was regarding utilization of home health aides, and skepticism was expressed about the appropriateness and safety of utilizing unlicensed personnel. Home health aides today, in most settings, provide more than half of the home care services, working closely in teams with professional staff.

Agency directors worked with Joyce Stickney at the Health Department in helping to extend services to surrounding towns in our service area, as well as providing consultation to local community groups who were interested in establishing new agencies to fill in some of the geographic gaps. The decision by the State Health Department to promote the development of community agencies was important in the evolution of the not-for-profit system in Vermont, which continues today to be one of the strongest statewide networks of organizations committed to meeting the needs of their constituents. Home health agencies and Visiting Nurse Association leadership worked to develop additional funding from town budgets, United Way, private funds, and volunteers. This supplemental funding continues to be a strong tradition in supporting the care of persons without health insurance or the ability to pay for care. Local governance of these agencies has also created an accountability for assuring access, as well as constraining costs, to the extent that Vermont continues to have the lowest home care cost in the nation.[14]

The nursing role also began to change as more disciplines became involved in the home care team. Nurses provided the supervision of home health aides, were responsible for developing the plans of care, and coordinated the other professional members of the team—which now included physical therapists, occupational therapists, speech pathologists, and medical social workers, as well as home health aides.

New nurse practitioners also expanded the role of nursing in the home care setting:

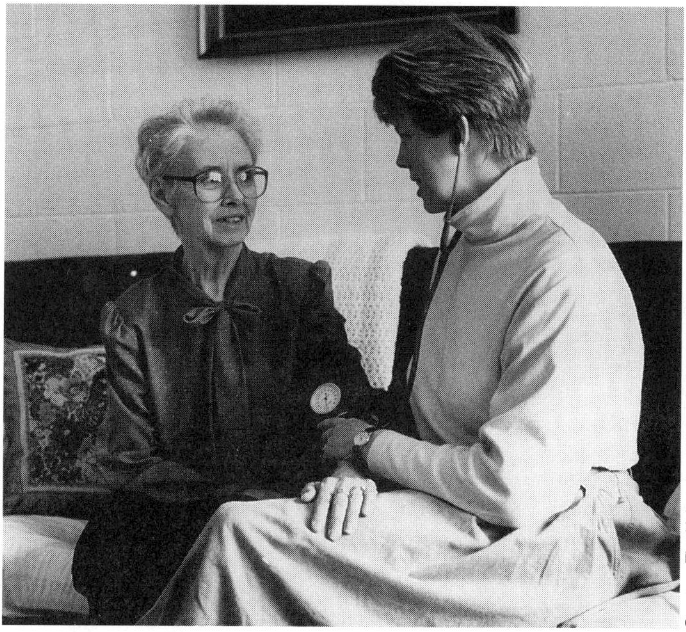

Courtesy The University of Vermont School of Nursing

Nursing home visit

Excited and enthusiastic about the new roles of nursing that have emerged in the last five years and with the new resources available to her profession is Berta Hess, RN, of Stowe.

Young, dynamic and totally involved in her work, Berta Hess covers some 50 miles daily on her motorcycle as an adult nurse practitioner for the Lamoille Home Health Agency and "loves every minute of it." She has worked in the area for four years. With one other registered nurse practitioner, she covers all of Lamoille County, "going into homes where families aren't able to get out to see their doctor but need some kind of follow-up medical treatment," through referral by their physician.

From Morrisville, besides working in the health center, she travels widely during a working day that often extends beyond her regular hours of 8 AM to 4:30 PM. Among her patients are stroke victims home from the hospital and "needing a lot of follow-up rehabilitation to learn self-care." There are also post-surgical patients, including those with cancer, accident victims, high-risk infants, diabetics, and many elderly persons.

"Restorative nursing is often a prolonged process and involves the whole family. It may include many emotional and mental problems as well as physical ones and we become very deeply involved in interpersonal relationships."[15]

But some things didn't change. The family has always been part of a holistic approach to care—and that includes the family pets!

> LINDA CULLEN: In home nursing it's not just the patient you're dealing with, it's often the family—and, of course, in the country it's also the animals. You meet raccoons, moose, ferrets, and geese.
>
> There was one man who lived up on a mountain with his wife and his geese. The wife was dying. He was pretty lonely, so I'd arrive at lunch time, sit at the table and eat with this man, but I'd also have to eat with the geese. The two geese would come in—they loved this man—they ate out of a pie plate, all pricked by goose beaks, and he'd say, "what have you got for Sam?" You'd have to give some of your lunch to the geese! After you'd fed the geese and talked with him for a while you could go in and see his wife—though at that point she wouldn't really know you were there.[16]

> MARTHA LUSSIER: I went on a case to visit an old farm woman who wouldn't let me in until I let the cows out to pasture. So I went out and climbed up on this wooden gate in full uniform, rode on it to get it open, and let the cows go by. Then she let me into the house, with my uniform all spattered with mud.[17]

In the early 1970s we encountered our first Medicare crisis. The expenditures in Medicare exceeded federal expectations, and we began to see denials for services once thought reimbursable under the Medicare program. Denials were based on more restrictive interpretations of "skilled" and "medical necessity." This created problems for the home health agencies in assuring access to adequate services. It was at that time that a group of home care directors got together, appealed to the governor and the Emergency Fund Board, and as a result of collective action, received additional funding. Recognizing that our strength was in our numbers, the Vermont Assembly of Home Health Agencies was organized to work together for statewide access to home health services, to work closely with the State Health Department, and to work collectively on a state level in communicating the issues in home health services to policymakers and state legislators. The nursing directors leading the way in that early organizational effort included Joan Blankinship from the Caledonia Home Health Agency, Marie Schoff from the Springfield Area VNA, Joyce Fellows from the Lamoille County Home Health Agency, Betsy Davis from the VNA serving Chittenden and Grand Isle Counties, Virginia North from the Bennington Home Health Agency, Mary Watson from the Central Vermont Home Health Agency, Nancy Warner from the Orleans/Essex VNA, and Evie Doyle from the Rutland VNA.

Although Medicare created considerable distraction and consumed energy in coping with an ever-increasing regulatory environment, home health agencies were able to extend services to broader regions covering most of the state by the end of the decade. Also during that period, VNAs and home health agencies turned their attention to building on the strong community health base and maternal child health services, continuing the well child clinics, home visiting services, and developing new programs. Nurse leadership developed new parenting education programs, giving nursing staff opportunities for advanced education in group process. Children and Youth Projects were funded in partnership with the State Health Department in the Springfield and Winooski areas, using nurse practitioners in leadership roles working closely with physician sponsors. A pediatric nurse practitioner, Sue Heath, employed by the Burlington VNA and with financial support from the State Health Department, instituted a mobile unit practice to serve the rural areas of Chittenden and Grand Isle Counties. From that mobile unit, the Champlain Islands Health Center—run by pediatric nurse practitioner Sue Heath and adult nurse practitioner Lyn Rothwell—was born, and served that county for a number of years. The nurse practitioners created strong linkages with physician practices in St. Albans and at Given Health Center in Burlington.

Home care stories continue to demonstrate the value of nursing services in the home:

> Sleet, snow, and bad roads are not deterrents to a nurse from the Orleans Essex VNA. The needs of the sick and disabled must be attended to, even if on occasion she has to walk a distance to get into a patient's home. Home Health nurses begin their day early, and often remain after hours to complete the frustrating, but necessary paperwork.
>
> The Agency employs 15 nurses with varied backgrounds and skills, but all have a common interest: caring for people in a holistic approach, and in their own home environment. Patients are encouraged to plan with the doctor and the nurse, and to understand the meaning and purposes of each individual program of treatment. Home Health nurses share problems, and patients become very special to the entire staff. A Home Health nurse is a "special" nurse, both in dedication and skills.
>
> The way the nurses are received in the homes is more revealing than volumes of printed pages—they are welcomed with smiles and words afforded only closest of friends or loved ones. You know immediately that they are more than just a nurse visiting the home twice weekly for duty only.
>
> Mr. Morin looked at me with an emotion packed face and said, "It's wonderful what these nurses have done for me. I didn't think I'd ever get out of bed again." But he has, and spends most of the day sitting in the pleasant living room of his home. Until the Home Health Care nurses started working with him, his only relief from time in bed was when his busy son Ron could come and help him.[18]

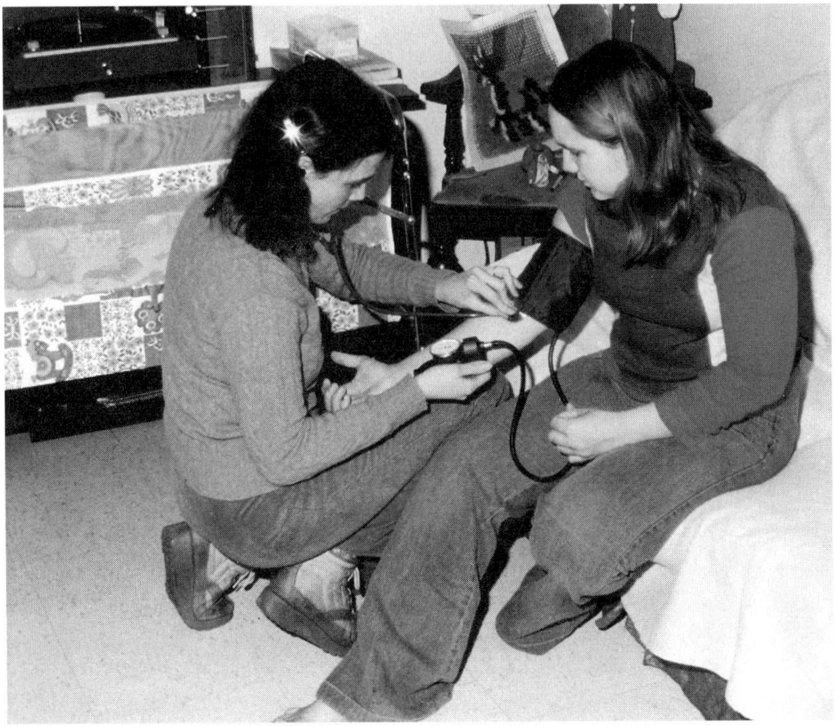

Courtesy Vermont Health Department

Nurse visits new mother and baby.

The late 1970s also witnessed another development in home-based services, that being care of persons with life-limiting illness. The hospice concept, originating in England, began to gain attention in the United States. The Branford, Connecticut, hospice was the first hospice to be organized in the U.S. Volunteer groups, with a growing interest in offering hospice support services, were organized in a number of communities in Vermont. In 1978, the federal government issued a request for proposals for pilot demonstrations of a home-based hospice model, integrating both clinical and volunteer services. Five agencies in northern Vermont, led by the nursing executives, came together to determine whether a joint proposal to the federal government would be feasible (Caledonia Home Health Agency, Orleans/Essex VNA, Lamoille County Home Health Agency, Franklin County Home Health Agency, and the VNA of Chittenden and Grand Isle County). It was an exciting few weeks when we worked hard (dashing through snowstorms to collaborate) to meet the deadline. The application was submitted, and we were selected as one of twenty-seven demonstrations in the country. The demonstrations proved so successful that Congress passed legislation in 1980 to create the Medicare Hospice Benefit. Again, nursing leadership from the VNAs and home health agencies, in partnership with the volunteer organizations, were able to develop collaborative models and extend Medicare hospice benefit services throughout the State of Vermont by the early 1990s.

There was yet another Medicare funding crisis in the 1980s, with increased denials again changing the interpretations of eligibility. Agencies worked together in seeking support to assure services for this very vulnerable population. Once more, we collectively approached the Legislature to seek funding, this time for homemaker services, and once again we were successful. This important program has continued to be state funded through the 1990s. In addition, the National Association for Home Care, with lots of support from most states, initiated a lawsuit against the Health Care Financing Administration and won. The result was that the interpretation of the regulations was once again clarified—and actually liberalized in relation to the eligibility criteria for home care services. This allowed for more care to be reimbursed for persons with long-term, complex chronic conditions.

The 1980s also saw the implementation of the DRG (Diagnostic Related Group) system in hospitals throughout the country, creating pressures to discharge patients sooner from those settings. VNAs and home care agencies responded to the challenge and were able to secure the skilled nursing staff needed to care for persons with more complex problems. This also meant more extensive weekend, evening, and night coverage, to assure 24-hour availability for nursing services 365 days a year. I remember meeting with one group of physicians, seeking their input and feedback regarding our services. One physician immediately responded, saying, "Your nurses are missionaries; it's incredible what they do and what fine care they provide for our patients."

> BARBARA KEOUGH: The Rescue Squad called me due to a patient vomiting profusely of frank blood. They could not start IV's, and the hospital wanted one started. So I escorted the Squad, started the IV and helped with the care of the patient. She survived.[19]

> CHERYL BARNARD: I saw a lady a while ago whose husband died while we were taking care of her, a sudden death. When I had seen them together before, it seemed there was a lot of coolness, but once he died I came to know how much she missed him, how much he meant to her, how important his just being there was to her.
>
> They had no children. She was alone now. Just—the things in the home that he did, now they had to be her things to do. Dealing with

the furnace, everything. I got thinking about my own parents—my father is 90, my mother is going to be 80 in another month.

We got the call, and I went out to her house that afternoon and sat with her for about two hours, didn't talk much, just sat. After a long time, she asked me if I would read the Bible. So I pulled a chair around and I read Psalms to her while she sat in the rocking chair by the window just rocking. I remember the crick of the rocker. Then she reached over and patted my hand.[20]

LINDA CULLEN: I became attached to a woman who was very much a recluse, though her husband had been prominent. She was nearly blind, and so arthritic she could barely move around. I found out about her from the milkman, who made deliveries to a little mudroom on the end of her house. He had noticed things he delivered would be moved but never placed inside the refrigerator. It turns out it was an old refrigerator that hadn't been defrosted in so long that the door had become a huge hunk of ice. She just stacked her cottage cheese and her milk against it. Her son would send a fruit basket once a month and she lived on that and what she could get from the milkman.

She never slept in bed because she couldn't go upstairs so her body had become pretty contracted. But she managed. She had made a pathway of stacked newspapers from her chair out to the dining room through the kitchen to the refrigerator. The edges of the newspapers were worn away; she had calluses on the sides of her feet, where they had rubbed against the papers.

We found a doctor to make housecalls, got a hospital bed in and put it in her living room so she could get into a bed at night. Once she was regulated on meds she was more of a social visit for me. I went to see her every single day and when I wasn't there I made sure somebody else helped her get into bed at night. She would only let maybe five people, volunteers like my daughter, come into her house.

With people like this I don't know if you win them over or if they win you over. It's a mutual thing. You develop relationships with these people; you learn things from them. What she did for me, more than anything, is teach me you do need to depend on people. You can't go through life just being alone. You need some kind of a relationship, to let someone get to know you, a best friend, somebody. I think about that a lot, I think about this woman.

We're always trying to work with the Aides on boundaries. Thanksgiving is coming and somebody doesn't have a tablecloth and they go out and buy one out of their meager wages or they buy them food. I know how that happens; I've been through all of that.[21]

BEV BROCK: We have a lot of back roads in our territory. Snow and mud roads are unreal. Somehow you manage to waddle through it. I carry a

> shovel, just in case of getting stuck, and we carry kitty litter. It's not unusual to have my staff running 75 to 100 plus miles a day.
>
> One of the nurses was showing me around. She handed me directions someone gave us and said to read them, she'd help me find the place. So we're going along: "Turn left, turn right. OK, now it says, go half-way down the road." She looked at me; I looked at her. "Well, that's what it says. I guess we have to go all the way down the road, then come half-way back!"[22]

Other serious challenges in the 1980s began to affect the nation—most significant were HIV disease and social dislocation leading to homelessness of individuals and families. HIV required advanced training of all staff for what was considered a fatal disease. Persons who were homeless often had significant physical, as well as mental, illness. A referral for VNA follow-up might mean visiting a family living in an abandoned car. Nurses were challenged to bring together the community's social support system to help families, as well as to coordinate their health care.

Also during the late 1980s and 1990s, there were growing pressures on nursing homes to reduce utilization in order to reduce state costs in supporting long-term care in that setting. The State of Vermont turned to VNAs and home health agencies to develop more extensive long-term care services, resulting in the development of the Medicaid Waiver Program. While nursing continued to have a lead role in the development of that program, new partnerships were being implemented with the area Agencies on Aging, hospitals, and the Vermont Center for Independent Living, etc. New opportunities for adult day program development and personal care services with nursing supervision were implemented. The challenges to community nursing and expanding career opportunities included case management roles, rehabilitation nursing, coordination of services, and development of partnerships with others to meet the special needs of the population with chronic conditions.

The Visiting Nurse Association of Chittenden and Grand Isle recognized what was ahead of them in 1981:

> There are numerous indicators that point to a growing demand for a stronger, more developed home care system in the '80s and '90s:
>
> - The remarkable increase in the aged population, particularly the over-75 age group that is projected to double in the next 50 years.
> - More efforts to integrate severely disabled persons into the community.
> - Growing public concern to control health care costs and reduce institutional care whether hospital or nursing home.

> - Greater emphasis on choices for families and individuals whether Hospice or long term care.
> - A desire to improve the health status, independent living and quality of life of seniors.
>
> This poses a significant challenge to local planning to take the initiative in building a comprehensive community-based long term care system—a system which includes not only home care, but other services such as sheltered housing, meals, transportation, adult day care, etc.
>
> It also poses a major challenge for creative funding and new organizational linkages between various health and social service providers. With new partnerships and community support, we will be able to respond to the challenge of a rapidly changing environment and meet the expanding home care needs of the people we serve.[23]

The comments of one Burlington quadriplegic illustrate the dependence of the patient and family on home care services:

> My wife has always felt very comfortable allowing VNA staff to enter our home. They have become part of the family as they hear and see practically everything the family is involved in. We have never felt that we had to hide anything from them, as we knew that what went on in our home was always kept in the strictest confidence.
>
> My wife has always been able to use the time during VNA home visits as a time to run errands, go grocery shopping, or do chores that I would normally do, such as going to the garage for car repairs, etc. It gives me a feeling of independence and a better self-image, as I don't feel so dependent on my wife and children. We feel that, because of the VNA, I have been able to live a somewhat normal life without being a burden to the members of my family.[24]

The pressures on hospitals to discharge patients as soon as possible continued through the 1990s. VNAs and home health agencies began to utilize more advanced nurse specialists, especially in the areas of wound therapies, infusion therapies, hospice nurses, care managers, pediatric specialists, psychiatric nurses—but still with the community and nurse generalists as the core of the team. Family health services and maternal child health nursing continued to be developed, as there was growing recognition of the critical phases of early growth and development of children relating to parenting skills. Research began to verify that home visiting by professional nurses was the most effective modality in influencing behavior change in parenting. State initiatives, like Healthy Babies and Success by Six, helped fund more of these services.

> Shortened hospital stays mean patients are arriving home "quicker and sicker." Advances in technology have allowed patients to receive anti-

biotic therapy, intravenous pain control and other high-tech care at home rather than in the hospital. "Equipment has been compacted and made much more mobile," explains Wendy Daley, RN, the high-tech coordinator for Rutland Area VNA.

These advances have shifted many of the daily care responsibilities away from the nurse and onto the home care aide, freeing up the nurse to coordinate the patient's overall care. This includes designing a plan of care in conjunction with the referring physician, supervising the activities of the home care aides, and educating family members on how to care for their loved one.[25]

VNAs and home health agencies throughout the country were once again devastated by draconian changes in Medicare funding resulting from the Balanced Budget Act of 1997. Medicare funding for home care services dropped by an extraordinary 45% over a two-year period, challenging all of us to assure essential services for those persons over sixty-five years of age whose payment by Medicare was denied. Once again the leadership of the VNAs and home care agencies mobilized. They met with members of Congress, organized petitions, promoted letter writing, and joined with the rest of the nation's home care agencies in pursuing amendments to the legislation. We (the State of Vermont VNAs and home health care agencies) even sued the Health Care Financing Administration. And while we didn't win in court, the suit brought national attention to the issue, and Vermont was recognized for its courage at one of the national meetings. The Vermont congressional delegation gave 100% support, and some victories were won providing some relief for the cost-efficient states like Vermont. State and community support helped offset some of the costs of care for patients over sixty-five who were no longer eligible for Medicare reimbursement. Once again, the system of not-for-profit agencies prevailed, ready to take on the next challenge.

The Rutland Visiting Nurse Association recorded in 1996:

One of the constant threads woven throughout the RAVNA history is the tremendous community support the agency has received. From the very first years, community members opened their hearts and wallets for this worthy cause. In a 1967 newspaper article, Dr. Benjamin Cook is quoted as saying "Frederick Chaffee was an angel. Every time we were $100 short, he would come in with a $100 bill."

That generosity is still evident today and ensures that RAVNA will be able to continue providing needed services no matter what changes are made to the Medicare and Medicaid programs.

We are committed to serving our community for many years to come," says Ronald Cioffi, RAVNA Executive Director. "As health care funding continues to be an issue, the demand for cost-effective home care services will continue to grow. Cooperation and collaboration will be the keys to building an integrated system of comprehensive health care for the Rutland region."[26]

David Reynolds, CEO of the Caledonia Home Health Agency, recently told of his experience in accompanying nurses on home visits. He spoke of the warm greeting and welcome the nurses always received, and gave examples of the kind of dedication he observed. One nurse, who had visited a very disabled man in his fifties, became aware of a special hobby/interest. Later, after hours, she took a copy of a magazine she knew would be of interest to him. "They really become like family." On another visit, while driving down a remote, very rough, long driveway with large boulders, the nurse told him that "this 98-year-old woman could be dead." After he expressed alarm, she said, "No, no—that's not a bad thing—she knows and wants it that way—she would never leave her family farm." He was amazed at how the nurse takes all this in stride and with compassion.[27]

The determination, the energy, the commitment, the perseverance, and the skill of nursing leadership throughout this period has made home care and hospice services throughout the State of Vermont one of the strongest in the nation. It was the values of those early town nurses and visiting nurses that were the seeds for growth of a system of care that has made all the difference in the lives of patients and families in our Vermont communities. It is that heart and skill, that art and science that they practiced, that I know is now and will continue to be the core of community nursing in the future.

Again, in the voice of a grateful family member:

> This is written on behalf of my brother and sisters and myself in appreciation of services provided for our mother by two of your nurses . . . Both women extended professional care of the highest standard . . . Beyond their medical attentions, they have provided sensitive assessments that are critical to our mother's emotional and psychological well being . . . Their insights have been very valuable in guiding us in a manner that will best serve our mother's recovery. The fact that they have been willing to initiate conversations to enlighten us, and then to spend time consulting with us, is a valuable and commendable feature of their true commitments to healing.
>
> Surely it is without doubt that medicine can produce amazing results for our bodies. However these two nurses have thoughtfully and caringly initiated a healing process of a more difficult nature. For them to care enough to pursue and guide us for our mother's sake is something we cannot ignore. We are grateful to you for providing staff of this quality. Medicine may treat the body. Only people with compassion can treat the spirit.[28]

—Elizabeth J. Davis, RN, MPH

NOTES

1. Beatrice Siegel, *Lillian Wald, Henry Street* (Macmillan, 1983).
2. Ibid.
3. Central Vermont Home Health Agency, "The History of CVHHA, Inc.," 75th Anniversary Brochure, 1986. CVHHA, Inc. office, Berlin, Vermont.
4. Lucille Waldo, interview by Nancy Serrell Coonley, "Mud Roads, Bed Baths, and Geese: An Oral History of Home Nursing in Rural New England," (masters's thesis, The University of Vermont, Burlington, April 2000), 1.
5. Martha Lussier, interview in Coonley, 3.
6. "History of Bennington Home Health Agency," courtesy of Julia Maroney, executive director.
7. Angela Johnson, interview in Coonley, 9.
8. Sheila Aubin, interview in Coonley, 10.
9. Angela Johnson, interview in Coonley, 10.
10. Frances Field, interview in Coonley, 6.
11. Sally Munro, interview in Coonley, 6.
12. Pat Harford, interview in Coonley, 7.
13. Martha Lussier, interview in Coonley, 7.
14. Health Care Financing Administration, "Trends in the Utilization of Certified Home Health Agency Services," HCFA reports of 1976 through 1995. U.S. Government Printing Office.
15. *Burlington (Vermont) Free Press*, 4 October 1974.
16. Linda Cullen, interview in Coonley, 12.
17. Martha Lussier, interview in Coonley, 12.
18. *Newport (Vermont) Daily Express*, 15 February 1979.
19. Barbara Keough, interview by author, May 2000.
20. Cheryl Barnard, interview in Coonley, 21.
21. Linda Cullen, interview in Coonley, 22.
22. Bev Brock, interview in Coonley, 13.
23. Visiting Nurse Association of Chittenden and Grand Isle, Annual Report, 1981.
24. Visiting Nurse Association, Burlington, Vermont, Special Edition, 1985.
25. *Rutland (Vermont) Herald.*
26. Visiting Nurse Association of Rutland, Annual Report, 1996.
27. David Reynolds, interview by author, May 2000.
28. Visiting Nurse Alliance of Vermont and New Hampshire, letter from patient, 1999.

Vermont Nurses in the Military: Harbingers of Peace, Care, and Humanity during Wartime

I SAT MESMERIZED by the remarks by General Colin L. Powell, Chairman of the Joint Chiefs of Staff, at the groundbreaking ceremony on July 29, 1993, for the Vietnam Women's Memorial in Washington, D.C.

> When this monument is finished, it will be for all time a testament to a group of American women who made an extraordinary sacrifice at an extraordinary time in our nation's history: the women who went to war in Vietnam. . . . I realized for the first time that for male soldiers, the war came in intermittent flashes of terror, occasional death, moments of pain; but for the women who were there, for the women who helped before the battle, and for the nurses in particular, the terror, the death, and the pain were unrelenting, a constant terrible weight that had to be stoically carried. It was a pain that had to be stowed away in a corner of your mind and put in an isolated piece of your heart or you wouldn't be able to continue your work. The nurses saw the bleakest, most terrifying face of war: the mangled men, the endless sobs of wounded kids . . . not just now and then, but day after day, night after hellish night. . . . It's to wonder at the strength you had to press on, the courage you had to fight to save yet another life, the fortitude to risk your feelings and compassion on yet another wounded soul that might spurn you by dying. It's to feel the invisible wound that you received every time that happened . . . And yet I see that yours is not a story only of loss and tragedy. It is, as well, a story of inspiration. It's a story of the triumph of the human spirit. I look into your eyes today; and I see there old pain, yes, but also great wisdom, tempered courage, deep wells of character. I find there the ability to clear the highest hurdles that life can put before any human being, the ability to take on the most terrible truths, and to prevail. . . . This monument will ensure that all of America will never forget that all of you were there, that you served, and that even in the depths of horror and cruelty, there will always beat the heart of human love . . . and therefore our hope for humanity.[1]

After listening to General Powell and to the celebration of patriotism and courage of nurses in the military, I felt proud—proud of my own twenty-seven years of service with the Navy Nurse Corps, United States Naval Reserve (USNR), and proud of being involved (during my annual two weeks of active duty) in the planning for the dedication ceremony of the Vietnam Women's Memorial which occurred on November 1993. The bronze statue, an exquisite work of art by sculptor Glenda Goodacre, celebrates the hope and strength, the tenderness and power, the kindness and passion that women in the military brought to the struggle for life. The statue shows three women and a wounded GI, touching each other, giving strength to one another, struggling with mortality, with human emotions, compassion, dedication, and with the pain and exhaustion of both their lives and their spirits. It is within this context of celebration of women's patriotism and courage within the military that the contributions of Vermont nurses are highlighted from World War II to 1996. As will be seen from their stories, Vermont nurses were harbingers of peace, care, and humanity, even during the darkness of war.

World War II

As the nation entered World War II, figures indicated that the state-accredited schools of nursing had admitted 41,397 for the 1940–41 academic year, approximately 5,000 short of the estimated need.[2] During the early years, nurses were often in a quandary as to whether they should stay in civilian positions or join one of the military nursing services.[3] Nurses who were single and under forty were encouraged to join the service, whereas a nurse that was an administrator, instructor, or in public health was encouraged to remain in his/her civilian position. The National Council for War Service was created to coordinate war nursing programs of voluntary and official agencies, Red Cross, army, and navy.

Nurses who joined the military early in the war received few benefits. Relative rank was bestowed upon nurses, which meant an officer's title and uniform without an officer's commission, retirement privileges, dependent's allowance, or pay. Not until June 22, 1944, did Congress enact a law providing members of the Army and Navy Nurse Corps with temporary officer's rank.

Nurses served in North Africa, Tunisia, England, France, Germany, and Italy in evacuation hospitals, which were intermediate links between the battlefield and the general hospitals in the United States. They also served in the Pacific theatre of war and in Hawaii after the bombing of Pearl Harbor. In 1942, a flight nursing school was created. Flight nursing consisted of a variety of duties in connection with the evacuation of the sick, wounded, and injured. Both the Army Air Corps and the navy utilized flight nurses to transport and treat patients.

As the war raged on, there was increasing competition for woman power in all segments of the workforce; nursing schools had great difficulties in attracting an adequate number of student nurses. To deal with this crisis, the Federal Security Agency arranged a series of conferences attended by representatives of major professional nursing and hospital associations, to explore possible solutions to the nursing shortage. The outcome of these conferences was a bill introduced into the House of Representatives by Frances Payne Bolton, a congresswoman from Ohio, that created the United States Cadet Nurse Corps. This bill became law on June 15, 1943. Under the Bolton Act, the U.S. Public Health Service subsidized the entire education of students. To receive these funds, the student had to promise to do nursing in either military or civilian arenas for the duration of the war. Candidates had to be between seventeen and thirty-five years old, with admission requirements, in good physical condition, and have a good scholastic record from high school. They submitted their credentials to the Red Cross, which categorized them as the first reserve, and therefore their credentials would be passed on to the army or navy. A senior cadet or graduate could be classified as the second reserve, which meant because of age, marital status, or physical condition, they were ineligible for the military service.

Enrollment quotas were established for the Cadet Nurse Corps: 125,000 for the first two years of the program. As of March 1945, 87% of all nursing students were in the Cadet Nurse Corps, with most patient care being given by students. Forty percent of senior cadets volunteered for service.[4] The quota for Vermont during the period July 1, 1943, to July 1, 1944, was 299 nurses. Vermont actually exceeded this quota by admitting 308 nurses into the service in this period. There were 335 graduate nurses in all assigned to the Army and Navy Nurse Corps since December 1942.[5] Quotas were exceeded in Vermont and nationally, establishing the Corps as the most successful nurse recruitment program of the war.[6] The major source of replacements for nurses from 1945 on were the senior cadets in the Cadet Nurse Corps.

During World War II, there were 75,029 U.S. nurses serving in the armed forces—12,239 in the navy and 62,790 in the army. Twenty percent had some college education, either before or after their nursing education. Almost ninety percent had received their nursing education after 1931, with a much larger percentage of younger nurses serving in the navy.[7] With the last Allied offensive in Europe in November 1944, American troops suffered their heaviest casualties—over 1,750 per day—and the need for nurses became acute. At the same time, a very serious shortage of both professional and nonprofessional nursing personnel in civilian hospitals coincided with a large demand for hospital care. This shortage

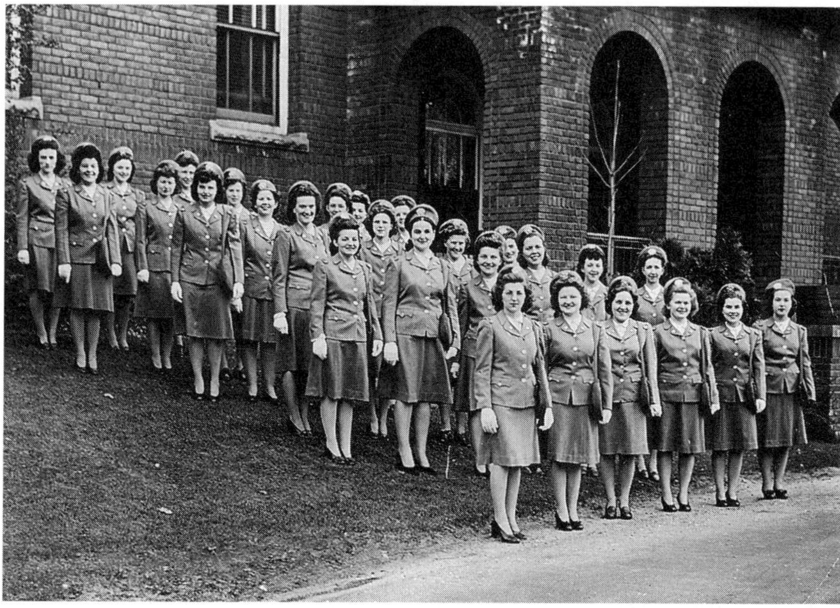

Courtesy Central Vermont Medical Center

Barre City Hospital members of the U.S. Cadet Nurse Corps, 1944.

resulted from the loss of 65,000 registered nurses in the civilian sectors to the army and navy. In an attempt to fill this gap, student nurses carried about eighty percent of the work of the 1,300 hospital-affiliated schools of nursing.[8]

Each state, including Vermont, established a branch of the Council on War Service to coordinate all activities that related to meeting nursing needs in the State in war time. The first chair of Vermont's State War Nursing Council was Miss Constance Galaise, later followed by Mrs. Hortense Harwood. The objectives of the state council were to aid the Red Cross in meeting military nursing needs; recruit student nurses; obtain and maintain a complete roster of all graduate registered nurses; to bring inactive nurses back to active practice; to relocate nurses from areas of oversupply to those of inadequate supply; to assure maximum utilization of nurses for professional duties only; and to bring about those necessary adjustments by nurses, employers, doctors, and the public, thus caring for civilian needs.[9]

On January 6, 1945, President Roosevelt requested a draft of women nurses in his State of the Union address. A bill quickly passed the House of Representatives, but got bogged down in the Senate. A letter was sent by Mrs. Abbie Starkey, RN, executive secretary of the Vermont State Nurses' Association, to Vermont Senators Warren Austin and George

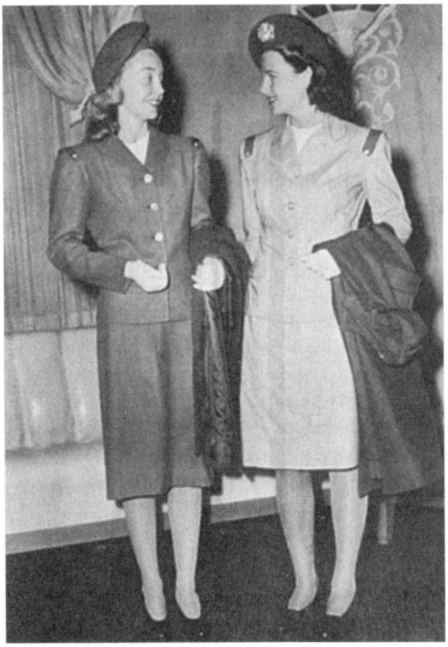

Uniform of the Cadet Nurse Corp
Reprinted from Vermont State Nurses' Association, *Fifty Years of Progress: Past/ Prospective* (Burlington, Vt.: VSNA, 1964).

Aiken as well as Congressman Plumley, concerning the bill as proposed and suggesting needed changes. These proposed changes were forwarded to the U.S. Committee on Military Affairs. The letter proposed that Vermont be given credit for those nurses already in service, otherwise additional quotas would lead to a severe shortage in Vermont. This was especially important because 70% of nurses in Vermont were married, leaving few available for future service. She also suggested that credit to states for voluntary recruitments should be given, and that there should be specific provisions against discrimination with respect to race, color, creed, and sex. Finally, the bill should not include preliminary draft of graduates of the U.S. Cadet Nurse Corps, as this would constitute a breach of faith with the Cadet Nurse Corps. The draft bill never came to fruition. Stimulated by the threat of the draft, the nursing profession responded with an overwhelming number of applications for commissions—10,000 during the three-week period of January 8–29, 1945. Also, sixty percent of the senior cadets chose the army instead of civilian employment. These efforts were so successful that efforts to pass the draft legislation ceased, and there were actually too many nurses that had joined the services.

The war ended with the dropping of the bomb over Hiroshima. By this time, about 29 percent of all active nurses were on duty with the armed services. 179,000 student nurses who joined the Cadet Nurse Corps had increased the enrollment in the schools of nursing since 1943 by thirty percent. In Vermont, there was a larger increase in student nurses who joined the Cadet Nurse Corps. There were seven accredited schools of nursing that enrolled cadet nursing students. These included Mary Fletcher Hospital and Bishop DeGoesbriand Hospital in Burlington, Fanny Allen Hospital in Winooski, Heaton Hospital in Montpelier, and Barre City, Rutland, and St. Albans Hospitals. Two other accredited schools of nursing, Gifford Memorial Hospital in Gifford and Brightlook Hospital in St. Johnsbury were not cadet-designated schools. In October

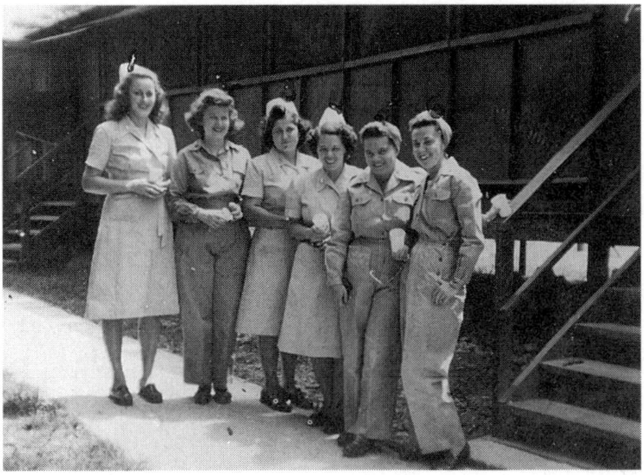

Second Lieutenant Lorraine Nelson, ANC (*second from left*) with "the gang in 7C," nurses' quarters, Fourth General Hospital, Manila, Phillipine Islands, April 1946.

1943, 127 of the 501 students enrolled in Vermont schools of nursing were cadet students. By March 1945, there were 414 cadet students out of 560 nursing students within Vermont schools of nursing.[10] The Cadet Nurse Corps stopped accepting applications after October 1945, and the program was terminated in 1948. Nursing's contribution to the war effort was unquestionable. More than sixteen million Americans served in the armed services. There were 292,131 killed and over 671,000 wounded; 96 of every 100 wounded were saved because of nursing care, effective first aid treatment, and early evacuation from the battlefield.[11]

There were many Vermonters who were recognized for their service. LT Eleanor Conti, Army Nurse Corps, from Barre, was attached to the Third Army in France, Belgium, Luxembourg, and Germany. She received a Bronze Star for meritorious service in connection with military operations from June 1, 1944, to May 7, 1945. She served as an assistant principal chief nurse, 109th Evacuation Hospital. Her citation stated that she "distinguished herself by her outstanding duty. The professional skill and resourcefulness she displayed, her untiring energy and loyal devotion to duty reflect great credit upon herself and the military service."[12] She was the only woman in the service from this area to receive a Bronze Star.

A Waterbury native, Second Lieutenant Lorraine Nelson, Army Nurse Corps, was a 1941 graduate of the Mary Fletcher Hospital School of Nursing. She served with the Fourth General Hospital in Manila, Philippine Islands. Describing her time in Manila, "she took quinine daily for prevention of malaria and salt tablets but soon stopped taking the antimalarial pills because it made her eyes yellow. She loved the Philippine people." The food left something to be desired: "They were served eggplant three times/day, breakfast, lunch, and dinner every day. It was the only vegetable served. . . .Wait until I tell you about the bread . . . buggy bread . . . they had to pick the bugs out of the slices of bread but it was better than the eggplant. The bugs infested the bin where the flour was stored. Protein was dried eggs—they didn't dare eat the meat . . . they ate dogs over there." Describing the hospital in Manila in which she worked, "there were huge rooms with seventy patients in a ward. "Ward boys" (U.S. Army personnel) would fill the syringes with penicillin; syringes were 50cc; nurses administered the drug (penicillin) three times/day by simply changing the needle as they moved from patient to patient with the 50cc syringe. The needles were removed and soaked in a basin of alcohol and reused." She worked twelve hours/day and six days/week. When describing how her service time affected her work life post-war, LT Nelson shared that she "had to learn all over; she was not allowed to do many of the nursing/medical activities that nurses must do in wartime."[13] Upon her return in 1946, she worked at Middlebury Hospital and did private duty in homes. In 1948, she married Arnold Clark,* whom she met before going into the service. They both went away to war—she to the Philippines and he to the European theatre. After the war, LT Nelson received a translation of a letter from a Japanese POW (prisoner of war) for whom she cared at the hospital in 1946. His letter recognizes the kindness and care of LT Nelson, as well as other American army personnel.

> Sound of music, chatters of people came in my ears faintly and pains in leg was coming back to my nerves and becoming severe and severe as time went on. And I came to be conscious at last. Looking to both sides of my bed, I saw many American soldiers in the big room of the ward and also several civilians among them and I felt it very strange to find myself there, the only POW in this room. An American nurse gives me injections at short intervals, and makes close watch to me, seeing my blood pressure, temperature and pulse in every other hour. She treats me kindly and carefully as if I were an American soldier. With a smiling face, she washes my back with soap and alcohol. No difference at all between food I eat and that Americans eat. No lack of any kind of things that I use daily. . . . I have been deeply impressed by kindness of the hospital personnel. I have been on bed and nothing I have done in this one month, and still I am treated and taken care very well. How could I say thanks for that?[14]

Another nurse, LT Christine Bostwick, from Bristol, graduated from Mary Fletcher Hospital School of Nursing in 1943. She served with the Army Nurse Corps during the last two years of the war. She first landed in

---

* Lorraine Nelson Clark now resides in Montpelier, Vermont.

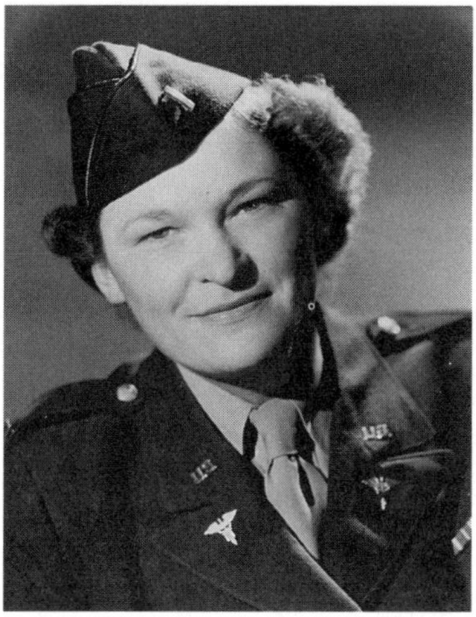

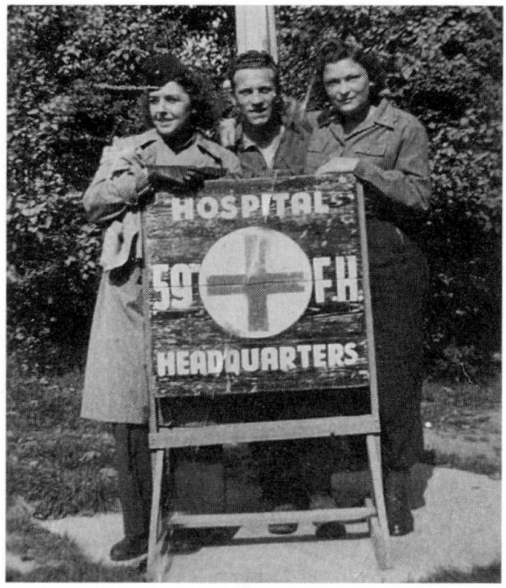

First Lieutenant Christine Bostwick, nurse veteran of World War II. *Left*, photo taken in France during the war. *At far right*, with co-workers at a field hospital in Germany during World War II.

Scotland, then went to England, where she was stationed in a hospital that was set up in small cabins. It was here that she first experienced blackouts. "With the D-Day invasion, the first casualties arrived in England in many ambulances. The ones sent to England were badly hurt, many belly wounds as well as shrapnel wounds. Patients with chest wounds didn't make it many times. We had plasma but little blood."[15]

She then left England soon after for France. She was soon transferred to an evacuation hospital, and ultimately to the 59th Field Hospital. Field hospitals were often set up in tents, school houses, or bombed out buildings. When she slept in tents, LT Bostwick put her clothes in a bedroll so they wouldn't get cold and damp. Field hospitals moved with the troops (contrary to Korea or Vietnam) and at one point, she moved every seven days during Patton's push through Europe. There were few luxuries in the field. "The tents weren't very warm, but we had little potbellied stoves in the middle. That heat didn't go very far." There was a large table for supplies. To wash their hair, the nurses dug a hole in the ground and put a helmet full of water in it so they could wash in warm water.

One of LT Bostwick's saddest experiences came soon after the Normandy Beach landing. "We had mail call, that was a big event. The GI who was mail clerk said, 'you must be a pretty popular girl,' because he saw all the letters." LT Bostwick got all her twin brother's letters back—they all had KIA (killed in action) stamped on them. That's how she found out her brother had been killed. "I was treating German prisoners at the time, even after my brother was killed. I know they were enemies, but to me they were patients." When the chief nurse asked her if she wanted to be moved, she refused. She obtained permission from her commanding officer to take a Jeep and to visit her brother's grave in France. "His dog tags were nailed in the middle of the cross. There were so many crosses. He was later sent home to Hinesburg and buried there."

When the war was over, "We were sent to . . . a concentration camp on the Austrian-Czech border (Mauthausen) to take care of the people who had seen atrocities. They were mostly Polish Jews, very emaciated. They had a mass funeral every morning for those who died in the night. Many had tuberculosis. That was very difficult." People at the camp were fed dried vegetables and bread twice a day. "That was all that was available. They ate our garbage—whatever we didn't eat. It was clean and they came and got it every day. It was unbelievable."

"I kept track of the names of those who died in my block. You expect war casualties but dealing in the concentration camps—it was impossible what human beings could do to others. One of the German officers had a twelve year old son who would have target practice on prisoners. I later got letters from kids who were displaced persons sent by the Russians to Ireland."

On her trip home in 1946, LT Bostwick became quite seasick. "About halfway across, they served Vermont turkey, but I couldn't even eat a saltine . . . I cried when I saw the Statue of Liberty. It was an awful good sight. We saw some terrible sights over there. Coming home was one of the best things." The transition from the war to home was difficult because "we were so over stimulated by the war. I didn't have a lot of patience with complaints about the lack of gas at home. Homes here weren't being bombed." Upon returning home, Bostwick did private duty in California, then returned home and got married. Her husband was called back into service during the Korean War and she worked in Chicago, where many of the railroad workers required lung and chest surgery.*

Korean War

On June 25, 1950, a short five years after the end of World War II, the Korean War broke out. At the beginning of the conflict, the total strength of the Army Nurse Corps was below 3,500 and the Navy Nurse Corps was below 2,000.[16] There was a relatively small number of active reservists upon which to draw.

---

* Gussie Bostwick Levarn retired from nursing at age 62. She now lives in Bristol, Vermont, where she has been active in the American Legion, the Middlebury VFW, and with hobbies such as carving apple dolls and making paper maché floats for the Bristol July 4th parade.

Aware that the civilian and military needs required cooperative planning, the Joint Committee on Nursing in National Security (American Nurses' Association, American Association of Industrial Nurses, Association of Collegiate Schools of Nursing, National Association of Colored Graduate Nurses, National League of Nursing Education, and National Organization for Public Health Nursing) recommended 1) the immediate recruitment of more students for schools of nursing, 2) calling back to active duty as many as possible of the 205,517 inactive professional nurses in the country, 3) increased training and employment of practical nurses, 4) systematic withdrawal of nurses from civilian services for military duty, 5) organizing state and local advisory boards of nurses and distribution of nurses and allied workers to assure that essential needs are met, 6) improvement of the nation's basic nursing education resources, 7) preparation of the necessary supervisory and administrative personnel to meet stepped-up educational and service requirements, and 8) stabilization of nursing service through sound personnel policies. The committee report also called for securing the active cooperation of physicians, hospitals, public health authorities, and the general public in rationing nursing service and according equal recognition to civilian and armed forces nurses.[17]

In compliance with the Joint Committee's recommendations, the Vermont State Nurses' Association established the Committee on Nursing Resources to Meet Civil and Military Nursing Needs, chaired by Constance E. Galaise. The functions of this committee were to:

1. secure cooperation in meeting civil and military nursing needs, through letters to directors of nursing service to ascertain the number of nurses on staff now in reserve with the Army Nurse Corps, Navy Nurse Corps, or Air Force, and the number of nurses needed to maintain essential hospital, public health, industrial nursing service and educational programs in schools of nursing; identification of replacements for each member of the staff in the event that they are called for military service; letters to professional registries to ascertain number of private duty nurses needed for essential services to hospitals and homes, numbers of nurses on reserve; and letters to schools of nursing to ascertain status of enrollment, present faculty positions;
2. build rosters of nurses in the state to meet civil and military needs;
3. maintain liaison with state directors of selective service in the event of a draft; and
4. prepare lists of private duty nurses who would be willing to serve other communities and would be interested in civil defense planning.[18]

The Vermont State Nurses' Association, through its newsletter, the *Vermont Registered Nurse*, asked members to think seriously on the question of national registration for selective service in 1951, although most state nurses' associations were not in favor of the selective service at the time.

Despite the fears of another acute nursing shortage like the one during World War II, there was a limited buildup during the Korean War—2,000 nurses volunteered or were recalled to the Army Nurse Corps. The Army Nurse Corps reached an end strength of 5,500, although only 10% received assignments in Korea.[19] Likewise, the end strength for the Navy Nurse Corps reached 3,238 (from 1,950 active duty officers). The Navy Nurse Corps officers were assigned to 26 naval hospitals and dispensaries, three hospital corps schools, three hospital ships (*Consolation*, *Repose*, *Haven*), and eight Military Sea Transport Service ships. In addition, one year prior to the Korean War, 1,199 army nurses had been transferred from the army to the new Department of the Air Force. By the start of the war, there were an additional 200 air force nurses actively engaged in the air evacuation of patients.[20]

At the beginning of the Korean War, a list of quotas for each state was distributed by the Army Nurse Corps based on the nurse population of each state. Vermont's quota for the Army Nurse Corps was 15 nurses, 11 general duty, 1 nurse anesthetist, 2 operating room nurses, and 1 psychiatric nurse. The quota was not filled for the state. Although information is scarce, there appear to have been approximately ten Vermont nurses who served in the Army and Navy Nurse Corps.

The experience of World War II demonstrated that early treatment and evacuation of the wounded significantly decreased fatalities. Despite the rugged terrain and extreme weather conditions of Korea, fatality rates were kept surprisingly low (about half that of World War II) with the advent of the Mobile Army Surgical Hospitals (MASH). These mobile hospitals provided the expert care of physicians, nurses, and technicians only 8 to 12 miles from the front lines. Most of the MASH unit was set up in tents, with patients first being admitted to a receiving ward where they were triaged, assessed, and treatment was begun. Treatment included the administration of blood, oxygen, preoperative preparation, and general support. MASH units contained fifteen medical officers specializing in general surgery, thoracic and orthopedic surgery, internal medicine, and anesthesiology. They also contained sixteen nursing officers, five nurses each for the preoperative and postoperative wards, four for the operating room, and two nurse anesthetists. This staff was supplemented by about 120 enlisted personnel to perform the supportive functions of the unit.[21] Attached to the MASH units was an army helicopter detachment that provided immediate evacuation for critically injured battle casualties or ill medical patients. If air evacuation could not be accomplished because of conditions, patients were brought to the hospital from the battalion aid stations via ambulances.

Air evacuation of the wounded from the battlefield to military hospitals in Japan was accomplished by the Military Air Transport Service. Nurses helped to save many lives by supplying prompt medical attention as well as advising pilots of the cruising altitudes suited to the individual medical needs of the patients. As more countries joined in the conflict, nurses used an informal sign language to communicate, although there were often some people on board who could help in the interpretation of language. Gradually a systematic air evacuation system evolved. Wounded men whose total hospitalization would require thirty days or less with return to duty were sent to Southern Korea. Those expected to be hospitalized for six months or less were taken by C-54 aircraft to Japan, and then later returned to Korea. Patients whose recovery would take greater than six months were airlifted back to the United States by the Military Air Transport Service to clear the hospitals in Japan for other wounded.[22] With the air evacuation methods during the Korean War, the hospital ship was rarely used for evacuation of the wounded. The Naval hospital ships off the Korean coast were used as mainly floating hospitals and were assigned to transport patients only en route to Japan for overhaul.[23] Two years of negotiations, during which the fighting continued, ended with an armistice agreement in July 1953. American losses during the three-year period totaled 142,091, of whom 33,629 were killed, 103,284 were wounded, and 5,178 were missing or captured.[24]

The following Vermont nurses served in the Army and Navy Nurse Corps during the Korean War:[25] First Lieutenant Bertha Ahern, First Lieutenant Ruth Reynolds, and Second Lieutenant Irene Moyse. Second Lieutenant Beverly Holt, from Gilman, worked stateside at Brooke Army Medical Center at Ft. Sam Houston, Texas. First Lieutenant Helen Gover, from Barre, served with the medical replacement training center also at Brooke Army Medical Center. She was the assistant chief of the hospital procedures training area for one of the Army's basic training schools for medical enlisted men. Second Lieutenant Hilda Winner, from St. Albans, worked at Camp Chaffee, Arkansas. Maj. Katharine Johnson, from Brandon, was chief nurse at the 128th Station Hospital at Zama and then became chief nurse at Sasebo. First Lieutenant Josephine Farmer, from Waterbury, was assigned to the 343rd General Hospital in Koizumi, Japan, and provided extensive medical care for UN casualties from the war. First Lieutenant Elizabeth Scheider, of Island Pond, joined the Army Nurse Corps in World War II, served in the South Pacific, and returned from overseas to accept a recruiting assignment of nurses. She traveled across the state speaking about the importance of serving our country and cutting through the red tape that discouraged nurses from joining the service. Another army nurse who entered the service during World War II was Capt. Rita Cleveland of Huntington Center. She graduated from Mary Fletcher School of Nursing in 1942 and entered the Army in 1943. During World War II she served in France, England, and Belgium until the war ended. She was discharged, and then attended The University of Vermont, receiving her BS in nursing education in 1950. She reentered the army during the Korean War, served with the 45th Hospital Mobile Army in Korea, and assisted with returning Korean POWs in Operation Little Switch. She was chief nurse at Brooke General Hospital, Ft. Sam Houston in Texas, at Irwin Army Hospital at Ft. Riley in Kansas, and with the 319th Station Hospital in Bussac, France. She received her master's degree in hospital administration from Baylor University and received two awards of the Army Commendation Medal.

Three Vermonters served in the air force as flight nurses. They were all Mary Fletcher Hospital graduates: Edith Griffith and Sylvia Drinkwine, who served at Sheppard Air Force Base in Texas, and Queenit Bird, who was assigned to Keeler Air Force Base in Mississippi. There were also three Vermonters who served in the Navy Nurse Corps. Ensign Betty Barr, from Sheldon Springs, joined in 1951 and served at the U.S. Naval Base, Newport, Rhode Island. LT Barbara Sumner, from St. Johnsbury, graduated from Bishop DeGoesbriand School of Nursing, and served in Korea. Lt.j.g. Elsie Lovely, from Waterbury, graduated from Gifford Hospital School of Nursing, and also served with the navy in the Korean War zone. She served on one of the navy hospital ships, USS *Haven*, arrived in Korea in September 1950, and was stationed at Inchon Harbor until she was transferred to Pusan.

Finally, excerpts from a letter written by LT Gertrude Clinton, who was stationed with the army in New Caledonia:

> On my birthday, we packed up and left the town we were in. We are now living in tents in the woods. The ride was a long one in trucks, and took us all day to reach our destination. We never had such a dusty, jolty ride in our lives. Each truck was furnished with cheese and ham sandwiches and each of us carried a canteen of water. The advance detail had gone ahead two days previous to set up the camp and as it was after dark when we arrived, it was a most welcome sight to see the campfire burning and smell coffee waiting for us.
>
> We enjoyed the ride in spite of being bumped through the ruts as we had an opportunity of seeing what the interior of the island looked like. We came through a pass where the road was so narrow that the truck barely made it. On one side was a sheer drop of about a half a mile. Some of the girls closed their eyes and wouldn't look until we had gotten

through. To me it was a beautiful sight and I didn't miss a thing. The horseshoe bend on the Mohawk trail had nothing on the curves we made. The trucks up above were waving to the ones below—cutting circles like a skater on ice. We passed native villages with thatched roof huts and the natives stood at attention as we whisked by. At the end of the trip we lost the road as it was quite a wilderness and darkness falling. But while waiting for the reconnaissance we were rewarded by unexpected entertainment. Off the road were some native huts and the natives started a real savage dance that was blood-curdling. They pounded on drums and when the searchlights were turned on them, we could see them dancing to the rhythm, working themselves into a frenzy. At the climax they let out a terrific yell and threw knives into the air. It was blood-thirsty to us who had never seen a real savage dance or heard a tom-tom.

The natives on this island have been civilized less than 100 years and were cannibals then. The ones we come in contact with are very childlike and are pleased with a kind word or a smile. They have taken a great liking to the Americans, probably because of the generosity that is characteristic of the boys. The French, who have had control of the island, and the blacks were hard task masters. Even the Tonkinese and Javanese who have come here under contract and work for the French government are partial to us. Their pay is 100 francs a month, which to us would mean starvation.

Our camp, when we arrived, was a mere skeleton, but it now has developed into a canvas village. The nurses and officers tents are set apart from the enlisted men's and the hospital area is a quarter mile away. Roads and paths have been worn through the woods because of the constant traffic of many feet and trucks.

It is now winter but the weather is similar to a Vermont fall. The days are sunshiny and beautiful but the nights are cold and damp. Bright colored parrots fly among the trees and the mountains rise up in purple hues on every side. It may be our imagination but the moon seems much brighter on this side of the world. While I was on night duty it was a delight to watch the morning star appear each morning. It is as bright in reality as the Star of Bethlehem has been pictured. Of course the days are not all sunshine. When the rain comes it gives no warning and when it is over our camp has been converted into a mud hole. We don't mind the weather, as we dress like the men. In fact, I'm afraid we'll have trouble fitting ourselves into civilization when this war is over. We are always hungry due to the fact that we are constantly in the fresh air. We've forgotten what a hot bath is like and the privacy and convenience of a flush toilet is a thing of the past. There is a creek close by where we bathe and wash our clothes. After the unsanitary conditions of the town we left, this is heaven in comparison.

We have no form of entertainment except what we make ourselves. We enjoy ourselves in small ways such as group singing, bridge and letter writing. We have no books to speak of and I miss them very much. I

> think my greatest enjoyment is working in the wards. The boys are jolly even when sick and only occasionally are their spirits low. They are respectful and good and I love them all. Our only hardships so far are mosquitoes, bugs and occasional low spirits when monotony and lonesomeness settle over us like a night of fog. We all feel it at times and is then that even an air raid would be almost welcome to break the spell. We have all wondered just how we would react under those circumstances and one night we had occasion to know. We didn't have a raid but just the scare of one and were informed we would have to be on the alert in the early morning. It seemed as if everyone else was excited and wakeful but I decided I'd better get some sleep beforehand so went to bed and never slept any better.
>
> I am writing this letter by the light of a kerosene lamp, using a foot locker as a table. I would enjoy a lot to hear from anyone in Brattleboro interested in writing. The distribution of mail is still the saddest and happiest day in the area.
>
> The vitamins you mentioned will be very welcome when they arrive. We are sadly lacking in them. Anything else you may send will be appreciated you may be sure and all packages are more or less common property. What is best of all is just a letter to say you remember and think of us who are away from family and friends. We have proved to ourselves that we can live a simple life and do without the luxuries but what none of us can do without is kindness and sympathy and love. It would be a desolate day indeed should we lose this war for that is what it would mean for us all. We won't lose for the courage of the boys is a grand thing to see.[26]

Vietnam War

Although the American interest in Southeast Asia began in the 1950s, it was not until the early 1960s that American military nurses arrived in Vietnam, along with increasing numbers of American military advisors. In 1960, North Vietnam announced the formation of the Viet Cong of the National Liberation Front, and increased terrorism in South Vietnam became increasingly evident. Thirteen army nurses were sent to the Eighth Field Hospital in Nha Trang in 1962, and the first Navy Nurse Corps officers were assigned to the Station Hospital in Saigon.[27]

Nurse recruitment was not an easy task at this time because of a chronic short supply of professional nurses. The military again had to compete with the civilian sector. The army and navy established incentive recruitment programs; the Army Student Nurse Program and the Navy Nurse Candidate Program. Student nurses received financial aid and in return served for a minimum of two years for a diploma in nursing, or three years for a bachelor's degree. Students could remain at their civilian schools until finishing their course of study, which then qualified them to take the state licensure examination. Four to six months prior to the completion of their programs, students were commissioned directly into the Reserve components of the respective military service. Once notified of licensure, they were sent on active duty. Despite the incentives, the strength of the Army Nurse Corps numbers declined. In addition to the competition from the civilian sector, there was increased specialization, demand for health services, increased civilian pay and benefits, and development of new practice areas during this time that made recruitment difficult.[28] With congressional funding, the U.S. Department of Defense approved the establishment of its own nursing school, Walter Reed Army Institute of Nursing, to increase the number of army nurses with a bachelor's degree in nursing.

The first large contingent of air force nurses was sent to Vietnam in February 1966, to the Twelfth Air Force Hospital, Cam Ranh Bay. The numbers of army nurses increased from 200 in June 1966 to more than 600 in 1967, and 900 in January 1969. As the war raged on, by April, 1966 more Americans were being killed in action (approximately 4,400) than the South Vietnamese. American nurses were not spared from these casualties with eight deaths by the end of the war. Four American navy nurses were wounded in the Viet Cong attack on the Brink Bachelor Officer's Quarters, becoming the first nurses to receive purple hearts in the Vietnam War. Hospitals from the northern highlands of Pleiku to the delta town of Vung Tau were always under threat of attack. Several, such as the 45th Surgical Hospital at Tay Ninh, the Third Field Hospital in Saigon, and the 12th Evacuation Hospital at Chu Chi, were hit one or more times.[29] Navy Nurse Corps officers were also assigned to the navy hospital in Danang, which had become the largest combat casualty treatment center in the world, comprising 600 beds and eventually treating over 70,000 patients.[30]

Two naval hospital ships, USS *Repose* and USS *Sanctuary*, also provided direct medical support, the *Repose* arriving in February 1966, and the *Sanctuary* arriving a little later in April 1967. Thirty naval nurses staffed each ship, along with naval medical corpsmen and physicians. These ships were floating modern hospitals with the most up-to-date equipment, and provided more flexibility and versatility in meeting the medical needs of the armed forces than fixed facilities.

Given the increasing demands for nurses, the number of casualties, and the difficulty in recruitment, a congressional bill authorized appointment of male nurses to the regular forces of the armed forces in 1966. By 1967, over 1,000 male Army Nurse Corps officers made up about 22% of the total nurses in the army, many in anesthesia, operating rooms, or neuropsychiatry.[31]

The nature of war in Vietnam was quite distinct from that of the more classic strategies of World War II and Korea. Because of guerilla warfare tactics used by the Viet Cong, there was no real "front" or large dramatic battles. Hospital care, therefore, required different strategies. Semi-permanent air conditioned hospitals were constructed in Vietnam. There was little ground evacuation of the wounded because there were no secure road networks.[32] Despite the problems of the terrain, climate, and guerilla strategies, 99% of the soldiers hospitalized for injuries or diseases recovered, with 90% returning to duty because of the skill of the medical personnel, sophisticated equipment and the helicopter personnel who provided rapid medical attention. It was clear that the care available in Vietnam was far better than what could be provided in previous wars, and the statistics bore this out. Of all those Americans wounded or hospitalized, 4.5% died in World War II, 2.5% in Korea, and 1.5% in Vietnam.[33]

In 1972, secret peace negotiations were conducted by Secretary of State Henry Kissinger and in 1973, a halt to all offensive actions was ordered by President Nixon, with a ceasefire becoming effective by January 1973. The last American troops left Vietnam in March 1973. There had been over 46,000 American deaths, with over 300,000 wounded. The national trauma brought on by the Vietnam War changed the public's perception of the American veteran, including those nurses who served in the military. Returning nurses not only had to deal with the horrors of war, but the ambivalence of the American public and conflicting feelings about U.S. involvement in Vietnam.

One Vermont nurse who served in Vietnam was Nancy Faller, an enterostomal specialist at Rutland Regional Hospital. A 1968 graduate of St. Joseph's College in Maryland, she went into the army (through its student nurse program) while in college. At that time, "one half of the class went into the army and navy."[34] When she was sent to Vietnam, she was first a staff nurse in orthopedics. The head nurse in orthopedics left soon after, but "another nurse became head nurse because her date of rank was one day earlier than mine and everyone in the military was promoted based on date of rank." She was named to the next available head nurse position—in the recovery room at an evacuation hospital in Qui Nhon, Vietnam. She had little recovery room experience, but she learned very quickly how to assess rapidly. She worked in this unit for about one year, from October 1969 to 1970. In 1970, she received the Bronze Star. After discharge, she did private duty, attended an enterostomal program in 1974, and became very active in its specialty organization in the 1980s. She received her master's degree in nursing in 1994, and completed her doctoral degree. She achieved the rank of Lieutenant Colonel in the Army Reserve.

Dr. Carol Green Hernandez, an associate professor at The University of Vermont School of Nursing, was a member of the Army Nurse Corps during the Vietnam conflict. She recounts a few memories from her experiences there:

> I graduated from D'Youville College on an Army Student Nurse Corps scholarship. I received my last two years of schooling on that scholarship. I had basic training in San Antonio, Texas and worked on the burn unit there until OR school at Madigan General in Washington state. I went from there straight to Vietnam (Da Nang). I am tearful just thinking about it. We worked 12 hour shifts—it was always just you and a corpsman—and 50+ cots with very sick kids. I remember at ampicillin time, my corpsman would start at one end and I at the other, adding sterile saline to ampicillin. Then (everyone got it, just about), we'd go up and down the rows and give the GIs who could, their bottle to roll to mix it up. Then we'd head back and draw it up and inject it. When I left Vietnam, I was sent to Ft Riley, Kansas. I truly loved that assignment; I met my husband there. I have wonderful memories of my time in the Army. I wouldn't trade that time for anything.[35]

Another Vermont nurse, Edie Poland,* who served during both the Vietnam War and Operation Desert Storm, shared her memories of more than twenty years of active duty in the U.S. Navy Nurse Corps (1970–1993):

> Following graduation from Mary Fletcher Hospital School of Nursing in 1968 and eighteen months of practice in Philadelphia, I joined the navy. In January, 1970, I reported to Officer Indoctrination School (OIS) at U.S. Naval Base, Newport, Rhode Island. During OIS, nurses received an introduction to the navy, its customs, traditions, rules, and regulations. Classes included marching, saluting, proper way to wear the uniform, the different kinds of ships and boats, and the differences between a ship and a boat. We also were fitted for our uniforms: dress whites, dress blues, summer blues, raincoat, and winter coat and gloves to go with each uniform. Back in 1970, Nurse Corps officers were still wearing white uniforms and caps when working in the hospital or clinics, so these uniforms and caps were included as well.
>
> While in OIS, we were required to wear our uniforms whether we were on duty or liberty—on or off base. You might remember that military service was not highly regarded during the Vietnam War. During a weekend visit to classmates practicing in Boston, I encountered some interesting comments. Many of those I met were anti-military, but had never considered that health care providers, like chaplains and lawyers, were also members of the services. I remember the conversations and finally the acceptance by these young adults who seemed to understand

---

* Edie Poland is presently a director of the Addison County district of the Vermont Department of Health.

that joining the navy didn't mean that I supported war, but rather felt that those in harm's way deserved medical care.

Following OIS, I was stationed at the National Naval Medical Center, Bethesda, Maryland. It was here that I first cared for sailors and marines injured in combat. These patients had been initially treated in Vietnam or onboard one of the hospital ships prior to being medically evacuated back home. Some were awaiting various stages of plastic surgery or for broken bones to heal. I learned never to touch a sleeping marine as they might strike out as they awakened . . . reflex reaction learned during combat. Some of my most rewarding memories come from the months that I spent on the orthopedic floors. These men were not sick, just waiting as bones mended. They were very sensitive to the moods of the staff and if any of us seemed down they made it their mission to cheer us up. They also spent a lot of time doing the same for one another. Occasionally, after lights were out, I found a young man huddled in a corner in the stairwell crying, trying to understand. On a lighter note, these same young men in full body casts on gurneys would race one another using crutches to maneuver, or they would get to the elevators and "escape" to the hospital compound.

In December 1971, I arrived at Naval Hospital, U.S. Naval Base, Subic Bay, Republic of the Philippines. It was during this tour of duty that I encountered all of those diseases that our textbooks told us that we would probably not encounter such as typhoid, typhus, and malaria. A visit to a hospital for contagious diseases provided us with the opportunity to observe how medicine and nursing were practiced as well as to see how patients with cholera, diphtheria, tetanus, polio, and tuberculosis were medically managed. This tour also provided an opportunity to explore the Western Pacific and visit various islands within the Philippines, Japan, Hong Kong, and Thailand. It was during this tour that the hospital ships were being decommissioned; patients and staff watched the POWs land back in the United States and we received a visit from the first nurse selected to the rank of commodore admiral.

From the high desert of California and the largest Marine Corps Base in the world, to Hospital Corps School, San Diego, to Okinawa, to the Naval Postgraduate School and Washington, D.C.—the following years brought more adventures, challenges, rewards and friendships. Each new assignment brought more responsibility, both as a nurse and as an officer. Our uniforms changed, we shed the "ward" whites and caps, and donned the uniforms of our fellow naval officers. A Nurse Corps officer was the first woman to be promoted to two-star admiral and others assumed positions never before held by nurses.

During the nursing shortage of the eighties, new education opportunities were created for nurses. As the result of phenomenal teamwork, in one year legislation for a new education program was introduced in Congress, enacted into law, and implemented, providing financial assistance to students willing to begin their nursing career in the Navy. Nursing students were added to those eligible for Naval Reserve Officer Training Corps (NROTC) scholarship. Certified nurse anesthetists were awarded specialty pay similar to the provisions available for years to physicians. A hospital ship with nurse corps officers of all services sailed on a humanitarian mission in the Pacific and during Operation Desert Storm, Navy Nurses served both on board hospital ships and ashore.

As I left active duty in September 1993, nurse corps officers were serving sailors, marines, and their families from the bedside in naval hospitals and clinics around the world to operational positions with the deployed services to the "front office" as commanding officers of hospitals.[36]

Operation Desert Storm

Iraq invaded Kuwait on August 2, 1990. In support of United Nations Resolution 660, the United States responded by sending troops to the Persian Gulf in what was named Operation Desert Shield. In late 1990, several thousand nurses were deployed to care for the 500,000 troops sent to Saudi Arabia and the Persian Gulf starting on August 22, when President George H. W. Bush issued the first executive order authorizing the call-up of 48,800 members of the Selected Reserve to active duty to force the Iraqi Army led by Saddam Hussein out of Kuwait. The call-up of reservists in support of Desert Shield/Storm marked the largest activation of reservists since President Johnson mobilized reserve forces during the Vietnam Tet Offensive in 1968. Many reservists filled large staffing gaps at military medical facilities, where manpower was cut to the bone to support Desert Shield. Other reservists served on hospital ships and at fleet hospitals in the theater.

More than five months later, on January 16, 1991, Operation Desert Shield became Operation Desert Storm as the United States and twenty-nine coalition countries began use of aircraft, guided cruise missiles, and ground forces to remove Iraqi occupation forces from Kuwait. Although Operation Desert Storm began with an air war against Iraq, a four-day ground war ensued thirty-nine days later. By the time of the cease-fire on February 28, 1991, the United States had 697,000 troops in the Persian Gulf. In contrast to previous U.S. conflicts, a larger proportion of participants were women (7% of the force) and Reserve/National Guard personnel (17% of the force). Medical preparations during Operation Desert Shield were extensive, with nurses equipped to handle over 15,000 casualties daily.

The few casualties[37] that occurred during this brief ground war were treated in the field, with sick and injured personnel being quickly moved up the medical treatment ladder as required. Battalion aid stations provided patients with skills and clinical judgement in a safer environment,

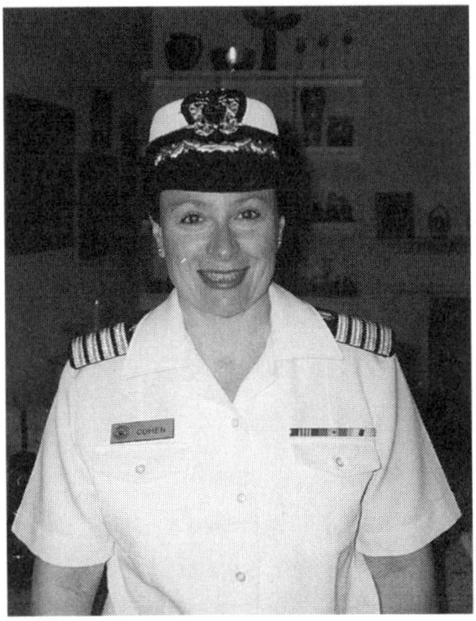

Captain Judith A. Cohen
Nurse Corps, U.S. Naval Reserve,
nurse veteran of Desert Storm

with sufficient time to accomplish a more complete examination. The next step up the ladder was a medical battalion surgical support company or a casualty receiving and treatment ship, where patients were treated by teams of physicians and nurses supported by a staff of medical technicians with more complete medical facilities—including a basic laboratory, holding wards, a pharmacy, and greater surgical capacity. Casualties requiring more extensive treatment were transported to either a combat zone fleet hospital or a hospital ship. While the fleet hospitals worked ashore, navy hospital ships operated in the waters of the Persian Gulf, Red Sea, and Gulf of Oman. Among the first ships deployed in support of Desert Shield, the USNS *Comfort* (T-AH 20) and USNS *Mercy* (T-AH 19) are the only hospital ships of their size in the world. These 1,000-bed floating hospitals stood at the ready throughout Desert Shield/Storm. Each hospital ship was equipped with fifty trauma stations that formed the casualty receiving area, twelve operating rooms, a twenty-bed recovery room, eighty intensive care beds, and sixteen light- and intermediate-care wards. The scope of treatment available at these facilities mirrored fully-staffed hospitals in the United States.

There were not only few casualties, but the incidence of nonbattle injuries and diseases was very low in comparison to other military campaigns. This attributed to preventive medicine efforts, minimal contact with local populations, and almost no access to alcohol.

Reserve staffing requirements for medical personnel were updated as a result of the war, and reservists initiated new procedures in the military hospitals that were already available in the civilian sector—such as same-day surgery programs.

From Vermont, there were six nurses from the Army National Guard and two nurses from the Navy Nurse Corps who served in Operation Desert Storm.

Linda Brier,* was commissioned as a captain in the Vermont Army

*Linda Brier is presently the nurse manager for rehabilitation services at Fletcher-Allen Health Care.

National Guard (VTARNG) in July 1980. She was assigned to Company B and was the only RN in the Army Guard for two years. In 1986, Captain Brier was appointed Health Services Liaison Detachment Chief Nurse and was promoted to Major in 1986. She recruited four to six RNs, and spent most of her time helping the field units with medic training. She also developed the first quality assurance program for the VTARNG. None of the field units had these programs, so she helped them compose some indicators/measurement tools.

In January 1991, during Operation Desert Storm, Major Brier and five other RNs were mobilized to Walter Reed Army Hospital in Washington, D.C. The five other nurses were Major Gary Boyce, Major Cindy Ross, Captain Joseph Megan, Captain Richard Weinberg, and Lieutenant Anne Marie Larose. They served as supplemental staff for the hospital until May, while the usual Walter Reed staff were serving in the Persian Gulf. Major Brier recounts her Desert Storm experience:

> I was assigned to the Neurosurgery Unit—all kinds of neuro injuries/medical problems. I was the senior officer and the head nurse was on emergency leave. I was put in charge for a short period of time. Several head-injured soldiers were returning from Saudi with needs for rehabilitation. The hospital had a physiatry medical team but no nursing expertise. The physical, occupational, and speech Language therapists and I instantly gravitated to each other. I was asked to join the weekly clinical rounds that were multidisciplinary.
>
> After two weeks, I suggested some in-service and arranged an eight-hour workshop for CEUs on Rehabilitation and Care of the Traumatic Brain Injured Person. I had boxes of my references and handouts sent down from Fletcher Allen Health Care (FAHC). I was "spotted" by Colonel Belandres, the Physiatrist Director and a psychologist in charge of a first-time-ever grant on getting soldiers back into service post TBI (traumatic brain injury). Prior to this, most head-injured soldiers were simply boarded out of the service. I was asked to coordinate the program development that was involved with the grant. Off the clinical unit I came into an office in the Therapy Department with the clinical team! I spent all my time designing treatment protocols, instructing staff, developing handouts and teaching the staff a rating scale to measure patient progress, developing follow-up clinics, and just having an all-around grand time, feeling I was involved with the first such project for the army. I also had Barb Murray and Nan Frymoyer, two nurses from home, fly down to Washington to work on a video we were developing for spine injured patients. I wanted it for both home and D.C., since I was also working with that population in D.C. I was asked if I would like to do this full time and become "real Army," but Washington, D.C. was not for my family, so I came home toward the end of May. My unit was sent

> home in April, but I stayed the extra month to get things going and to develop a job description for a replacement.
>
> Cindy was assigned to Occupational Health, Anne Marie was in cardiology, Richard was in the OR, Joe was in ICU, and Gary was in Labor and Delivery. We all had apartments in Silver Springs. Roommates of course. I took the bus or the subway for my entire stay. I loved not needing a car.
>
> My family and I had vacation at Easter in D.C. and it was our most memorable time together. I really enjoyed it. John, my husband, was wonderful with Macaela, our six-year-old. We kept in touch several times a week with letters, packages, and calls. It helped me see I could really pull myself together and help even in such stressful times.
>
> The hospital was really good and I thought the civilian hospitals could learn a lot from some of their systems. The documentation process made me nuts because it was so old. I spent a lot of time teaching the problem oriented form of documentation and despite many naysayers, made some decent headway with that. I was told by the nursing director that she'd never seen a newcomer make so many things happen in such a short period of time. She also offered me a job. Great place to be to get lots of nursing experience.
>
> It was clear from my experience at Walter Reed during Operation Desert Storm that the Reserve medical staff were very skilled and oriented to new situations very quickly. Good care happened in many places. The Army systems were working in many ways—Lots of people with different backgrounds all came together to help sick and injured soldiers and that was great! I think the American public is sadly lacking information about the good things the military accomplishes.[38]

In the years following the Persian Gulf, Major Brier was promoted to lieutenant colonel (1992) and was assigned as the State Chief Nurse. She worked with the State Surgeon for Medic education on the development of the Combat Lifesaver Course for nonmedical soldiers. She continued to expand the quality assurance program to statewide.

The two Navy Nurse Corps officers who were recalled to active duty during Operation Desert Storm were LT Kathleen Smith, a psychiatric clinical nurse specialist, and myself, LCDR Judy Cohen. Both of us were recalled to the National Naval Medical Center in Bethesda, Maryland. The following is my personal story as a nurse in the military.

> I had joined the navy as a junior at The University of Vermont (UVM) School of Nursing in 1973 through the Navy Nurse Corps Candidate Program, which was initially designed as a financial incentive for recruiting students from nursing programs into the navy during the Vietnam War. As a junior, I was considered on active duty, given the equivalent of an enlisted rank, although I had no contact with the navy until graduation after the Vietnam War had ended. I was given tuition, book fees,

and $500/month for my enlisted rank. This was a fair amount of money in those days, so I never really had any student money worries. Six months before I graduated, I was commissioned as an officer—an ensign—and received $700/month. Needless to say, I did a lot of traveling during my student days, often visiting family in Israel. In July 1975, after graduation from UVM, I went to Newport, Rhode Island, to the Naval Officer Indoctrination Program for physicians, dentists, nurses, and lawyers. I'm sure that the marine drill instructor who tried to teach us how to march was well aware that although we were professionals, we had two left feet and did not have that crisp military bearing that they were used to! We learned military history, rules of conduct, how to wear a uniform, how to march, how to salute—all the essentials.

I had been given a choice of active duty stations, which for new graduates in nursing, tended to be the larger military hospitals. I got my first choice, the National Naval Medical Center in Bethesda, Maryland, the showcase hospital for the navy at that time, and where the president and congressmen often received care. I'm not sure that my education could have ever prepared me for my first professional position. Every month, I did one week of day shifts, one week of evening shifts, and one week of night shifts. On day shift, I was the only nurse for a thirty-bed medical ward of patients. On evenings and nights, I was the only nurse for three thirty-bed wards of medical and surgical patients. I was very lucky to have good corpsmen who worked with me, but needless to say, I learned a lot about crisis management, prioritization, and delegation! I only wish that I had the same expertise, knowledge, and experience then that I do now! After a year-and-a-half on these wards, I was moved to the cardiothoracic surgery unit where I supervised just one unit. At UVM, I especially enjoyed my clinical rotations on cardiology, and having experience on the surgical side of cardiology was just what I wanted.

I finished my three-year military commitment on active duty here, but realized I wanted to go on to graduate school, so I chose to leave active duty and continue my connection with the military in the Reserves. The GI Bill paid for my graduate school tuition, and I completed my master's program in medical-surgical nursing at the University of Michigan in 1981. I returned home to Burlington to teach at UVM in the associate degree nursing program. I drilled monthly at the Naval Reserve Center in Burlington, holding various positions with the medical unit, including training officer, executive officer, and ultimately commanding officer.

In 1989, I started my doctoral program in nursing. The navy had just started a stipend program for health professionals who were in graduate work. Although most of the monies went to attract medical residents into the Reserves, I technically met the criteria and once again the navy played a large part in paying for this phase of my education. Vermont did not have such a program in nursing and at the time, summer programs were offered in several institutions whereby coursework could be done while off from UVM each summer. I returned to Michigan, Wayne State University, each summer for four years to complete my coursework. I also transferred into a flexible drilling unit which made it possible for me not to drill each month, thereby making meeting my academic requirements more reasonable.

I had just completed my second summer of doctoral coursework when the mobilization of reserve forces began in August 1990, for Operation Desert Shield. I was a lieutenant commander at this time in the Naval Reserve. I was just about to start the new academic year. I was trying to switch gears from being a student to being a faculty member at UVM. Throughout the semester, as I listened to the news and watched more and more of my colleagues being mobilized, I realized the question was not if I was going to be mobilized, but when. The semester ended, followed by the holidays, and just as the spring semester began, the Allied air forces began to attack Iraq and to forcibly remove Iraqi troops from Kuwait. I remember being glued to the television set as I watched the Iraqi Scud missiles attack Israel, and wondering if members of my family living in Israel were safe. The ground forces began their operations about a month later, and I was heartened in that it appeared that there would be few casualties and there was beginning to be talk about starting to send troops home. Needless to say, I was somewhat surprised that I was phoned at the School of Nursing on Valentine's Day, February 14, saying that I was to be mobilized even though the war was almost over. I received orders from California to provide support for the naval hospital there while the West Coast staff were deployed on one of the hospital ships. The East Coast staff at Bethesda had been deployed to the other hospital ships, so I called Washington to see if I could get my orders changed so at least I would be closer to home. I was also hopeful that since the hospital ships were on their way home, that my orders could be cancelled. This was a very difficult time in the semester to have to leave and get a faculty replacement, especially in light of the few casualties and the returning staff. Although my orders were changed to Bethesda, they were not cancelled.

UVM was very supportive during my mobilization. I received a call from the Benefits Office assuring me that they would make up the difference in my salary between my faculty pay and my military pay. I started to laugh because what I was making as a Lieutenant Commander with almost eighteen years of service was almost twice what UVM was paying me. I asked if they would continue to make up the difference between my military pay and my faculty pay when I returned, but they politely declined. I was also given a memorable goodbye party by faculty and students along with a UVM sweatshirt to remember Vermont.

Probably the most memorable nursing that I provided during this time was at the Blue Line Diner at breakfast with friends and faculty before driving to Washington. An elderly man sitting at the counter eating scrambled eggs had a massive heart attack. Lorri Clarke (Welch) and

I proceeded to do CPR on the man before the emergency personnel arrived, but unfortunately the heart attack was so massive that he never recovered. A memorable beginning to my involvement with Operation Desert Storm.

I worked on a surgical unit to provide staffing for those who had left, providing education, and setting practice standards. It was soon thereafter that the hospital staff started to return from the hospital ships. There were only a few wounded to care for and with double staffs, we were tripping over each other. It was interesting to see the staff return who had been away for almost nine months. During that time, the reservists had taken over the hospital and introduced many new innovations that were found to be in the civilian sector but had not yet been instituted in the military. One of these was the introduction of the same-day surgery program at Bethesda, and reservists demonstrated how this could produce significant savings and better care for the patients. There were some tensions between the returning staff, who recognized that the operation of their facility was not as they had left it, and the reservists, who approached problems of care with new insights. It was clearly recognized that for future medical mobilizations, the reservists should be a significant component of those being mobilized with their active duty counterparts, rather than completely replacing staff at a hospital with reservists.

I spent approximately eight weeks on active duty before being discharged and returning to UVM. I am now a Captain in the Navy Nurse Corps and have served as Commanding Officer of the flexible drilling unit which is based in Albany, New York. I counsel nursing students who are interested in the military and serve on the Military Studies Committee at the University. The Navy has afforded me a bachelor's, master's, and doctoral degrees in nursing and opportunities for me to grow in ways I could never imagine. For those opportunities, I am truly grateful.

I am also grateful for the opportunity to contribute to this historical contribution to the literature, bringing visibility to those Vermonters who served as nurses in the military during wartime. My research for this chapter has reaffirmed what we, as nurses, already know—nurses are harbingers of peace, care, and humanity, even during the cruelest moments of wartime.

—Judy Cohen, PhD, RN

NOTES

1. Colin L. Powell, remarks at the groundbreaking ceremony for the Vietnam Women's Memorial, in Vietnam Women's Memorial Project, "Celebration of Patriotism and Courage, November 10–12, 1993."
2. P. A. Kalisch and B. J. Kalisch, *The Advance of American Nursing*, 3rd ed. (Philadelphia: J.B. Lippincott, 1995), 326.
3. Ibid.

4. *Evening Argus* (Montpelier, Vermont), 26 July 1945. Vermont State Nurses' Association Special Collection, Research Library Annex, The University of Vermont, Burlington (hereafter cited as VSNA Archives), clippings folder.
5. VSNA Archives, box 15.
6. Kalisch and Kalisch, *The Advances of American Nursing.*
7. Ibid.
8. Ibid.
9. Nursing Council for War Service, 1945 folder, VSNA Archives, box 12.
10. Nursing Council for War Service, 1945 folder, Report of Student Recruitment Committee, 1 June 1945, VSNA Archives, box 12.
11. Kalisch and Kalisch, *The Advances of American Nursing.*
12. Vermont Nurses in Military Service folder, 1942–1944, VSNA Archives, box 12.
13. Lorraine Nelson, interview by Pat Allen, 30 May 2000.
14. Ibid.; worn translation of letter in possession of Lorraine Nelson.
15. Recollections of Christine Bostwick are from J. R. Morin, "Army Combat Nurse Supports National WWII Memorial," *The Addison Independent*, 11 May 2000, 12.
16. Kalisch and Kalisch, *The Advances of American Nursing.*
17. ANA Civil Defense Directors, 1950–1951 folder, VSNA Archives, box 12.
18. Reports/meetings, Civil Defense, 1950–1955 folder, State Nurse Association Committee on Nursing Resources To Meet Civil and Military Nursing Needs, VSNA Archives, box 12.
19. Kalisch and Kalisch, *The Advances of American Nursing.*
20. Ibid.
21. Ibid.
22. Ibid.
23. Ibid.
24. Ibid.
25. These nurses were identified through research at the VSNA Archives. See especially box B, VSNA scrapbooks, 1950–1953.
26. Letter from Gertrude Clinton.
27. Kalisch and Kalisch, *The Advances of American Nursing.*
28. Ibid.
29. Ibid.
30. Ibid.
31. Ibid.
32. Ibid.
33. Ibid.
34. Nancy Faller, taped interview, fall 1997, VSNA Archives.
35. Carol Green Hernandez, personal communication.
36. Edie Poland, personal communication.
37. Kalisch and Kalisch, *The Advances of American Nursing.*
38. Recollections of Linda Brier are from written narratives, June 2000.

THREE

Nursing Organizations

Nursing Organizations and Associations

NURSING ORGANIZATIONS and associations quickly followed the inception of nursing education in the United States in the late nineteenth century. From those early days, it was clear that establishing the validity of the profession, impacting care, controlling and standardizing education and practice, effecting change, and improving working conditions required the unified work of the growing number of individuals practicing nursing.

The first general nursing organization was the National League for Nursing Education (NLNE) begun in 1893 to foster development and improvement of nursing services and education. In 1897, the American Nurses' Association (ANA) began. As we begin our story in the 1940s, these two organizations continued to be the dominant organizations for nurses; however, the first specialty groups had arrived. The Public Health Nursing Section of the American Public Health Association started in 1923, the American Association of Nurse Anesthetists began in 1931, and the American Association of Occupational Health Nurses began in 1942. Three groups related to leadership and scholarship had also begun: Alpha Tau Delta, National Fraternity for Professional Nurses (1921), Sigma Theta Tau International Honor Society of Nursing (1922), and Chi Eta Phi Society (1932).

At the beginning of the 1940s in Vermont, there were only two nursing organizations: Vermont State Nurses' Association, Inc. (VSNA), part of the American Nurses' Association; and the Vermont League for Nursing Education (VLNE). In 1952, the VLNE, following the leadership of the National League for Nursing Education (NLNE), became the Vermont League for Nursing (VLN), with a formal affiliation with the National League for Nursing (NLN). Although informal groups of specialty nurses began meeting earlier, most did not develop formal associations until after the 1960s.

An association such as the ANA and VSNA has a general focus on all of nursing. ANA and VSNA have a global approach. They have a strong emphasis on policy development related to the practice of nursing and enhanced health care. They develop standards and ethics of practice and promote excellence in nursing care. All activities—for example, those related to work, or practice, or reimbursement, or education—are on behalf of nurses in all roles and facets of the profession.

Specialty organizations focus on education of their members related to their specialty practice. Other issues are addressed if they relate to their targeted membership. For example, emergency nurses are interested in helmet laws, school nurses are interested in air quality in schools. Most specialty groups now develop standards of practice for their specialty, either independently or in collaboration with ANA.

A variety of types of organizations and associations have developed in Vermont, and have formal or informal ties with their national counterparts:

- General membership associations (e.g., Vermont State Nurses' Association)
- Specialty organizations (e.g., Vermont State School Nurses Association)
- Honorary organizations that require invitation for membership (e.g, Sigma Theta Tau)
- Associations which cross state lines (e.g., Vermont New Hampshire Association of Peri Anesthesia Nurses)
- Organizations which include nurses and nonnurses (e.g., Vermont League for Nursing Education)
- Associations for nurses as well as other health care professionals (e.g., Vermont Association of Diabetes Educators)
- Organizations of nurses with strong links to nonnurse organizations (e.g., Vermont Organization of Nurse Leaders, related to the hospital association)
- Organizations created for a limited period of time related to a grant (i.e., the Vermont Nursing Initiative)
- Organizations of organizations (e.g., Coalition of Vermont Nursing Organizations, COVNO).

A phenomena which has been particularly prevalent in Vermont is the development of clusters of specialty nurses who may be individual nurses of a national group, but have no formal chapters in the state, often because of the small numbers of nurses in the state.

This section of the history will feature the following organizations/associations: Vermont State Nurses' Association, Inc.; Vermont League for Nursing Education; Vermont State School Nurses Association, Inc.; Vermont Emergency Nurses' Association; Vermont New Hampshire Association of Peri Anesthesia Nurses; Vermont Association of Occupational Health Nurses; Kappa Tau Chapter of Sigma Theta Tau International, Inc.; and Vermont Nursing Initiative. And now we begin the journey, to follow Vermont nurses working together to improve health care and the profession of nursing.

—Lynne Ann Dapice, MS, RN

Vermont State Nurses' Association

WRITING THE HISTORY of the Vermont State Nurses' Association is a daunting task. The association is fortunate to have an extensive collection of documents in its Special Collection at The University of Vermont, Burlington. The material presented in this section and in the Appendix is only a small sample of the activity. It is intended to give a flavor of the enormous effort of thousands of nurses over the years on behalf of all nurses, and on behalf of quality health care delivery for Vermonters.

The 1940s began with nurses working twelve-hour shifts, six days per week. Eight-hour shifts had been discussed and implemented in some places, but they were not a part of the Vermont reality. Nursing education occurred in varying types of programs housed in hospitals that we now refer to as diploma schools. Students still staffed hospitals. Many graduate nurses practiced outside the hospital—in homes as private duty nurses, as public health nurses, and as educators and administrators. The fifty-five years from the beginning of this history have seen great changes in education, the sites where nursing is practiced, and the scope of practice. Through all these changes the purposes of the association have stayed relevant, and so undergird the profession of nursing that many forget that the work is ongoing. No other association encompasses those purposes that define the profession of nursing.

Purposes

Since its inception, Vermont State Nurses' Association, Inc. (VSNA) has shared the purposes of the American Nurses' Association (ANA):

1. Work for the improvement of health standards and the availability of health care services for all people
2. Foster high standards of nursing
3. Stimulate and promote the professional development of nurses and advance their economic and general welfare

Vermont has the following additional purpose:

4. Serve Vermont nurses as the constituent association of the American Nurses' Association

"VSNA . . . fights for the right of nurses to provide nursing care . . ."
—Margaret Luce[1]

Looking at the fifty-five years as a whole, there are themes which reemerge with varying degrees of frequency: nursing shortages, quality of services, appropriate education for entry into practice, the Nurse Practice Act, workplace issues, and the ability to provide quality care. An ongoing activity of the association has been providing and approving continuing education for nurses. Constant themes underlying all other activity have been the continuous struggles for members and money to accomplish the overall goals and deal with the problems which emerged. Even in 1946, when the membership totaled 1,021 nurses out of 3,700 registered nurses, it was felt that more nurses needed to be members to project one strong voice. To sort out all of these themes, we will use the purposes of VSNA to organize the activities of the fifty-five years. But first, we will set the stage to provide a context for the events.

The Historical Context: Happenings in the Rest of the World

The forties were dominated by World War II and the advent of the atomic age. When the actual war was over, there was a period of recovery. Images include that of women participating fully in the workplace, symbolized by "Rosie the Riveter." Frank Sinatra was the heart-throb of the bobbie-sockers. It was a time of Big Bands. Nylon was a great new commodity. In medicine, antibiotics were widely used for the first time. (VSNA had a special program on the new medication—penicillin.) Nurses' scope of practice broadened as they took an active role in the care of the wounded, as well as caring for those on the home front.

In the fifties, we knew that "rock and roll was here to stay!" Televisions became commonplace. The MASH units which were later to become the theme of a popular television show were the real thing in the Korean Conflict. The first satellites were put into orbit. Alaska and Hawaii become states. Segregation was challenged. Polio vaccines were developed that relieved families of the fear of the disease that particularly struck the children.

In the sixties, even the Beatles and the Supremes couldn't drown out the controversy over the Vietnam War. Nurses were there again to try to save the dying, and they continue to carry the memories of those they touched. My "good friends John, Martin, and Bobby" were slain. Acid was no longer only a chemical term.

In the seventies, Helen Reddy sang, "I am woman, hear me roar." Man walked on the moon. Kent State students were shot. The Watergate scandal led to Nixon's resignation. No wonder The Carpenters sang about rainy day feelings getting them down! Microwave ovens became a staple in many kitchens.

In the eighties, typewriters began to give way to computers. The internet didn't begin until the 90s so we weren't yet worried about computer viruses, but another virus began to take its terrible toll—the AIDS virus.

VSNA Structure

VSNA has had a variety of structures to facilitate the implementation of its purposes. While the structure will not be reviewed in detail, a few comments may make it easier to understand the rest of the history of VSNA.

VSNA has always had the structure of most organizations: a board that has a core of a president, at least one vice president, one or more secretaries, trustees or directors, and a treasurer most of the time. Various positions have come and gone. Sometimes chairs of committees and officers of constituent groups have had formal seats on the board, sometimes not.

At the beginning of the forties there was a core board. In addition, there were groups called sections, standing committees, a nominating committee, delegates elected to attend the ANA annual meetings, and various special groups that today we would call task forces.

One committee that has always had a place in the structure is the Legislative Committee. Sections which existed in 1941 included the Private Duty (PD) Section (1921) and the Public Health (PH) Section (1921). There was also an Education group, a Publicity and Press Committee, and a Membership Committee. Over the years the following sections were added: the General Duty (GD) Nurses (1949), the Nursing Service Administrators (NSA, 1950; also called the Institutional Nursing Service Administrators, INSA), and the Educational Administrators, Consultants, and Teachers Section (EACT, 1952). In 1945, an Industrial Section was referenced in VSNA board minutes from that year. Each section had its own officers and budget.

Membership consisted of individual members (who graduated from out-of-state schools) and members of Vermont School Alumnae Associations. Dues were collected by the treasurers of the alumnae associations. In November 1946, VSNA voted to reorganize by geographical districts instead of by school alumnae groups. Five districts were formed:

District I	Addison, Chittenden, Franklin, and Grand Isle counties
District II	Lamoille, Orange, and Washington counties
District III	Caledonia, Essex, and Orleans counties
District IV	Rutland and Windsor counties
District V	Bennington and Windham counties

In 1952, the number of districts was decreased to four by combining District II and III; in 1961, they were reduced to three with the combination of Districts IV and V—the current number. The boundaries have been adjusted slightly. Each district had its own officers and budget.

A large variety of committees, beyond those mentioned, also met during the same period. As the years went by, the sections had increasing difficulty recruiting officers and members. The nature of nursing changed, requiring different ways to approach the primary work of VSNA. In 1967, VSNA was markedly restructured. The sections were eliminated. District presidents had a formal seat on the board; a Council of Nursing Practice was added; the standing committees of Bylaws, Nominating, and Legislation continued with the addition of the Economic Security Committee; and a means was formalized to create special interest groups, e.g., nursing education. Although there have been other changes since then, none have been as all-encompassing.

The work of the Association is accomplished at the Annual Meeting, which is held as part of a convention. A list of the conventions as well as the presidents and executive secretaries/directors are listed on pages 349–351. In the forties, there was usually a semiannual meeting as well. As years progressed, special meetings could be called, but one meeting was the usual number. The annual convention is used for continuing education and celebrations. In 1964, VSNA celebrated its fiftieth anniversary.

Through all of the years until 1974 there was no seal, or logo, for VSNA. In 1974 there was a contest to design a seal. The winning design, submitted by VSNA historian Mary Thompson, utilized the shape of the pin that nurses who were registered in Vermont could purchase until about 1940. It was essentially two concentric circles superimposed on a triangle. In the VSNA seal the outer circle which forms a rim for the inner circle holds the words Vermont State Nurses Association. The inner circle pictures a lantern (representing the lantern carried by the founder of modern nursing, Florence Nightingale); has the Latin words lux *meaning light,* studiis *meaning endeavor or study, and* unitas *which means oneness or unity; and has the date of the founding of VSNA, 1914.*

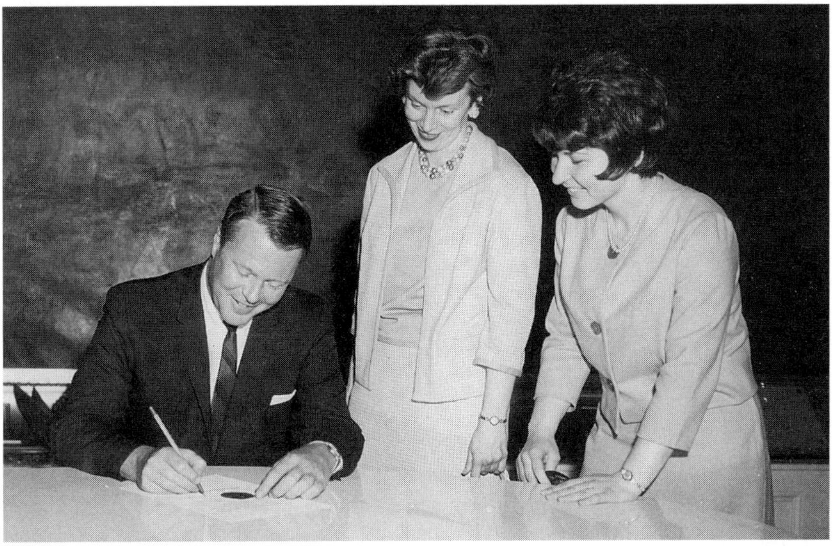

Governor Philip Hoff signs "Salute to Nursing," honoring the fiftieth anniversary of the Vermont State Nurses' Association with Jean Milligan, VSNA president, and Sandra Gillespie, president of the Student Nurses Association of Vermont, 1964

"Working for the Improvement of Health Standards and the Availability of Health Care Services for All People"

Work to support this purpose has taken two major forms. One major focus has been on nursing practice, with the goal of delivering high quality nursing care to Vermonters. The other area which has been vigorously pursued is the effort over the years to influence policy that actually impacts the health care system, leading to improvement of health standards and health care services. That effort has been spearheaded by the Legislative Committee and special task forces.

Nursing Practice

Nursing practice has been an umbrella for many types of activities.

- Nursing shortages
- The scope of practice (i.e., what is appropriate practice for nurses), including
  - Treatments
  - Medication administration

Technical activities
Expanded practice roles
Diagnostic samples for legal reasons
Certification of nursing specialties and of continuing education

- Licensure
- Appropriate practice for others (e.g., nurses' aides and practical nurses)
- Inservice education
- Grants (e.g., the Tri-State Quality Assurance Grant)
- Educational issues related to entry into practice
- Clinical sessions for convention
- Standards of Practice
- Peer review

It is always enlightening to look at what nurses have done as a part of their practice; that is covered in great detail in Section Two of this book. Immediately after World War II, physicians were willing to give up taking blood pressures, so that became a registered nurse's responsibility. There has long been a dynamic tension over what is medical practice versus what is nursing practice; the definitions have constantly changed. In turn, there has been discussion about what varying health care assistants and technicians can and should do. Areas that have been discussed by the VSNA include:

1960s

- Emergency preparedness and disaster nursing was a focus of the EACT Section
- Adding blood to transfusions
- Cardiopulmonary resuscitation (CPR; could only be done until a physician arrived to take over)
- Examination of the patient in labor
- Venipuncture
- Insertion of intravenous (IV) catheters (could only be done in the presence of a physician)
- The role of the RN in the emergency room (ER)
- Isolation technique

1970s

- Drug management
- Blood drawing for alcohol
- Series of educational sessions on the Problem-Oriented Medical Record (POMR), 1973
- Accepting orders from physician assistants (rejected)
- Licensure of midwives

- Nurse anesthetists
- IV drug administration for RN/LPN
- Administration of meds by unlicensed personnel
- Prescription writing

1980s

- Nursing diagnosis
- Diagnostic related groups (DRGs)

1990s

- Practice needs for reformed health care system
- Occupational safety, e.g., prevention of needle stick injuries
- Health care environments that do not create problems; providing health care without creating new health problems for patients and care givers
- Staff to patient ratios
- Cost-effective quality care

Other important practice issues included

- Development of a statement of the scope of practice and qualification of nurse practitioner/clinicians/clinical nurse specialists (1978)
- A study of salaries, scope of practice, educational preparation, distribution of nurse practitioners, certified registered nurse anesthetists, and nurse midwives (1985)
- A survey related to "down" substitution (use of lesser prepared individuals to do the work previously done by nurses, 1985)
- Practice issue survey (1994)

Adequate Supply of Nurses to Provide Care (Nursing Shortages)

Throughout the period covered in this history there have been periodic nursing shortages, with a variety of causes. During World War II, it became difficult to fill the need for nurses to care for the wounded; and back at home, the shortage was even more severe. It was clear that more nurses would have to be educated, and the Cadet Nurse Corps was begun. The struggle to keep up with the demand is well documented in "Fifty Years of Progress: Past/Prospective," published on the occasion of Vermont State Nurses' Association fiftieth anniversary in 1964.[2]

The minutes of the VSNA meetings of the early 1940s relate the efforts at recruitment. In 1942, there was discussion about the difficulty of recruiting nurses into the Red Cross. The impact of the sacrifices of the war were also evident. In minutes from the council (board) meeting preceding the annual meeting, June 22, 1943, there was discussion about whether to have a fall meeting. At the time, the regular practice was to have the annual meeting in June and to have a semiannual meeting in the fall. The discussion centered around gas rationing and what the contingency plan should be. It was decided that the issue would be brought to the annual meeting. In the event that the fall meeting could not be held, members of the board would meet with representatives of the alumnae groups throughout the state. There is no record of a fall meeting being held.

As 1943 progressed, the activity of the Association increased. At the September 1943 meeting of the Executive Committee for the State Nursing Council for War Service, the ten military districts, had already been designated by the states, to organize the effort to recruit nurses. A Procurement & Assignment Committee was formed to fulfill the military quota. One hundred and eight nurses were needed by January 1, 1944. As of January 1, 1943, fifty-nine nurses had enlisted. Meetings were also held jointly with the Red Cross. November of 1945 saw the final report of the Procurement & Assignment Committee; i.e., that committee and the State Nursing Council for War disbanded.

In the postwar period, the shortage in Vermont was exacerbated by expansion of hospitals, expansion of public health nursing, and the introduction of more complex treatments. These treatments included antibiotic treatments consisting of numerous injections administered in a hospital setting. The shortage continued.

> . . . in 1957, the General Assembly established an Interim Commission to study nursing made up of one representative from the Vermont Medical society, the VHA, VSNA, PNAV, and VLN, and two from the House of Representatives and one from the Senate. Their recommendations were: that legislation be introduced to establish a two-year school of nursing leading to the associate degree in nursing; that the $15,000 annual appropriation for nursing scholarships be increased to $45,000; and endorsement of mandatory licensing for both professional and practical nurses.[3]

The keynote speaker of the 1958 VSNA convention was Mildred Montag, PhD, who spoke on "Preparation of General Duty Nurses in Junior College 2-year Schools." Dr. Montag is considered the "mother" of associate degree education.

The presence of another nursing shortage was sufficiently well established that a resolution was passed in 1987 to recommend that the Practice Committee and the Manpower Task Force study the problem, make recommendations, and share them with concerned parties.

In June 1989, VSNA representatives were called to a meeting with Governor Madeline Kunin, who asked VSNA for specific recommendations related to the Department of Health and Human Services Secretary's

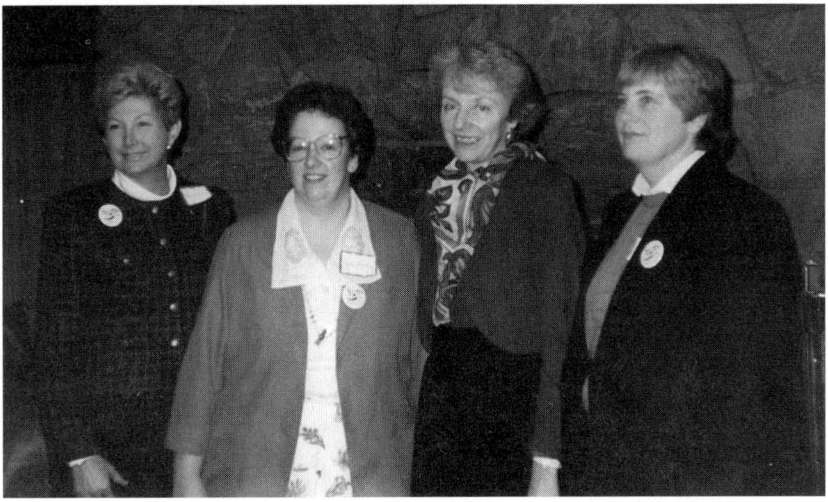

Governor Madeline Kunin (*second from right*), was honored with an award for outstanding contributions to nursing by a nonnurse at the 1989 VSNA Convention. She is shown here with VSNA President Margaret Luce, Carol Green Hernandez, and Bonnie Stiles.

Commission on Nursing report completed in 1988. A paper responding to her request was completed in July 1989 by the legislative aide, members of the Legislative Committee, and the executive director.

In 1989, VSNA adopted a resolution supporting the recommendations of the Department of Health and Human Services Secretary's Commission on Nursing, summarized

I. Utilization of Nursing Resources: It was recommended that the nurse should concentrate on direct care of the patient and family with assistance from other health workers under the nurse's supervision.

II. Nurse Compensation: Recommendations included increase in salary and development of innovative compensation packages.

III. Health Care Financing: Reimbursement levels needed to be sufficient that organizations could recruit and retain adequate numbers of nurses.

IV. Nurse Decision Making: Nurses should have representation on policy making organizations and in the governance, administration, and management of the organizations where they are employed. It also emphasized collaboration among members of the health care team.

V. Development of Nursing Resources: Financial and nonfinancial barriers to nursing education needed to be eliminated to encourage more people to enter nursing.

VI. Maintenance of Nursing Resources: There should be a five-year commission which acts in an advisory capacity to the Secretary to monitor the implementation of the recommendations. There was also a call for research on the relation between health care financing and nursing practice.[4]

Task Force on Entry into Practice

The first task force was established in 1978 as a mandate from the VSNA Education Committee to

1. Study the issue of preparation for entry into professional nursing practice as it affects the state of Vermont;
2. Make recommendations to the VSNA Board of Trustees regarding a position for VSNA on the issue of entry into professional practice.[5]

After the resolution on Entry into Practice was passed at the 1978 convention, the first group was dissolved and a new task force was appointed. By 1984, the focus of the task force had changed to defining competencies for two levels of nursing practice—professional and technical.

The report of the task force was published in 1985 and stated its purpose: ". . . to differentiate associate degree practice and baccalaureate degree nursing practice."[6] The report listed assumptions about the roles of both types of graduates, and assumptions about the differences. The report then compared and contrasted the practice in sections related to parts of the nursing process, i.e., assessment, planning, implementation, and evaluation. It also had sections on communication, leadership, and research.*

Registration and Licensure of Nurses

In 1944, an Executive Committee was appointed to meet with the Vermont State Board of Registration of Nurses to explore and implement a recommendation whereby "all nurses who work for hire could be registered within the State of Vermont."[7] This is the first of many activities of the association relating to the registration of nurses.

The end of the 1950s and the beginning of the 1960s were dominated by consideration, development, passage into law, and interpretation of the

---

*The entry into practice issue is discussed in more detail in Section One, Nursing Education.

first mandatory licensure law. In 1957 the State Legislature established an interim commission to examine issues related to nursing education, the shortage of nurses, the type of nursing care that was being given, state and federal support for nursing education, mandatory licensing for both professional and practical nurses, and advanced educational opportunities for graduates of basic programs.

Consideration of a mandatory licensure law began in 1958. The purpose of the VSNA Committee on Legislation for 1959–61 was to study the pros and cons of mandatory licensure for both professional and practical nurses in Vermont, and to prepare for discussion of a Nurse Practice Act defining the practice of nursing and that ". . . will require all those who nurse for hire, as defined in the law, to be licensed in the state."[8]

In 1960, the proposed Mandatory Licensing Act was completed by the legislative committee. Legal counsel was critical to the development, writing, and passage of the bill. Because it included practical nurses, VSNA worked closely with the Practical Nurses' Association and they shared the legal fees. The bill was introduced in 1961. All of the preparatory work paid off. The Nurse Practice Act was signed by Lieutenant Governor Foote on June 28, 1961. The task over the next several years was to interpret the Act to the public and to nurses.

In November of 1973, a joint committee of the VSNA, two practical nursing organizations, and the Vermont State Board of Nursing, recommended revisions to the practice act. The impetus for the revision was a legal opinion that the expanded practice of nursing (e.g., nurse midwifery), was not legal under the current practice act. Terms added to the practice act included "diagnosis" and "treatments."

The major changes to the Nurse Practice Act brought before the legislature in 1974 included ". . . new definitions of practice to allow for expanded role of the nurse, changing qualifications of board members, and adding a public member . . ."[9] VSNA needed to have—and was able to have—a continued presence at the statehouse to ensure passage of the revisions to the Practice Act in 1974.

The body that licenses and regulates nurses has been a concern to VSNA. The history of the Vermont State Board of Nursing is examined in detail in another section of this history, but we would be remiss if we did not mention the role of VSNA. Although the work of the Board is to protect the public, nurses have felt that the composition of the board should be such that the members can understand nursing practice; and that nurses, not other professions, should control the practice.

VSNA believed that the Board should have adequate staff and financial resources to do the work the Legislature had mandated that it do. One example of a time when VSNA has been active on behalf of the

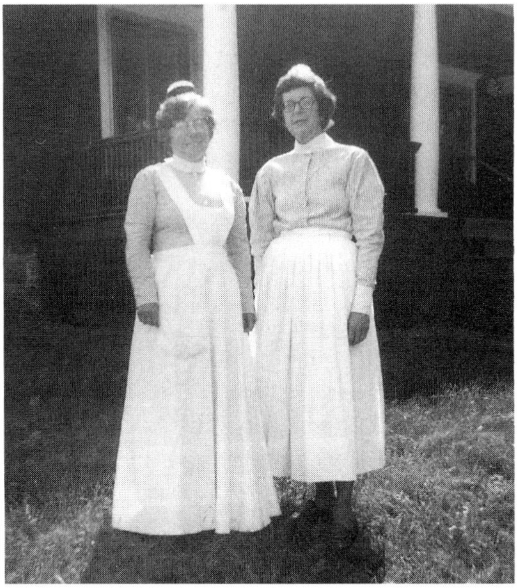

VSNA celebrated its 60th anniversary in 1974 at the Lake Morey Inn, Fairlee. Pat Allen, Convention Committee, and Ann Janney, Executive Secretary, in nurse uniforms of an earlier time.

board was in 1975, just one year after passage of the revised practice act. There was a 15% reduction in appropriations for the Board of Nursing. The effort was to get the Legislature to restore the funding to meet the mandate of the law. Nurses were encouraged to write letters to their legislators and to call them. At the same time, VSNA also had an active presence in the statehouse, and funding was restored.

In 1994, there were major changes in the practice act that affected advanced practice registered nurses. These included nurse practitioners, clinical nurse specialists, certified registered nurse anesthetists, and nurse midwives. For the first time, their practice was regulated solely by the Vermont State Board of Nursing, and did not require joint review of practice guidelines. This was a major legislative activity which built on and moved beyond the work that had been done by advisory groups to the Board of Nursing. It required major negotiations between representatives of the Boards of Nursing and Medicine, the Medical Society, nurse practitioner groups, and the VSNA, with VSNA playing a leading role. Over the next year the effort switched to the regulatory arena as the rules and regulations were developed. This legislation also granted licensure to nursing assistants in an effort to more closely control the practice of this group of care givers and to better protect the public.

Legislative Activity

Throughout the years, VSNA has had an active presence in the Vermont State Legislature. In the early years the effort was particularly related to working conditions, including how many hours a nurse should work. Work conditions continued to be a part of the mix, especially during the active collective bargaining years. Legislation related to the Vermont State Board of Nursing, registration of nurses, and then mandatory licensure consumed an enormous amount of effort. Even if something was not occurring at the moment, the potential was always there, not just at the times when the practice act would sunset. Another area of activity was related to appropriations for scholarships or loans. That activity often mirrored the cyclical nursing shortages.

From 1973, when Priscilla (Pat) Allen became the first legislative aide (lobbyist), to the present, with the Executive Director of the organization serving in that role, VSNA has had visible and effective presence in the policymaking arena. There often have been years without legislative activity of particular interest to nurses, or years when legislation has been introduced but not moved; other periods of time (e.g., in the nineties), have been extremely busy and productive. Even in the years with little activity, members of the Legislative Committee faithfully screened and studied legislation that had been introduced, and developed a stance in the event the bills became active.

As the years moved closer to the time of the writing of this history, the number of bills introduced has exploded. Trying to carefully analyze each one in the committee became an overwhelming challenge. Gradually, the committee shifted focus to one of developing a platform which could serve as a reference point for the legislative aide.

Legislative activity in the 1990s was guided by resolutions passed by VSNA in convention which formed the basis of the legislative platform. As a sample, the following resolutions were passed in 1992. (Related actions in which VSNA had an active role, whether it happened in 1993 or in subsequent years through the present, are also listed.)

- Nursing's Heritage: Recognition; Appreciation; Preservation (although it is not legislative, this book is related to that resolution)
- Discouragement of Economic Support for the Tobacco Industry (Clean Indoor Air Bill passed)
- Support of Rural Health Care (participated on Vermont Department of Health Primary Care Steering Committee to assure primary care providers in rural areas; was part of successful lobbying effort to get loan repayment for primary care providers including nurse practitioners)

- Sexual Harassment in the Workplace (actively supported successful legislation including provision of some of dialogue for introduction of the bill for the vote)
- Environmentally Responsible Practice Resolution
- Protect the Title "Nurse" (work on the revision of the practice act)
- Discrimination Against Gays and Lesbians by the Military
- Regulation of Advanced Practice Nursing (work on this is cited elsewhere in this section of the history)
- Single Payer Systems and Nursing's Agenda for Health Care Reform (testimony at the state and federal level. Although a single payer system was not passed, VSNA actively supported successful initiatives on insurance reform and helped craft successful legislation in a multi-disciplinary retreat on health care reform.)
- Health Care Reform in Vermont (see previous resolution)
- Gun Control (tabled and passed the next year; actively supported gun control legislation, including appearing in dialogue on cable television).
- Reinvest In a Healthier America
- Occupational Health, Safety, and Wellness Resolution (actively supported successful mercury control law and was on the coalition)

Another important activity of the Legislative Committee has been the sponsorship of Legislative Educational Sessions to help nurses understand the process and how to become involved in helping to shape policy. Efforts have also been aimed at legislators: VSNA began holding Legislative Days at the statehouse. Initially, they were several days long and consisted of displays at the statehouse about nursing and nursing care. Today, the limited space at the statehouse is in fierce demand, and groups are lucky to be able to get even one day. Legislative Day has evolved to become an educational day for nurses as well as an opportunity for nurses to connect with and inform their legislators.

A central part of the work of the Vermont State Nurses' Association and ANA has become policy. It is harder for nurses to relate to this piece than it is to relate to practice-oriented activity; yet, it is this work that allows nurses to practice and enables nurses to have a say in the design of the health system in which we practice. It is a difficult arena to work in because everything is in shades of gray. One must become skilled in the arts of negotiation and compromise. And it is costly in terms of human resources. Yet VSNA has always done, and continues to do, this work for all nurses in Vermont.

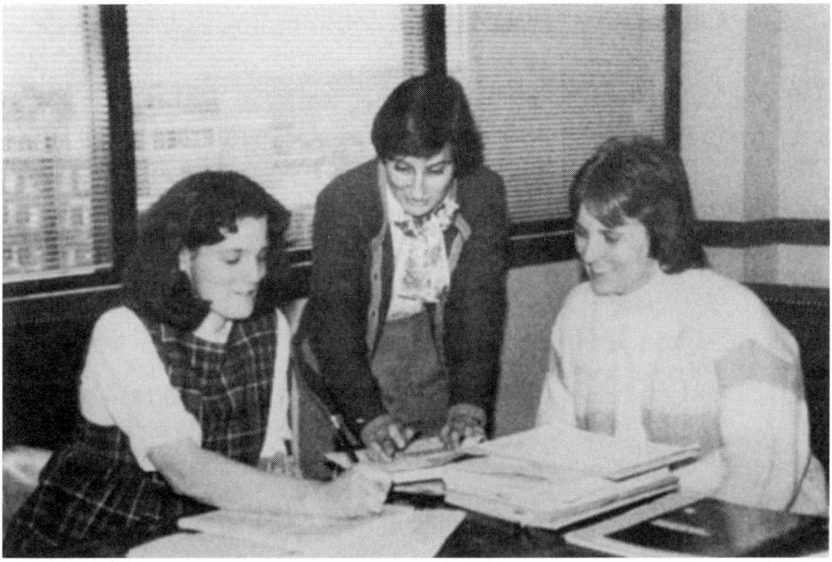

Kathleen Ready, legislative aide, VSNA Executive Director RoseMarie Bagioni, and Marge Douglass, chair of the legislative committee, 1985.

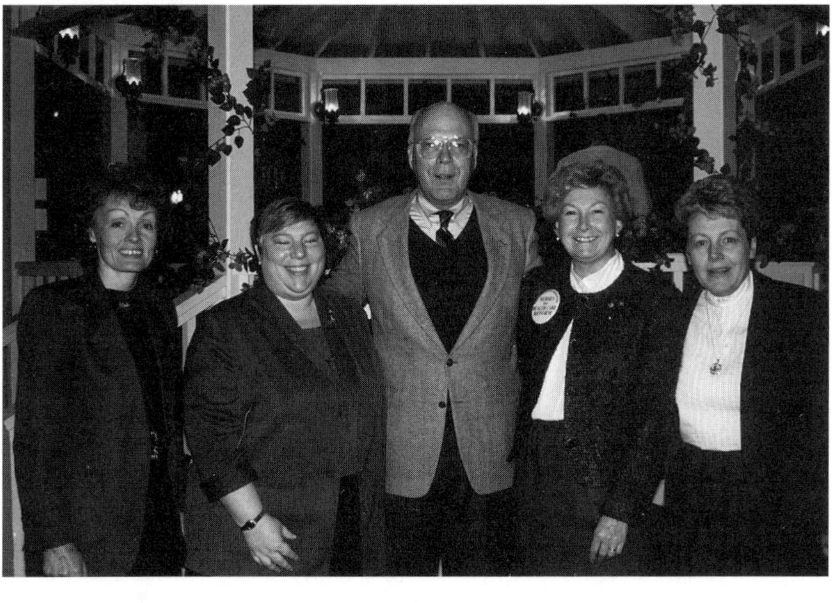

The ANA made a PAC award to Senator Patrick Leahy in 1992. *Left to right*, Marcelle (Mrs. Patrick) Leahy, Michelle Walker, Senator Leahy, Margaret Luce, and Lynne Dapice.

VSNA Political Action Committee

The Vermont State Nurses' Association Political Action Committee (PAC) had its beginnings with Sue Reilly's efforts to hold organizational meetings in 1983. Carol Hernandez was able to move the group to the point of being officially recognized by the VSNA board in 1986. In 1984 Hernandez wrote:

> Political Action has as its goal the election-support of candidates who will view legislation in the way the group wishes them to view it . . . Our purpose [for the VSNA PAC] is not to raise and contribute money *per se* to candidates as much as it is to provide other forms of campaign support . . . Our primary purpose . . . is education.[10]

The VSNA PAC was particularly active in 1986 during the election campaign of Senator Patrick Leahy. The activity decreased markedly after that. There have been intentions of reactivating it; however, those volunteers who have been active have focused their activity on following pending legislation.

"Foster High Standards of Nursing"

Nursing Education

There are two types of education which have been a focus of the association: basic education that prepares an individual to become a registered nurse, and continuing education that is designed for the practicing nurse to assist in maintaining and increasing knowledge related to the practice arena. Both of these areas have had a variety of homes in the association. Basic nursing education has been under the purview of the EACT Section, the Practice Committee or Council, the Legislative Committee, the VSNA–VLN Coordinating Council, and a variety of special task forces. During the period we have seen the demise of diploma schools in the state—the primary source of nursing education in the forties—and the development of associate, baccalaureate, and master's degree education.

In 1961, two major activities related to education were happening. The VSNA–VLN Coordinating Council developed a questionnaire related to developing programs for graduate nurse education to go to all nurses in the state. The other activity centered on Standards, Functions, & Qualifications. These issues were discussed throughout the structure of the Association. VSNA President, Philip Day, served as chair of the ANA Committee on Standards, Functions, & Qualifications of the ANA Nursing Service Administration Section. He spearheaded the activity in VSNA as well. The Nursing Service Administration Section discussed their responsibility to staff to keep them informed and prepared to meet their changing role. They also discussed the responsibility for nursing education to supplement initial education. The concept was also discussed by the General Duty Section.

VSNA has not only discussed what the education should be, but it has consistently supported the education programs for nursing in the state. Sometimes those serious efforts and discussions have taken on a lighter note.

> In November 1974 VSNA was one of the prime factors in helping to save the AD Nursing program at UVM. How many remember the night when nurses all over Chittenden County *Ironed on* mailing labels by hand because the heat transfer machine at UVM was tied up?[11]

An in-depth review of nursing education is covered in Section One of this book. It must be noted that VSNA was active in all the changes related to basic nursing education.

Continuing Education

The work of providing continuing education has been a part of nursing sections that developed educational opportunities for their members, convention committees, special committees, the Practice Committee and Council, and through special grants, for example, the TRICE Program. Approval of continuing education began in the practice committee, but it became evident that most educational activity, and especially the approval process, needed to be in a separate structure within the association.

Work began in 1972 on development of a proposal for initiating a systematic program for continuing education for nurses in Vermont.

> The Practice Committee recommended that VSNA advocate the development of a pilot program which would use the continuing education unit as a uniform basis for recognition of participation in organized continuing education programs . . .
>
> The essential components of such a program will include consideration of the following: administration, budget, teaching staff, curriculum, facilities, educational methods and evaluation . . . The Council on Practice proposes that task forces be established to study and develop specific recommendations for implementation of this program.[12]

In January of 1974, a two-year pilot of the Continuing Education Approval and Recognition Program (CEARP) was begun. The definition of a CEARP was included in a report by the director of the program in 1977, Sylvia Morse:

> . . . We quote the first three sentences on page 410 in the March 1977 issue of the *American Journal of Nursing.* "A system in which all nurses in this country will be able to obtain recognition for continuing education

> . . . Part of this system is the review of continuing education activities so that nurses will know, before they spend their time, effort, and money, which activities have the profession's stamp of approval. Today, in almost all states, nurses' associations are conducting programs which record and/or recognize CE offerings."[13]

Nurses enrolled in the program. After recording forty contact hours of approved continuing education in a given period of time, the enrollee received a certificate from VSNA. The service was free for members; initially nonmembers paid a $40 fee.

The VSNA was ready to apply for ANA accreditation in 1977, except for the fact that it did not have an ongoing structure for financial support. The three-step process for final accreditation began. The first step was to receive regional accreditation which allowed credit to be given.

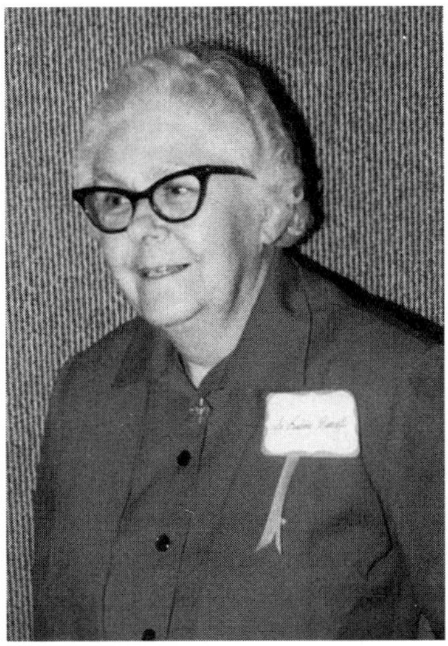

Sister Evaline Barrett, 1984
longtime chair of the
VSNA Education Committee

Accreditation was not the only work of the Committee. That same year the committee was asked by the Vermont State Board of Nursing to assist in developing guidelines for refresher courses for nurses who had been out of practice for five or more years.

At last in 1984, the Vermont State Nurses' Association received accreditation from the American Nurses Credentialing Center. In 1988, using new guidelines, VSNA was accredited for four years as an approver of continuing education for nurses. The model for the accredited organizations changed. VSNA only approved programs. They no longer kept records for individual nurses. The approved programs distributed the contact hours. Accreditation occurred again in 1994 for six years.

Continuing Education in the Tri-State: Model for Nursing Care (TRICE)

In 1975, the Council on Nursing Practice began work to secure a grant to focus on quality. The states of New Hampshire, Vermont, and Maine received a joint grant for the period of July 1, 1978, to June 30, 1981, with the purpose to

> . . . provide the means for nurses in all education and practice settings . . . (in the three states) . . . to become proficient in the use of the American Nurses' Association's model for Quality Assurance. The . . . model is a mechanism through which stable and changing factors can be assessed, outcomes planned and care designed so that nursing actions contribute to the attainment of a maximum level of wellness. It provides a methodology for measuring and evaluating the many components of nursing care to individuals, families and communities. It provides for the introduction of changes based on information supplied by the measurements.[14]

The grant was to be implemented by providing workshops and consultations to nurses in their employment settings, and through public and professional communications. The consultants, based in their geographic areas, would become expert and then be available to assist other nurses. Three staff members were a part of the grant. The grant was funded by the Department of Health, Education, and Welfare as a special project of the Nurse Training Act and was directed by Sylvia Morse, a VSNA member. Initially, seventy-three nurses (out of 155 applicants) were educated to be consultants in their local settings. "The intent . . . [was] . . . to make a transition from individual staff support to interdependent group support."[15] Those interdependent groups began to form within the first year.

The work of TRICE continued as planned and projected. Based on the activity, the TRICE project presented a program at the 1980 ANA conference in Boston on "Quality Assurance: Programs in Action."

In the December 1980 *Vermont Registered Nurse*, Morse related that the focus of the ANA model was on the profession of nursing.[16] Participants in the Vermont TRICE project decided that the focus should be on health status, and voted to form a separate corporation to continue the work at the end of the grant period. During the second year, the focus turned to evaluation of clients and the client outcome, and pilot projects were under way.

The grant was scheduled to conclude at the end of June of 1981; final meetings were held in July of 1981 to complete the process. A review of the total project led to the conclusion that the goals had been achieved; indeed, many of the people who participated in the program went on to be involved in quality assurance in their institutions.

Special Interest Groups as Part of the Structure of VSNA

Sections, which were a form of special interest groups, were discussed above in "VSNA Structure." One of these sections was the School Nursing subgroup of the Public Health Section. Prior to its dissolution in 1962, school nurses recommended that Vermont should have a School Health Director. Other sections continued through 1966; by this time, many nurses began joining specialty nursing organizations. Some practice areas, however, had either not developed independent organizations, or issues related to the specialty seemed better handled within the state. There was a need to provide a way for these groups to have support to pursue their special needs.

The first special interest group to organize within VSNA was the Nurse Practitioner Group. By the 1980s, that group was inactive. A formalized process within the bylaws was created for special interest groups.

The Psychiatric and Mental Health Nursing Interest Group was formed by resolution at the 1986 convention to support a core group of psychiatric clinical nurse specialists who were working together to secure third-party reimbursement for services, to provide peer consultation and support, and to formalize their meetings and have the support of VSNA. Throughout its history, Lorraine Impey and Bill Windels have spearheaded its continued activity. It continues to meet two or three times a year, and continues to focus on these issues. Attention has also been given to Nurse Practice Act changes and clinical practice updates.

Coalition of Vermont Nursing Organizations

The need for a coalition among the numerous nursing organizations first became evident in February of 1982, when VSNA established a task force on the Vermont State Board of Nursing at a time when there was a threat to the existence of the Board of Nursing. The Secretary of State's office published "Structural and Organizational Recommendations in Vermont's Occupational Licensing Boards," that advocated an umbrella board under which many professions would be regulated. The book was alluded to as "the green book." Part of the activity of that VSNA task force was a call to action, which resulted in a temporary coalition of nurses from all disciplines and associations. The perceived threat temporarily subsided, and that group did not continue to exist.

The benefits of having all nursing organizations working together were recognized, and the VSNA passed a 1984 convention resolution supporting a multi-nursing organizational group to meet "for the purpose of providing a unified nursing approach to health and nursing issues."[17] The effort was initiated by Janet Patterson and Priscilla (Pat) Allen. The first meeting was held March 15, 1985, with two or three representatives from each of thirteen Vermont nursing groups. And thus was born the Coalition of Vermont Nursing Organizations (COVNO). By November of 1985, there were eighteen Vermont Nursing Organizations in the new coalition. It was hoped that the joining together would give nurses greater power. It was recognized that no one nursing organization

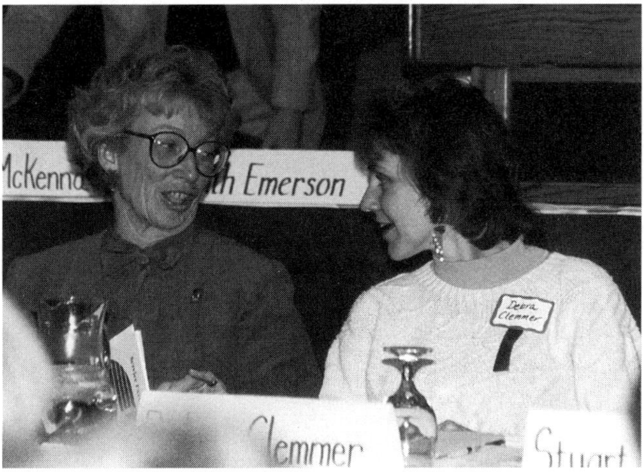

Sally Sample and Debra Clemmer at the annual meeting of the Vermont State Nurses' Association, 1990.

had the numbers to impact on policy, but together they had a better chance of being heard—especially in the legislative arena. VSNA became the "home" for COVNO, and provided support for the work of the coalition. The structure was set up to be very informal, which is the way it continues to function.

COVNO meets two times a year: in the spring during the legislative session and in the fall for update and planning on other nursing issues and initiatives. The collaborative work of the members has been instrumental in successes related to legislation, including practice act issues and health issues (for example, the Clean Indoor Air Act, passed in 1993, which prohibits smoking in indoor public areas). Nowhere was that united activity more apparent then at a Nursing Summit hosted by VSNA in 1991. Speakers included Governor Howard Dean and representatives from the ANA, the Vermont Hospital Association, the Vermont House and Senate, the State Medical Society, and Blue Cross/Blue Shield. The visible presence of nurses from eleven nursing organizations as well as VSNA demonstrated that we do speak with one strong voice.

Vermont Recovering Professionals Program

The VSNA Task Force on Impairment Among Nurses began meeting in April 1985. In 1986, a resolution was introduced to "Continue and Expand the Charge of Task Force on Impairment Among Nurses." The charge included:

> To continue a cooperative effort with other health professionals, state authorities, licensing boards, and nurse employers in the development and promotion of uniform Peer Assistance Programs and accessible, affordable resources for treatment of impairment.[18]

The task force grew out of the Vermont Policy Group of the Prescription Abuse Data Synthesis (PADS) Project, on which VSNA had official representation.

In 1989, the Vermont Recovering Professional Program (VRPP) became an official nonprofit organization. Members included representatives of boards and associations from the following health care groups: physicians, dentists, pharmacists, nurses, and veterinarians; the Office of Drug and Alcohol Abuse; and legal counsel from the Secretary of State's Office. The VSNA Task Force on Impairment Among Nurses was integral to the development of VRPP. Once VRPP was formally organized, the task force was disbanded. The member organizations provided the financial support to allow the organization to function. VRPP was "an alternative to disciplinary action for that professional whose ability to practice is impaired due to dependence on, or abuse of, drugs or alcohol."[19] An additional goal was to provide a stronger support system.

From its inception, VRPP served more nurses than any other profession. This was partially a function of the fact that far more nurses are in practice than in any of the other professions represented. There also seemed to be a reluctance for professionals to acknowledge before members of other professions that they had a problem.

An executive director position was created in 1994. As the organization continued, philosophical differences developed over funding of care for those professionals seeking assistance, and how programs were being implemented. Funding decreased, although VSNA maintained its continuous—albeit limited—financial support. Although VRPP provided a valuable service in a small state with relatively small groups of professionals needing assistance, the lack of funding finally caused VRPP to cease operations at the end of 1996.

Vermont State Nurses' Foundation

Work began in 1995 on a sister organization to VSNA, the Vermont State Nurses' Foundation. Priscilla Allen and Lynne Dapice developed draft bylaws to begin to move the process forward. At the 1995 VSNA annual convention, the Articles of Association of VSNA were amended to permit a foundation. Founding purposes for the foundation were put forth as follows:

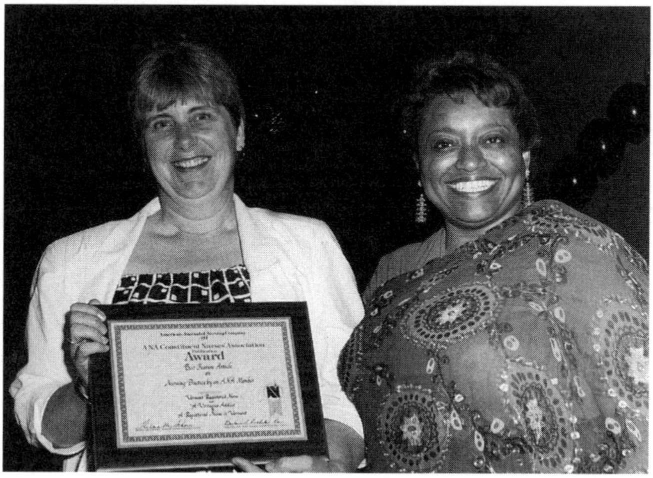

Bonnie Stiles, member of the editorial board of the *Vermont Registered Nurse*, accepts a national award from American Nurses' Association President Barbara Nichols, Louisville, Kentucky, 1988.

a. To make outright scholarship grants to nurses and students of nursing.
b. To expend funds for research in the public interest by nurses.
c. To increase public knowledge and understanding of nursing and the nursing profession and of the sciences and arts on which human health depends.
d. To support publication and distribution of reports, treatises and other literary works on nursing subjects.
e. To solicit, establish, maintain and administer funds necessary to accomplish these purposes.[20]

In 1996, a preliminary board of trustees was appointed to facilitate the process of incorporation and to achieve tax-exempt status.

Vermont Registered Nurse

The *Vermont Registered Nurse* (VRN), has been the primary means of informing members about the activities of VSNA and nursing in Vermont. It has been the official publication of the Vermont State Nurses' Association since 1935, growing from a four-page leaflet, to an eight-, to a twenty-page booklet; some convention issues were even larger. The format has ranged from professionally-prepared publications to mimeographed copies. There was a time when all the issues were pasted-up by hand, a laborious process that began by typing out the content to be printed in the typeface to be used in the publication. Then the articles were cut and pasted into the booklet format before taking it to the printer. That required a steady hand, a sure eye, and lots of time. With the computer age, the copy is desktop published and delivered to the printer. However the work was done, the end result was communication to the members and a valuable record of the work of the association.

The VRN has been the proud recipient of two special awards for outstanding feature articles. The first was in 1988 for "The Virtuous Addict," April 1987, by an anonymous author. The article recounted the author's journey into drug use while practicing nursing, and her recovery. In 1994 the award was for "To Russia with Love," June 1993, by Patricia Donehower. That article described the program developed by a Medical Center Hospital of Vermont registered nurse to travel to Russia with supplies and expertise to assist Russian nurses.

"Stimulate and Promote the Professional Development of Nurses and Advance Their Economic and General Welfare"

The history of workplace advocacy is central to understanding the dynamics of the Association. Nothing else the VSNA has been involved in has elicited the gamut and complexity of emotion as has this focus. Workplace issues and the concept of economic and general welfare encompass a wide range of activities. The most obvious are the economic pieces, with salary and benefits being the primary components. Included in general welfare are things like the length of shifts, occupational safety, staffing, and insurance coverage.

In the mid 1940s, movement related to workplace advocacy was gaining some momentum nationally. The issue was collective bargaining for nurses. On November 21, 1946, at the VSNA semiannual meeting, the gathered members were asked to consider a program on Economic Security as proposed by ANA. Anne Collison was reported as ". . . warning them to proceed cautiously and urging a complete survey of personal [sic] policies and practices throughout the state . . ."[21] Discussion centered around the idea that nursing would cease to be professional if a union told them what to do. As part of the examination of practices throughout the state, a survey was initiated. It found that the majority of hospitals in the state did utilize an eight-hour shift/48-hour week, as opposed to a twelve-hour shift/60-hour work week.

In the forties and fifties, discussion of workplace issues centered in the sections. The Private Duty Section made recommendations for fees that should be charged for varying shifts. Private duty nurses functioned both in the home and in the hospital. In 1956, the Private Duty Section recommended that private duty nurses should receive $18.00 for a twelve-hour shift, or $2.00 for the first hour, and $1.50/hour thereafter. Sections for General Duty nurses and Nursing Administrators were also active. There was no move toward collective bargaining during this period. It was a time of evaluation of work conditions; however, there were issues to pursue.

Bylaws changes in 1960 added, as a standing committee, the Economic and General Welfare Committee. Its functions included studying the ANA Economic Security Program, creating and reviewing policies and procedures for conducting a state program, formulating objectives and making recommendations to the board, preparing educational programs and materials, and making recommendations on related legislation. A statewide, coordinated approach with accountability to the VSNA Board of Trustees was formally launched.

In 1961, the Nursing Service Administrators (NSA) Section stated in their annual report that "The Section would like to go on record as fostering growth of an Economic Security Program."[22] The following year, although there was strong interest in related activities, VSNA withdrew a request to ANA for assistance in establishing consultation service from ANA related to the economic security program, because of staff and financial limitations. Financial and human resource limitations would continue to plague the development of economic and general welfare activities throughout the rest of the century.

In spite of the lack of resources to engage in bigger projects, in 1963 the NSA Section took on a project related to economic security by working on minimum employment standards as guidelines for all hospitals in the state in drawing up their own policies and salary scales. That work continued into the next year-and-a-half. Prior to the release of the standards, the General Duty Section reviewed them and had some points of disagreement. After a Committee of Conference between the General Duty Section and the Nursing Service Administrators, the differences were resolved and a statement of Employment Standards for General Duty Nurses and for Nursing Service Administrators, Supervisors, and Head Nurses was released May 1, 1965, with the date of October 1, 1965, as a date of effectiveness.

In the meantime, in 1965 the Private Duty Section released its latest salary recommendations: pay for an eight-hour shift should be $20.00, with an hourly rate of $5.00 for the first hour and $2.50/hour thereafter.

All workplace-related activities in the early 1960s were pursued in the sections. In 1967, as noted earlier, the sections were dissolved. The Economic and General Welfare Standing Committee was also eliminated from the structure.

The ongoing needs of nurses did not disappear. In 1969, an Ad Hoc Economic Security Committee met with the charge to explore the role of

VSNA in maintaining and improving the economic security of nurses in Vermont. The Economic Security Committee was added to the list of standing committees. It recommended that a permanent Economic Security Committee be formed with the following duties:

a. Establish a functioning mechanism to keep the committee informed of personnel policies and wages of all nurses, updated annually.
b. Recommend employment standards.
c. Set up grievance procedure.
d. Serve as Consultant.
e. Plan educational programs on Economics for Vermont nurses.[23]

The board approved a permanent committee which was composed of both staff nurses and nursing administrators. In fact, the chair of the committee, Ann M. Terhune, was an administrator at North Country Hospital.

In 1969, a resolution was passed related to salaries:

> BE IT RESOLVED that the Vermont State Nurses' Association make all effort to implement the ANA 1968 salary pronouncement of $7,500 per year for graduates of associate degree and diploma programs and $8,500 per year for graduates of baccalaureate programs.[24]

The work of 1970 was to implement the resolution. There were also workshops to educate the members and to develop standards for employment for nurses in Vermont.

In 1971, the Economic Security Committee became the Economic and General Welfare Committee (E&GW). Nurses at Medical Center Hospital of Vermont (MCHV) and Rutland, Brightlook, and Springfield Hospitals had petitioned hospital administrations for payroll deduction of SNA membership dues. It was recommended to the VSNA Board that Professional Performance Committees (PPCs) be formed on local levels. Executive Secretary Ann Janney was hired and assisted in the work of the E&GW Committee that developed a grievance procedure and guidelines for PPCs. A resolution was presented to the membership in 1971 to approve PPCs and also to allow those PPCs to act as bargaining representatives in the agencies. That resolution was passed unanimously. In 1972, PPCs were also developed for Directors of Nursing and supervisory personnel. To have a PPC, 51% of nurses had to approve and all 51% had to be members of ANA/VSNA. This provision had a positive impact on the numbers of VSNA members, which moved toward 700 members after decreasing to less than 325 in the middle 1950s. In 1972, Brattleboro Retreat Hospital formed a PPC. Rutland County agencies were forming a PPC. Efforts were also proceeding at the Springfield Hospital, Rutland Hospital, and North Country Hospital.

In 1974, the ANA E&GW supported the employment of the Director of the Massachusetts Nurses' Association E&GW to function as a consultant to Vermont. In the state, the VSNA membership voted the E&GW Program to be its top priority, and agreed to back the program financially as much as possible. At this juncture, the E&GW Committee became semi-autonomous of the VSNA board and funds for the committee were segregated from the VSNA budget. The board no longer appointed the members.

By 1975, there were PPCs at the following five hospitals: Brattleboro Memorial, Brattleboro Retreat, Northeast Vermont Regional (NVRH, St. Johnsbury), MCHV, and Springfield. VSNA membership climbed to 833. Membership dues were increased to $93.50. Petitions for certification to represent all registered nurses were filed with the National Labor Relations Board (NLRB) for NVRH, MCHV, and Brattleboro. The vote at Brattleboro was successful; however, votes at NVRH and MCHV were not.

In 1976, VSNA began having financial difficulties related to collective bargaining activity and tried unsuccessfully to get major grants. It was able to get a loan from ANA ($5,270). Membership dropped to 504 members. The E&GW Committee developed a policy that 51% of a bargaining unit must be members of VSNA.

VSNA assisted the nurses at Brattleboro Memorial Hospital in the development of their first contract in 1977. A consultant from New York State Nurses Association, who had also helped Vermont in 1975 and 1976, assisted. The financial straits of VSNA carried into the E&GW program. An application for a grant from ANA was turned down. While it was felt that the program was vital, concerns began to be voiced by even the E&GW Committee about the continuation of the committee. The financial problems led to there being no staff person for the program in 1978. Forty percent of the bargaining unit not only were not members, but paid no administrative fee.

In 1979, the Economic and General Welfare Committee recommended that VSNA consider affiliation with a traditional union for services. ANA continued to be unable or unwilling to assist the state. In 1980, VSNA voted to continue its commitment to collective bargaining, but stipulated that

1. at least 75 percent of those in any unit represented by VSNA had to be members of the association,
2. the units of nurses represented by VSNA be assessed a per capita tax to help defray some of the costs of collective bargaining, and
3. the E&GW Committee needed to look for ways to be self-sufficient.

In 1981, a labor relations consultant was hired to develop a proposal to fund collective bargaining. In the spring of 1981, ANA awarded Maine, New Hampshire, & Vermont a one-year critical assistance Tri-State Grant of $2,000 to partially pay the cost of contract negotiations. When application for a continuation of that grant was considered, VSNA decided to withdraw from the Tri-State grant. It was apparent that it would require progressive VSNA financial involvement up to $32,000 by 1987. The difficulties were exacerbated by the fact that VSNA had no Executive Director. Relations with the Brattleboro Unit were strained with few members of the unit being VSNA members, and agency fees were in arrears. At the May 1, 1982 meeting, the board unanimously agreed that it was opposed to representing Brattleboro in future negotiations.[25]

All collective bargaining activity of VSNA ended with a motion passed at the board meeting in January of 1983, effective on September 15, 1983. Retrospectively, members recall a process which was far more costly, difficult, and acrimonious than anticipated. The time involved in the intense workplace activity was a journey of hope, excitement, frustration, anger, and sadness. As a very small state association, VSNA had neither the financial and human resources nor the expertise to accomplish this important work.

Although VSNA was unable to sustain collective bargaining, ANA and VSNA bylaws indicate that it is a service that should be available to members. After much consideration, the VSNA passed a "Shared Services between State Nurses' Associations" resolution in 1989 that included the following section:

> RESOLVED, that on the occasion that a nurse or a group of nurses within Vermont request(s) a service from VSNA that VSNA does not provide that nurse or group of nurses shall be referred to another SNA. These services may include but not be limited to legal services, peer assistance, collective bargaining, research, provision of continuing education, grant writing, and other services.[26]

New York State Nurses Association (NYSNA) initiated action at Medical Center Hospital of Vermont in 1991. NYSNA requested that VSNA endorse their presence; however, the VSNA Board of Directors felt that it was inappropriate to support that activity, but they also did not oppose it.

The controversy about VSNA's role in the workplace subsided only briefly. For VSNA board members, it was increasingly clear that workplace advocacy was much more encompassing than just collective bargaining. It included occupational safety, patient rights, ethics, and even practice (e.g., adequate staffing). In 1996, calls related to assistance with workplace issues began increasing from nurses throughout the state. The dilemma once again surfaced about how VSNA should meet its bylaws'

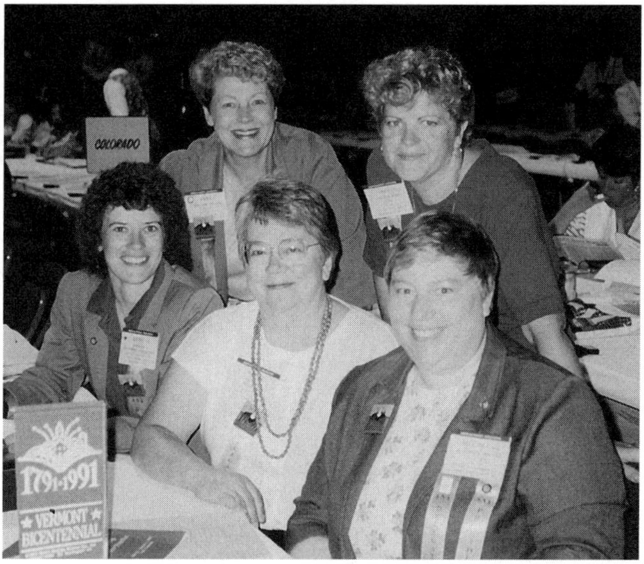

1991, ANA House of Delegates, Kansas City
Left to right, back row: Lynne Dapice, Laurie Murray; *front row:*
Deborah Hayward Sanguinetti, Rachael Burroughs, Michelle Walker

responsibilities to facilitate collective bargaining services for its members. The story is not over; in fact there is every indication that it will become more complex. The only thing that is clear is that VSNA is no more able—financially or in appropriate human resources and expertise—to manage collective bargaining on their own now, than they were in the seventies. The answer has to lie in another direction.[27]

"Serve Vermont Nurses as the Constituent Association of the American Nurses' Association"

Representation to the ANA House of Delegates throughout this period has been based on the number of members. Vermont has always had at least three delegates with one of those delegates being the president. Minutes and reports in the *Vermont Registered Nurse* often note people being referred to as delegates to the House of Delegates. For example, minutes of many of the sections allude to a member of the group being sent as a delegate. Whether they were delegates only of that group to have someone there, or whether they had official standing is unclear. In 1976, when the membership was 833, VSNA had five official delegates. For at least the last 20 years, VSNA has had four official delegates.

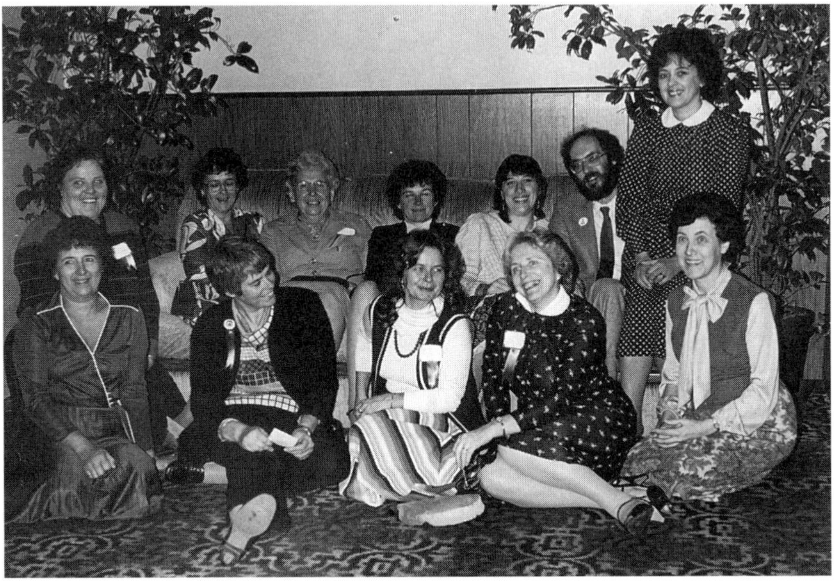

Vermont State Nurses' Association, Board of Directors, 1983.
Back row left to right, Linda Ellis, Anne Logsdon, Virginia North, Audrey Swarkowski Larrow, Catherine Howland, Alan Sousie, and Anita Ristau; *Front row,* Carol Livingston, Hilary Smith, Janet Patterson, Caroline Frey, and Barbara Beeker.

Delegates understand that they represent the general membership of VSNA when they participate in the ANA House of Delegates. Issues which impact nursing and health care are discussed and supported or negated. The decisions are used to guide legislative and policy work for ANA during the coming years. Most states also adapt many of the activities which are locally relevant. No other nursing association has the policy power that ANA has developed over the years.

Conclusion

When reviewing the documents related to the history of the Vermont State Nurses' Association, several things impressed me. There has been an enormous amount of important activity that was begun, but that could not be sustained because of the ongoing fragile financial status of the association. The activity of the Association has always been for the benefit of all nurses, not just those who pay membership dues. Although VSNA now represents only about 5% of the nurses in the state, its presence still provides representation for all nurses in matters of public policy. It advocates for quality health care for all Vermonters. It ever guards the right of all Vermont registered nurses to practice their profession in many different arenas and in many different ways.

The numbers of nurses through the years who have donated an extraordinary amount of time and energy to VSNA are overwhelming. As executive director, I found it amazing that a remarkably high percentage of members found time each year to participate in the association. When that is multiplied by fifty years, it is even more impressive. We salute and thank them all. There are names which appear again and again. Some names appear for a period of many years—eternal flames. Others burn brightly and intensely for a shorter number of years. A few burn intensely for many years. They keep the light of nursing bright. May the light of the lantern represented in the VSNA seal ever stay lit.

—Lynne Ann Dapice, MS, RN

NOTES

1. Margaret Luce, interview by Bonnie Stiles, 19 May 1998, audiotape in Vermont State Nurses' Association Office, Winooski, Vermont.
2. Vermont State Nurses' Association, *Fifty Years of Progress: Past/Prospective* (Winooski, Vt.: VSNA, 1964).
3. Ibid.
4. A copy of the entire resolution can be found in the "VSNA 75th Jubilee Convention Program," 1989, 19.
5. *Vermont Registered Nurse* (newsletter of the Vermont State Nurses' Association) (November 1978), 29.
6. "Task Force on Entry into Practice," *Vermont Registered Nurse* 51, no. 4: 9–10, 12.
7. Minutes of the Meeting of VSNA Board of Directors, 28 June 1944. Vermont State Nurses' Association Special Collection, Library Research Annex, The University of Vermont, Burlington (hereafter cited as VSNA Archives), box 11.
8. *Vermont Registered Nurse* (September 1959): 25.
9. *Vermont Registered Nurse* IV, no. 4 (1974): 34.
10. *Vermont Registered Nurse* (June 1984): 10.
11. *Vermont Registered Nurse* (November 1975): 18.
12. Kathryn Lambert, "Vermont State Nurses' Association, Inc. Statement and Proposal on Continuing Education for Nurses in Vermont," *Vermont Registered Nurse* (Fall Convention issue, 1972): 21–22.
13. Sylvia Morse, *Vermont Registered Nurse* (April 1977): 27.
14. Department of Health, Education, and Welfare, Public Health Service Training Grant Application, Vermont State Nurses' Association Council on Nursing Practice, 1978. VSNA Archives, box 10.
15. "Convention '79" *Vermont Registered Nurse* (1979): 33.
16. Sylvia Morse, *Vermont Registered Nurse* (December 1980): 6.
17. Pat Allen, "President's Message," *Vermont Registered Nurse* 51, no. 2 (1985): 5.
18. *Vermont Registered Nurse* 52, no. 5 (1986): 9.

19. *Vermont Registered Nurse* 55, no. 4 (1989): 17.
20. *Vermont Registered Nurse* 61, no. 4 (1995): 1.
21. Minutes of Meeting of Vermont State Nurses' Association, 21 November 1946, VSNA Archives, box 11.
22. "Official Call: 47th Annual Convention," *Vermont Registered Nurse* (1961): 11.
23. Ann M. Terhune, "Official Call–55th Annual Convention," *Vermont Registered Nurse* (1969): 12–13.
24. "VSNA Convention Call: Partners or Puppets," *Vermont Registered Nurse* (1970): 15.
25. *Vermont Registered Nurse* (July 1982): 6.
26. *Vermont Registered Nurse* 55, no. 5 (1989): 8.
27. Resources for this section include an unpublished manuscript by Alan Sousie, former VSNA President.

Vermont State Nurses' Association, Inc.

		Annual Meeting			
Years	*President*	*Date*	*Place*	*Theme*	*Executive Secretary/ Executive Director**
1940–1941	Helen Marsden	June 25–26, 1941	Burlington City Hall		Abbie L. Starkey
1941–1942	Jessie Grant	June 17–18, 1942	Barre		Abbie L. Starkey
1942–1943	Mary Harty	June 23–24, 1943	Mendon Jr High, Rutland		Abbie L. Starkey
1943–1944	Mary Harty	June 28–29, 1944	Brooks, Brattleboro		Abbie L. Starkey
1944–1945	Hortense Harwood	June 7–8, 1945	Hotel Putnam Memorial Hospital, Bennington		Abbie L. Starkey
1945–1946	Hortense Harwood	June 13–14, 1946	Fleming Museum, Burlington		Abbie L. Starkey
1946–1947	R. Anne Collison	June 2–3, 1947	Barre City Armory		Olga Dittig
1947–1948	Gladys Hinds	Sept. 24–25, 1948	Bellows Falls		Olga Dittig
1948–1949	Esther Martinson	Sept. 26–27, 1949	Fuller Hall, St. Johnsbury		No Executive Secretary
1949–1950	Esther Martinson	Oct. 16–17, 1950	Mary Fletcher Hospital		No Executive Secretary
1950–1951	Grace Buttolph	Sept. 13–14, 1951	Armory Rutland		No Executive Secretary
1951–1952	Rosa Zeller	Oct. 20–21, 1952	Knights of Columbus Hall, Bennington		No Executive Secretary
1952–1953	Rosa Zeller	Sept. 29–30, 1953	Redstone Campus, UVM, Burlington	Calling Vermont Nurses to Action	No Executive Secretary
1953–1954	Florence Tyler	Sept. 27–28, 1954	Barre Municipal Auditorium	You and Economic Security	No Executive Secretary
1954–1955	Florence Tyler	Sept. 26–27, 1955	Grange Hall, Middlebury	Cooperative Planning for Patient Care	No Executive Secretary
1955–1956	Florence Tyler	Sept. 24–25, 1956	Community Building, Brattleboro		No Executive Secretary
1956–1957	Joyce B. Riddel	Sept. 30, Oct. 1, 1957	First Congregational Church, Burlington		No Executive Secretary
1957–1958	Joyce B. Riddel	Sept. 29–30, 1958	Pavilion Hotel, Montpelier	The General Duty Nurse: The Backbone of Nursing	M. Patricia Chase, RN
1958–1959	Joyce B. Riddel	Sept. 28–29, 1959	Mead Community House		M. Patricia Chase, RN
1959–1960	Joyce B. Riddel	Sept. 26–27, 1960	Bennington		M. Patricia Chase, RN

* In 1983, the position of Executive Secretary was retitled to Executive Director.

Vermont State Nurses' Association, Inc.

Years	President	Annual Meeting: Date	Annual Meeting: Place	Annual Meeting: Theme	*Executive Secretary/ Executive Director**
1960–1961	Philip E. Day	Sept. 25–26, 1961	Hotel Vermont, Burlington	Improved Nursing Practice: Better Patient Care	M. Patricia Chase, RN
1961–1962	Philip E. Day	Sept. 24–25, 1962	Barre Municipal Auditorium		M. Patricia Chase, RN
1962–1963	Jean Milligan	Sept. 23–24, 1963	First Congregational Church and the Hartness House, Springfield		M. Patricia Chase, RN
1963–1964	Jean Milligan	Sept. 28–29, 1964	Edmunds High School, Burlington	Fiftieth Anniversary The Past—Fifty Years of Progress The Future—Commitment or Complacency?	M. Patricia Chase, RN
1964–1965	Sr. Evaline Barrett, RHSJ	Sept. 27–28, 1965	North Congregational Church, St. Johnsbury	VSNA—A Long, Hard Look	M. Patricia Chase, RN
1965–1966	Sr. Evaline Barrett, RHSJ	Sept. 19–20, 1966	Lodge Motel & Restaurant, Bellows Falls		M. Patricia Chase, RN
1966–1967	Sr. Evaline Barrett, RHSJ	Oct. 16–17, 1967	Town & Country Motor Lodge, Stowe	Soul Searching for VSNA	M. Patricia Chase, RN
1967–1968	Sr. Evaline Barrett, RHSJ	Sept. 23–24, 1968	Tavern Motor Inn, Montpelier	Is the Role of the Vermont Nurse Changing?	M. Patricia Chase, RN
1968–1969	Ruby C. Carr	Oct. 27–28, 1969	Stratton Mountain Inn, Stratton, VT	Are Vermont Nurses Nursing In Space Or In A Vacuum?	No Executive Secretary
1969–1970	Ruby C. Carr	Sept. 28–29, 1970	Basin Harbor Club, Vergennes	Partners or Puppets	No Executive Secretary
1970–1971	Marie Schoff	Sept. 27–28, 1971	Sugarbush Inn, Warren	Quality Patient Care	Anne Janney
1971–1972	Marie Schoff	Oct. 19–20, 1972	Fox Run, Ludlow	$67.50: Your Investment in Your Future	Anne Janney
1972–1973	Fernando A. Duran	Oct. 24–25, 1973	Bolton Valley	Practice and Politics	Anne Janney
1973–1974	Fernando A. Duran	Oct. 24–25, 1974	Lake Morey Inn, Fairlee	Winds of Change	Anne Janney
1974–1975	Jeanette (Jan) Folta	Oct. 16–17, 1975	Cortina Inn, Rutland	Florence's or Rosamund's Web	Anne Janney
1975–1976	Jeanette (Jan) Folta	Nov. 5–6, 1976	Montpelier		Anne Janney
1976–1977	Jeanette (Jan) Folta	Oct. 21–22, 1977	Fox Run Inn, Ludlow	Survival	Anne Janney

* In 1983, the position of Executive Secretary was retitled to Executive Director.

Vermont State Nurses' Association, Inc.

Years	President	Annual Meeting: Date	Place	Theme	Executive Secretary/ Executive Director*
1977–1978	Jeanette (Jan) Folta	Nov. 3–4, 1978	Radisson Hotel, Burlington		No Executive Secretary
1978–1979	Mary Ellen Henry	Oct. 19–20, 1979	Stowehof Inn, Stowe	Looking at Lifestyle: Listen; Talk; Learn; and Enjoy!	No Executive Secretary
1979–1980	Mary Ellen Henry	Oct. 17–18, 1980	Cortina Inn, Rutland	Harmony for the Future: Let's Take Ourselves Seriously	No Executive Secretary
1980–1981	Alan Sousie	Nov. 6–7, 1981	Middlebury Inn	Challenge: Shaping Health Care For the Future	No Executive Secretary
1981–1982	Alan Sousie	Nov. 5–6, 1982	Tavern Inn, Montpelier	Nursing In Vermont: Who's in Charge?	No Executive Secretary
1982–1983	Janet Patterson	Oct. 28–29, 1983	Quality Inn, Brattleboro	Convention '83: Voices of Nursing	Vacant/Eileen Lauer
1983–1984	Janet Patterson	Oct. 26–27, 1984	Radisson Hotel, Burlington	Creativity in Nursing	Eileen Lauer
1984–1985	Priscilla (Pat) Allen	Nov. 1–2, 1985	Lake Morey Inn, Fairlee	Focus on Families	Eileen Lauer
1985–1986	Priscilla (Pat) Allen	Oct. 31–Nov. 1, 1986	The Centre of VT at Holiday Inn, Rutland	Ethics: A Dilemma For Nurses	RoseMarie Bagioni
1986–1987	Kathleen Mariak	Sept. 25–26, 1987	Radisson Hotel, Burlington	Unity in Nursing Today and Tomorrow	RoseMarie Bagioni
1987–1988	Kathleen Mariak	Oct. 20–21, 1988	Bolton Valley Resort, Bolton	Nursing: Empowering, Surviving, Progressing	Lynn Hardee
1988–1989	Margaret Luce	Oct. 19–20, 1989	Stratton Mountain Inn	75th Anniversary Look to the Past: Plan for the Future	Hollace Reed
1989–1990	Margaret Luce	Nov. 1–2, 1990	Radisson Hotel, Burlington	Nursing: 1990s and Beyond	Hollace Reed
1990–1991	Michelle Walker	Nov. 7–8, 1991	Topnotch Resort, Stowe	Excellence in Practice	Hollace Reed/L. Dapice
1991–1992	Michelle Walker	Nov. 5–6, 1992	Cortina Inn, Rutland	Change, a Positive Force for Nursing	Lynne A. Dapice
1992–1993	Debra Clemmer	Oct. 28–29, 1993	Sheraton Hotel, Burlington	Nursing—Advancing Health Care in Vermont	Lynne A. Dapice
1993–1994	Debra Clemmer	Oct. 27–28, 1994	Topnotch Resort, Stowe	The Changing Faces of Nursing	Lynne A. Dapice
1994–1995	Judith Cohen	Oct. 26–27, 1995	Cortina Inn, Rutland	Nurses: One Voice, One Goal	Lynne A. Dapice
1995–1996	Judith Cohen	Oct. 24–25, 1996	Radisson Hotel, Burlington	Striving and Thriving in Times of Transition	Lynne A. Dapice
1996–1997	Elizabeth Carney	Oct. 23–24, 1997	Capitol Plaza Hotel, Montpelier	Ride the Healing Wave: Create New Environments	Lynne A. Dapice

* In 1983, the position of Executive Secretary was retitled to Executive Director.

The Vermont League for Nursing

EARLY IN THE TWENTIETH CENTURY—1913 to be exact—Vermont nurses and consumer members of the National League for Nursing Education came together to form the Vermont League for Nursing Education (VLNE).[1] Over the ensuing years, the group was primarily representative of nurse leaders from hospitals, schools of nursing, and public health agencies; however, it was not recognized by the National League for Nursing Education (NLNE) as a "constituent" state league until May 1946.[2]

On March 15, 1946, twenty Vermont members of the national organization met in Burlington, Vermont for the first organizational meeting of the Vermont League for Nursing Education.[3] In May, the VLNE was recognized as a bonafide constituent league. In-state activities were carried out through five committees:[4]

Curriculum Committee	Grace Buttolph, Chairman
Membership Campaign	Eleanor Dyke, Chairman
Psychiatric Nursing	Catherine Terrien, Chairman
Measurement and Educational Guidance	Mary Ferry, Chairman
State Board Problems	Not Identified

The VLNE clearly stated its relationship with the Vermont State Nurses' Association: "The Vermont League functions as the department of education of the State Nurses Association."[5]

Various archival documents indicate a transition in 1952 from the VLNE to the Vermont League for Nursing (VLN). Nationally, the National League for Nursing had replaced the NLNE by vote of the membership in 1952. The July 7, 1952, issue of the VLNE newsletter reports activities directed toward dissolving the VLNE and forming the VLN. This structural change was occurring throughout the nation with guidance from the national organization. Anna Fillmore's letter of July 30, 1953 to Geraldine Labecki, president of the VLN, reports a total of forty-five reorganizations and welcomes VLN as a branch of the National League for Nursing (NLN).

Organization purposes are reflected in the VLN constitution and by-laws:

> The object of this organization will be to foster the development and improvement of hospital, industrial, public health, and other organized nursing services and of nursing education through the coordinated action of nurses, allied professional groups, citizens, agencies and schools, to the end that the nursing needs of the people will be met.[6]

The by-laws outlined the following functions:

1. To assess resources and needs and to develop programs for the improvement of nursing services and nursing education.
2. To cooperate with . . .
   The NLN in implementing its national program through the VLN;
   the VSNA, Inc. in working for unified support of nursing education and service in all fields of nursing;
   other services and professional groups
3. To represent organized nursing services and nursing education in Vermont and in regional planning.
4. To cooperate with other services, professional and governmental groups, and with the public in regard to matters related to the purpose of the Vermont League for Nursing.[7]

Many members of the VLN were also members of the VSNA. The primary difference between the organizations was that the VLN provided for and encouraged consumer/nonnurse membership. Unfortunately, large numbers of consumers were not attracted to membership in the VLN; and the small Vermont nurse population presented problems of duplication of activity and dual membership resulting in time and energy problems for some members.

A coordinating committee of the VLN and the VSNA was created to facilitate organizational activities and to avoid duplication and competition. In December of 1962, the VLN-VSNA Coordinating Committee appointed a committee to study the amalgamation of the two organizations.[8] The findings of the study committee are reflected in the resolution adopted by VLN members in 1964:

> In view of the geographic distribution of membership and lack of manpower, and to more effectively utilize personnel, the Nursing Service Division of the Vermont League for Nursing does hereby make a resolution to inactivate the Vermont League for Nursing and recommends that we direct our energies to the professional nursing organization in the state.[9]

The vote for dissolution was by mail ballot. The official date of dissolution was October 15, 1964. VLN funds were equally divided and given to each of the four VSNA district organizations to be used for educational programs within the district.[10]

Although its tenure was limited to twelve years, the accomplishments of the Vermont League for Nursing were important ones, with long-term impact on nursing in Vermont; that impact is still apparent in this last decade of the twentieth century. The Vermont Plan improved communications between schools of nursing and Vermont high schools. The Conference on Nursing Education considered the merits of the associate degree program in nursing. The Council on Practical Nursing was formulated by the VLN in 1960, and refresher courses for nurses were planned and provided throughout the state in 1962 and 1963.[11]

The Vermont Plan, initiated by the VLN in 1964, became the "Committee on Nursing Careers [that] is administratively responsible to the VLN but is sponsored and assisted financially by the VSNA and other allied organizations."[12] Future Nurses Clubs were organized in Vermont high schools; hospital tours were offered to students interested in nursing as a career; a Speakers Bureau targeted the high schools; and a directory of Vermont schools of nursing was developed as well as a brochure describing Vermont nursing programs and featuring the nursing caps of each.

The purpose of the VLN's Conference on Nursing Education was:

> To encourage the establishment of schools of nursing at the junior college and practical nurse level as one step toward increasing the supply of nursing personnel; encourage increased scholarship assistance to all nursing students including graduate nurses who wish to prepare for ward administration and teaching and to encourage studies relating to the utilization of nursing personnel.[13]

The Vermont Conference on Nursing Education was sponsored by the VLN and the Vermont Board of Registration of Nurses in cooperation with NLN, Inc., Vermont Medical Society, Vermont Hospital Association, and the VSNA, Inc. The Conference was held at the Pavilion Hotel, Montpelier, Vermont, April 25–27, 1956.[14]

The ongoing work of the members of the Conference resulted in the development of associate degree and practical nursing programs in Vermont. Coincidental to these intensive efforts was the passage of the mandatory nursing law in 1961, and the move of the Vermont State Board of Nursing from 323 Pearl Street, Burlington, to Riverside Annex in Montpelier.[15]

—Priscilla (Pat) Allen, RN, MSN

NOTES

1. Vermont League for Nursing Education, reports of officers, 1913. Vermont State Nurses' Association Special Collection, Library Research Annex, The University of Vermont, Burlington (hereafter cited as VSNA Archives), VLN box 2.
2. National League for Nursing Education, *53rd Annual Report*, 82. VSNA Archives, VLN box 2.
3. National League for Nursing Education, *52rd Annual Report*, 75. VSNA Archives, VLN box 2.
4. See note 2.
5. Ibid.
6. Vermont League for Nursing By-laws, 1962, Article I. VSNA Archives, VLN box 2.
7. Ibid., Article II.
8. Vermont League for Nursing–Vermont State Nurses' Association Coordinating Committee Report, 1963. VSNA Archives, VLN box 2.
9. Vermont League for Nursing, Minutes of Board of Directors, 11 September 1964. VSNA Archives, VLN box 2.
10. Vermont League for Nursing Newsletter, June 1964, 4. VSNA Archives, VLN box 2.
11. Vermont League for Nursing President's letter, 1 October 1964. VSNA Archives, VLN box 2.
12. Vermont League for Nursing, Minutes of Annual Meeting, 2 June 1964. VSNA Archives, VLN box 2.
13. G. Labecki in letter to Senator W. Prouty, 2 July 1956. VSNA Archives, VLN box 2.
14. Program of Vermont League for Nursing, Conference on Nursing Education, April 1956. VSNA Archives, VLN box 2.
15. Vermont State Board of Nursing, press release January 1963. VSNA Archives, VLN box 2.

School Nursing and the Vermont Experience

SCHOOL NURSING has evolved from Public Health Nursing, which had its origin in Liverpool, England, in 1858. In Liverpool, the first "district" nurses were employed to provide home care for the sick. As early as 1837, France mandated health supervision of school children and enforcement of sanitary conditions by school authorities. Brussels, Belgium, was the first city to employ a regular school physician to establish a system of school health inspections. The first employment of a nurse in the schools was in London in 1892, when Amy Hughes was hired for the purpose of investigating the nutritional status of school children. The first health services in the United States were medical inspections begun in the Boston schools in 1894. These inspections were to identify and exclude students with communicable diseases.

Lillian Wald was instrumental in directing the focus of both public health and school nursing in this country. Having helped to establish New York City's Henry Street Settlement, she visited England and saw the possibilities of school nursing. She approached the New York City School Board and offered to place a public health nurse in selected schools to combat communicable diseases, thereby reducing absenteeism. In September 1902, Lina Rogers Struthers became the first American school nurse. Following the impact of her work, additional school nurses were soon hired in New York and elsewhere. Miss Wald is recognized today for her efforts on behalf of school nursing. The Lillian Wald Research Award is awarded annually by the National Association of School Nurses.

In the 1920s and 1930s, school nurses primarily assisted physicians in curbing communicable disease. They introduced health education aimed at developing responsible health behaviors in students and parents.

In the 1940s during World War II, there was increased emphasis on school health. It was discovered that a large number of supposedly healthy young males needed for the draft had physical deficiencies. There was increased interest in the vision- and hearing-impaired child, as well as in the handicapped children's classes for children experiencing the after-effects of polio. Dental health gained prominence, as did health counseling. This expanded role of the school nurse necessitated additional educational preparation. By 1949, sixteen states required certification of the nurse to work in the school.

Family life education in the school setting involved the school nurse in the 1950s. There was a renewed interest in sound nutrition, thus the school lunch program was born. Positive mental health was stressed. Health education, formal and informal, was viewed as an important role for the school nurse.

The 1960s and 1970s brought an era of rapid social change. Health and welfare programs abounded, though many were short-lived. The emphasis on the needs of the handicapped child within the regular school program had a definite impact on the life of the school nurse. At the same time, the health needs and concerns of the traditional school-age child were changing. The increased problems of drug abuse, teenage pregnancy, delinquency, divorce and the decline of the family structure, the legal mandate PL94-142—all required the school nurse to expand skills. To increase the preparation of school nurses, attention was paid to certification. The school nurse was encouraged to earn a baccalaureate degree. In the 1970s, the School Nurse Practitioner Program was developed. This required an extensive post-educational program for nurses, and an ongoing preceptorship with a pediatrician.

Beginning in 1986, the school nurse could become certified (CSN) by the National Board of Certification of School Nurses after successful completion of an examination. There is an active national organization of school nurses (National Association of School Nurses) composed of state and individual memberships. The association publishes a quarterly magazine and newsletter.

Vermont State School Nurses' Association, Inc.

On October 13, 1944, twenty-three Vermont school nurses met in Burlington as a part of the Vermont Association for Health, Physical Education, and Recreation. Mrs. Hortense Harwood from the Vermont Department of Public Health served as temporary chairperson. The following October, school nurses decided to meet one day annually and to assess dues of fifty cents.

In 1949, there was the first indication that the Department of Education recognized the need for a health concerns consultant. There were a handful of school nurses in Vermont; a Director of Health and Physical Education was established and a joint school health committee formed.

November of 1961 saw the formation of the Vermont School Nurses' Organization. Plans were made to write a constitution and to request affiliation with the Vermont Education Association. Dues had increased to two dollars per year by April of 1962. Speech therapists and dental hygienists were included in the organization by 1964.

Title I funds came into existence in 1966. Many school districts hired school nurses under this federal program, thereby increasing the number of school nurses to eighty-five. During this year, the Department of Education sponsored a working conference for new school nurses. The Department recommended that a Supervisor of School Health Services and School Health Instruction was needed to improve and coordinate these services. The increased numbers of school nurses employed by Vermont schools made the Vermont School Nurses' Association a stronger organization. The Association was notified that the National Education Association now had a School Nurse Division.

In 1970, the Association sent a letter to the Vermont Commissioner of Education requesting a School Nurse Consultant. In response, the Vermont Department of Education placed the school nurses in the Pupil Personnel section of the Division of Special Education and Pupil Personnel Services. Shortly thereafter, the Vermont Department of Health approached the Education Department about creating a cooperative School Nurse Consultant position. In October of 1971, Mrs. Carolyn Harris was introduced to the organization as the School Nurse Consultant for the State of Vermont, working under the Department of Education and Department of Health, and in cooperation with Shirley Reid, Pupil Personnel Services Consultant.

In 1971, Beginning School Nurse workshops were organized by Claire LeFrancois of the Department of Health. This program continues today as a three-day program, two days in August and one in October, and provides a school nurse mentor for each new school nurse. A cooperative effort of the Vermont Department of Education and VSSNA, the program works toward maintaining a quality school health program in Vermont schools.

Carolyn Harris wrote and secured a major grant utilizing HURA (Health Underserved Rural Areas) funds to train school nurse practitioners. Twelve school nurses were selected and completed the program over a period of three years.

A subcommittee of VSSNA met and in 1972 developed a document, ("School Nurse Functions") for the purpose of delineating Vermont school nurse functions within the schools and thereby improving the quality and consistency of health services. This document was revised, printed in booklet form, and distributed to all Vermont school nurses, superintendents, principals, and special educators. This document continues to be updated as needed, and is monitored through the Association's Strategic Planning Process.

The School Nurses' Association divided the state into five districts, and in 1974 each elected a representative to the Executive Board. Districts were encouraged to meet on their own during the year. This structure improved communication among the school nurses.

Audrey Poole replaced Carolyn Harris as school nurse consultant in

1978. A major effort was mounted for passage of a Vermont immunization law that was finally implemented in 1979. Vermont was one of the last three states to have such a law.

In 1972, the name Vermont School Nurses' Association was changed to Vermont State School Nurses' Association (VSSNA). Constitution revisions were approved by the Association in 1972, 1979, 1987, and 1996.

In 1981, due to funding restrictions, the position of school nurse consultant in the Department of Health was eliminated, and Shirley Reid, Program Specialist for Guidance and Health Services in the Department of Education, took over the position of school nurse consultant. In October 1981, a VSSNA logo was chosen. Also, at this time, a budget was presented to the membership and accepted, with dues being raised to five dollars annually.

In 1983, presidents of the New England school nurses' state organizations met, setting up a rotation of conferences around the New England states. A committee of representatives from each state presently coordinates this New England Regional School Nurse Conference that continues to rotate among the states annually each May. Also in this year, several school nurses completed the School Nurse Achievement Program (SNAP), a course from the University of Colorado which included instruction in serving students with handicapping conditions and use of health care plans and the nursing process.

A School Nurse Evaluation Committee was established in 1984. It enabled superintendents, principals, or school nurses to ask for a school nurse evaluation to be done by a trained group of school nurse peers. This exists today as the Professional Standards Committee, and it has performed evaluations of school health service programs for school districts who request such evaluation. Their recommendation includes an in-depth program evaluation of services and staff coverage within a district, not an individual assessment of a school nurse's job skills. Additional duties of the committee revolve around professional development and ethical issues.

An Eye Bank (money fund) to be used for eye care costs for children in the primary grades was established by the Vermont Order of Odd Fellows–Rebekahs and administered by VSSNA. This program went out of existence in 1997, when the Rebekah organization was unable to continue funding.

In addition, Vermont revised its school standards (Public School Approval Process) for all schools in 1984 with input from school nurses for the school health services component. This revision had a positive impact on the quality of school health services in Vermont.

In 1985, VSSNA became an affiliate of the National Association of School Nurses (NASN), forming a network with school nurses across the country. Each state has one representative to the two board meetings held each year. NASN also holds an annual membership meeting and convention. Vermont has had active representation to NASN. Cynthia Rugg was the first representative and Elaine Taboskey-Wade served as the national president in 1992–93.

A Time Study of participating Vermont school nurses was also done in 1985, giving the school nurses data with which to measure priorities and to plan for standardizing school nurse practice in Vermont.

In 1986, a major contribution to school nursing was made by the printing of the "Vermont School Health Services Standards of Practice Manual." This document was drafted by the School Health Services Task Force, a committee of VSSNA members, who worked with the Vermont Medical Society–School Health Committee. This task force was convened by Shirley Reid, program specialist for guidance and health services with the Department of Education. The task force went on to be established as an Advisory Committee to the Vermont Department of Education. The manual was endorsed by the Vermont State Board of Education, the Vermont Board of Health, the Vermont State Board of Nursing, and the Vermont Medical Society–School Health Committee as the standard for school health services in Vermont schools. Annual updates were distributed by the Advisory Committee and the Vermont Department of Education to keep each school manual current. A full revision of the "Vermont School Health Services Standards of Practice Manual" was completed by the Committee in June of 1997, and submitted for approval to the Vermont State Medical Society–School Health Committee, the Vermont Board of Health, the Vermont Board of Education, and the Vermont State Board of Nursing. New manuals will be available to schools by 2000.

The Advisory Committee has established a three-year rotating representation process and includes school nurses and nurse educators from area institutions of higher learning. This committee, which meets regularly throughout the year, addresses issues relating to school nursing practice. It works closely with the VSSNA to remain proactive in addressing school health issues.

From 1988 onward, VSSNA has worked extensively with the Vermont State Board of Nursing to support and clarify the nursing rules as they relate to school nursing practice. Board opinions have been elicited on delegation, unlicensed personnel, and medication administration.

VSSNA conferences continue to be held twice a year, in October at the time of the Vermont–NEA (National Education Association) Convention and in April. These conferences are hosted by districts following a rotation schedule around the state. Program workshops are held following the business meetings. VSSNA sponsors other workshops, conferences, and courses throughout the year, including the popular three-day "Introduction to School Nursing Practice" in August. Programs pertinent to school health practice are chosen as topics for conferences and vary with the focus or concerns of the time. Judy Igoe, a national leader in school nursing, was the featured presenter for the Spring 1997 conference. Relicensing credit is recommended according to the number of hours of participation.

The Association promotes the professional development of its school nurses. Two Vermont school nurse practitioners, Debbie Christie-Maples and Karen Reedstrom, were sent to training offered by NASN for a physical assessment course entitled the PASS Project. They returned to Vermont and made the PASS Project Assessment Course available to school nurses in the state. This program has undergone revision and updating and new versions are offered periodically.

The Association, in conjunction with the Department of Education, promotes programs for assistive personnel training. Schools are providing services for students with multiple handicaps and many social, emotional, and behavioral disorders. Delegation of duties is necessary to provide services to these students and others, and to provide coverage for school nurses serving multiple schools or schools with part-time nursing services. The need for training unlicensed assistive personnel to properly carry out the delegated duties was recognized and addressed.

Shirley Reid served in the capacity of Program Specialist for School Health Services and Guidance until her retirement in 1991. She was honored by VSSNA members for her support to Vermont schools for a quality school health program, and her role in organizing the task force to bring about one of the first national school health services standards-of-practice manuals. After her retirement, Sara Simpson assumed this role for the Department of Education. This position underwent a variety of changes as the Department struggled to meet the needs and demands placed upon it by government and changes in our society. The position went unfilled for a period of time when Sara left in 1993.

In March 1995, this position was partially reinstated and Mary Gill, a Vermont school nurse, was employed as School Health Services Program Specialist for one day a week. This was subsequently increased to two days a week by additional funding from the Department of Health. VSSNA developed a position paper on the need for this position, and submitted it to the Commissioner of Education. The Association continues to actively promote the establishment of a full-time school nurse in such a position.

In addition, the Association has developed a Strategic Plan and an Action Plan which direct Association activities and address the needs of the organization and its members. This plan was last updated in 1996.

VSSNA Board of Directors meetings are held periodically throughout the year, and individual districts meet as time permits, from one to five times a year. The membership list has been computerized, and storage space for records is provided at the Vermont–NEA office in Montpelier. The Association is incorporated and is a tax-exempt organization.

During this period, the association enlisted VSSNA member Linda Kane to develop a video in conjunction with the Lyndon State College Communications Department that demonstrated the role of the school nurse as a valuable resource within the health care system. This video was successfully marketed nationally as a resource to nurses, schools, and communities for promoting health service programs within schools.

The Vermont School Nurse Newsletter is printed three times annually. Association dues are currently thirty dollars a year. The Association acknowledges the fourth week in January as National School Nurse Week, with the fourth Wednesday in January being designated specifically as School Nurse Day. In 1985 and 1987, school nurses presented programs on Vermont Educational Television's "Open Studio" in conjunction with School Nurse Day.

VSSNA is represented on various state committees including:

- Vermont Medical Society–School Health Committee
- Coalition of Vermont Nurses Organizations (COVNO)
- Teenage Pregnancy Task Force
- Nutrition Education and Training Coalition
- Vermont Children's Forum
- Vermont National Education Association
- Vermont Diabetes Coalition
- Vermont Safe Kids
- Vermont Campaign for Tobacco-Free Kids

A Vermont School Nurse of the Year Program has been revised and implemented on an annual basis. The following individuals have received this recognition: Beverly Hatch, A. Dorothy Desrochers, M. Elizabeth Solari, Susan Cota, Virginia Incerpi, and Joan Smidutz. A rotating plaque is placed in the school of the present school nurse of the year. The presentation of this honor occurs annually at the fall conference. The candidates are nominated by their district members and the School Nurse of the Year Selection Committee reviews the curriculum vitae of the nominees. The selection is made based on the accomplishments and contributions of each nominee to school nursing.

An annual scholarship was established in 1996 to assist school nurses currently working in Vermont to further their professional education.

A legislative program was started with representatives of the Association attending the Nurse in Washington Internship, a training program for school nurses to become legislatively proactive in school health issues. The Association representatives follow the legislative bills pertinent to school health and advise Association directors and members on the need for action.

In the mid 1990s, a collaborative effort began among the Association, the Vermont Department of Health, the Vermont Department of Education, and the Vermont Human Services Department to coordinate services for children.

In 1996, Vermont's Framework of Standards and Learning Opportunities was introduced as a guide to student learning to be used by school districts in Vermont. The Association established a committee to work on these educational standards as they relate to the Vermont School Health Services Program.*

Budgetary concerns and changes in health care locally and nationally have begun to impact school nursing positions in Vermont, as school districts attempt to contain school costs. To assist nurses facing possible job elimination or changes in staffing patterns, a School Nurse Action Kit was compiled under the direction of Janice Whitaker, VSSNA President (1997–99), with input from many Vermont school nurses. This tool would be used to strategize ways to advocate for school nursing practice.

VSSNA continues to grow in status and in size. In 1996, there are 303 school nurses, assistants, and others interested in school nursing in Vermont, with 149 active VSSNA members. Over the years, many school nurses have given years of service to make this an active educational organization and to promote school health services in all Vermont schools. The Association attempts to remain a proactive professional organization which promotes high quality school health services that meet the needs of our students, families, and school communities in these ever-changing times.

—Virginia A. Incerpi, RN, BS, NCSN
Janice L. Wimmer, RN, BS

BIBLIOGRAPHY

Vermont State School Nurses' Association, "A Brief History of School Nursing and the Vermont Experience," 1 June 1989.

Vermont Department of Education, "Vermont School Health Services Standards of Practice Manual," 1986.

---

* These are educational standards, not to be confused with the school nursing Standards of Practice previously mentioned.

Vermont Emergency Nurses Association

THE VERMONT Emergency Nurses Association (VTENA) is an affiliate of the national Emergency Nurses' Association headquartered in Chicago. VTENA was chartered in 1979 and currently has a membership of 116, the largest number in its history. ENA's mission is to provide visionary leadership for emergency nursing and emergency care. ENA's mission encompasses the following values:

1. All individuals have a right to quality emergency care delivered with compassion.
2. Respect for diversity of patients and colleagues is inherent to emergency nursing practice and emergency care.
3. Prevention of illness and injury and promotion of wellness are essential components of emergency nursing practice and emergency care.
4. The discipline of emergency nursing includes a defined and evolving body of knowledge based on research.
5. Continuing education and professional development are fundamental to emergency nursing practice and emergency care.
6. Emergency nursing practice is both independent and collaborative.

Emergency nurses in this demanding and quick-paced specialty must have a broad knowledge of disease processes that afflict all age groups. It requires good assessment skills, judgement, and decision making. There are a wide range of technical skills needed as well as a sense of humor. As with all of nursing, it is beginning to move out of the confines of the hospital setting and into the community. Emergency nurses can be found in a variety of settings.

ACLS (Advanced Cardiac Life Support) is a required certification in most emergency departments, but increasingly TNCC (Trauma Nursing Core Course), ENPC (Emergency Nursing Pediatric Course), and CEN (Certified Emergency Nurse) are also becoming required or desirable.

This chapter is excerpted from Bonnie Strand, "Emergency Nurses: Emergent/Urgent and Preventive Care," *Vermont Nurse Connection* 1, no. 4 (December 1998). Reprinted with permission.

The VTENA provides a number of educational programs throughout the year. The Trauma Nursing Core Curriculum (TNCC), Emergency Nursing Pediatric Course (ENPC), and Concepts in Advanced Trauma Nursing (CATN) are three courses offered several times each year. In addition, VTENA combines its annual meeting with an educational day, usually held in November.

In addition to educating nurses, ENA provides community projects to promote safety and well being. Both Southwestern Medical Center in Bennington and Porter Hospital in Middlebury have sponsored gun safety events. ENA and Masterlock Gun Lock Company have teamed to promote gun safety. Masterlock donates 100 gunlocks to each event to be distributed free. This program is available nationwide. ENA is also involved in bicycle helmet and highway safety programs. Emergency Nurses CARE is the injury prevention arm of VTENA. This group of emergency nurses is engaged in educating community groups, particularly teenagers, about alcohol-related injuries and prevention methods.

Nationally, ENA's convention and scientific assembly is held in September, and Vermont has been able to send four delegates. In February, VTENA sends one or two members (usually the president and president-elect) to the ENA's President's Meeting and Leadership Symposium.

More information about the Emergency Nurses' Association is available at their Web site, www.ena.org.

—Bonnie Strand, RN, MA, CEN
VTENA Treasurer and
"Shared Visions" (newsletter) Editor

Vermont New Hampshire Association of Peri Anesthesia Nurses

RECOVERY ROOM NURSES in Vermont and New Hampshire identified the need to have their own professional organization and to define standards of practice. The Vermont New Hampshire Association of Post Anesthesia Nurses (VT NH APAN) had its beginnings on June 13, 1981, at Cheshire Hospital, Keene, New Hampshire, by a steering committee of post anesthesia nurses from Vermont and New Hampshire.

The goals of the association are:

1. To develop standards of care compliant with the standards of care set forth by the American Society of Post Anesthesia Nurses (ASPAN)
2. To maintain optimum efficiency and quality in post anesthesia recovery care
3. To update techniques for more effective practice
4. To promote a greater understanding of post anesthesia recovery nursing
   a. To increase collegial relationships with other professionals
   b. To increase public awareness of the specialty
5. To promote professional accountability
6. To encourage membership in ASPAN

On July 11, 1984, the association received Vermont certification of incorporation. Certification of nonprofit status was obtained November 7, 1984, in New Hampshire, and September 13, 1985, in Vermont. In 1985, the Vermont New Hampshire Association of Post Anesthesia Nurses became a chartered component of the American Society of Post Anesthesia Nurses.

From the initial membership of twelve, the organization has grown to 126 members in 1996—in Vermont, New Hampshire, Massachusetts, Maine, and Alaska. A board of directors elected by the membership determines the organizational decisions of the association. Representatives of the association are sent yearly to the national conference sponsored by ASPAN. The Association holds educational seminars for nurses twice yearly, in the spring and fall, either in Vermont or New Hampshire.

The Board of Directors voted in 1987 to officially change the name of the association to the Vermont New Hampshire Association of *Peri* Anesthesia Nurses, following the lead of the name change of the national association (American Society of *Peri* Anesthesia Nurses). This was done to reflect the various areas of perianesthesia care represented by the national society.

—Jocelyn H. MacDonald, BSN, RN, CPAN
President, VT NH APAN, 1998

Vermont Association of Occupational Health Nurses

VERMONT NURSES specializing in occupational health banded together in 1989 with the objectives of enhancing their professional network and fostering continuing professional education, and with an overall goal of improving the standard of care rendered to individuals at the work site. With a population of roughly 500,000 and a rural makeup, Vermont surprised the American Association of Occupational Health Nurses (AAOHN) in 1990, when Vermont nurses further organized to form a new state constituency, the Vermont Association of Occupational Health Nurses (VAOHN). The addition of Vermont as a state constituent completed state membership in the Northeast Regional Association of Occupational Health Nurses (NEAOHN).

While the national association had estimated that only sixteen registered nurses were in clinical practice in work-site settings statewide, over forty-five nurses in occupational practice were identified through direct contact with area businesses, hospitals, and the State Health Promotion Office. Charter members included nurses from General Electric, Simmonds Precision, IBM, Fletcher Allen Health Care (Medical Center Hospital of Vermont and Fanny Allen Hospital locations), National Life of Vermont, Eveready Battery, and Wyeth-Ayerst, to name a few.

This was not the beginning of occupational health nursing in Vermont, however. In 1895, nearly 100 years before the formation of the VAOHN, industrial health nursing was being pioneered at the Vermont Marble Company in Proctor, Vermont. Ada Mayo Stewart, a nurse trained by the Waltham Training School for Nurses, was the first nurse hired in New England to provide services to workers.* In addition to provision of nursing care to employees of Vermont Marble Co., Ms. Stewart also provided preventive health services and health education to family members, traveling by bicycle or horse and buggy to deliver these services

---

*Jane E. Parker-Conrad, "A Century of Practice: Occupational Health Nursing," *AAOHN Journal* 36, no. 4 (April 1988).

in the community. She is widely recognized as a leader in the development of the specialty practice now known as occupational health nursing.

Today, occupational health nurses in Vermont continue to provide a wide spectrum of services at the work site. These include delivery of direct clinical services for work- and nonwork-related injuries and illnesses; development and implementation of health education, screenings and disease prevention programs, case management for work- and nonwork-related disabilities, provider access and clinical referral services, and health benefit design and administration. The association meets roughly five times annually, rotating meeting locations in an attempt to reach as many members as possible given the statewide membership. Annual meetings are often organized in tandem with other associations, including safety personnel and school nurses, depending on the topic of interest. Additionally, with formation of the Vermont constituency, the president of the VAOHN is now a member of the Board of Directors for the Northeast Association of Occupational Health Nurses, further enhancing our opportunity for professional networking and access to continuing professional education seminars at the annual regional meeting.

—Eileen Girling, RN, MPH, COHN

Kappa Tau Chapter
Sigma Theta Tau International

IDEAS THAT RESIDE in the minds of a few individuals often exist long before they evolve into action. Such is the case with the founding of the Kappa Tau Chapter of Sigma Theta Tau International, Nursing's Honor Society at The University of Vermont (UVM). Early in the 1970s Norma Woodruff, the director of the School of Nursing, approached students to explore their interest in forming a nursing honor society. At the time, students felt that those who excelled academically should not be singled out from their peers. By the early 1980s, however, there was a change in perspective by some of these same students, now alumni. They now believed that an honor society was the means to foster nursing excellence, scholarship, and leadership. So begins the story of the establishment of the Chapter—a story that reflects nursing's commitment to work through local, regional, and international efforts to support and contribute to the well-being of people throughout the world.

The Center for Nursing Scholarship, the headquarters for Sigma Theta Tau International, Inc., is located on the campus of Indiana University Purdue University Indianapolis (IUPUI). It is also the location of the Virginia Henderson International Nursing Library. Sigma Theta Tau International is an organization started by six nursing students in 1922 at the Indiana University Training School for Nurses. It has a membership that has grown to more than 220,000 members in some seventy-five countries.

After nearly a year and a half (November 1982 to April 1984) of meetings with local members of Sigma Theta Tau International, a Steering Committee was established that would guide a fledgling organization through to chapter initiation. With the guidance of University faculty members Ellen Ellis and Hollace Reed, the Nursing Honor Society, a chapter prerequisite organization, was formed. The Steering Committee steadily worked toward establishing a firm foundation for a new chapter. With the strong support of Dean Jean Milligan, undergraduate students, and members of other chapters of Sigma Theta Tau International, the UVM Nursing Honor Society was developed. Finally, in the summer of 1987 (as noted in the Nursing Honor Society's Executive Committee

Annual Report, July 1986–July 1987) the petition for a charter was sent to Sigma Theta Tau International.

Once the charter petition was reviewed, an on-site evaluation visit was scheduled to provide guidance to the Steering Committee and determine readiness for chartering. In March 1987, Dr. Vickie Lambert, a member of the consultation team for petitioning chapters, made a visit to UVM. Dr. Lambert highly recommended approval of the petition for a charter. She was very complimentary about the members' level of interest, the growth of the organization over the three-year period, and the organization of the Nursing Honor Society. The Executive Committee continued its work by developing a prescribed committee structure (Program, Nominating, and Eligibility Committees) and establishing the organization's financial base.

In June 1987, the Governing Council of Sigma Theta Tau International voted favorably to have the petition presented to the House of Delegates at the next Biennium Convention. In the fall of 1987, Holly Reed, president of the Nursing Honor Society and Judy Cohen, chairwoman of the Eligibility Committee and faculty advisor, presented the petition at the Biennium Convention taking place in San Francisco, California. Upon action of the House of Delegates, the Kappa Tau Chapter, the 257th chapter of Sigma Theta Tau International, was established. In a moving ceremony witnessed by delegates of the more than 250 previously established chapters, the Chapter was welcomed.

As each chapter begins its life it is assigned a mentoring chapter. The Delta Gamma Chapter at the State University at Plattsburgh, New York, was Kappa Tau's mentoring chapter. The mentoring relationship can take many forms and the nature of the relationship changed over time. In the beginning, Delta Gamma was a resource for information and a supportive presence. In subsequent years, the two chapters have cosponsored activities and sent delegates together to Biennium Conventions.

The next milestone of the Kappa Tau Chapter was the induction of all members of the UVM Nursing Honor Society into the Kappa Tau Chapter in a chartering ceremony held in the spring of 1988. The names of these members reside on display at the UVM School of Nursing.

Developing the Kappa Tau Chapter

The chartering ceremony made Kappa Tau the first chapter of Sigma Theta Tau International in the state of Vermont. Building a chapter means establishing a network of local, regional, national, and international connections, which fosters nursing excellence, scholarship, and leadership. It is a broad perspective of these multiple relationships that best represents the goals of Sigma Theta Tau International. The Chapter initially was concerned with excellence, scholarship, and leadership at the local level, but the broader network of regional and international efforts soon emerged. Leadership of the Chapter passed from presidents Holly Reed (1988–90), to Dr. Laurie Murray (1990–93), to Kathy Clark (1993–94), to Dr. Lorraine (Clarke) Welch (1994–96), and to Dr. Mary Botter (1996–2000). Dr. Janet Brown is the current president for the 2000–2002 term. Under the leadership of each president, the Board of Directors has set a course which has broadened and enriched the scope of chapter involvement.

Local Activity

The first five-year strategic plan established by the chartering officers was the initial guide for the organization. Sigma Theta Tau International is set upon a tradition that recognizes excellence. It was fitting then that one of the earliest chapter achievements was an award to recognize an outstanding senior nursing student. The recipient of the Kappa Tau Chapter Award is selected annually by the senior nursing class at UVM. With the initiation of the master's program at The University of Vermont, a graduate student award was added. Other awards recognizing excellence in nursing education and practice were established. The Folta-Deck Award, established by Edie Deck in 1996, recognizes members' published nursing research. Dr. Brenda Hamel-Bissell was the recipient of the first award. Subsequent Folta-Deck award winners were Nancy Sowan (1998), Jeanine Carr (1999), and Pat Winstead Fry (2000). Each year the Awards Committee also calls for nominations of members who represent excellence in nursing education and practice. The Excellence in Practice award has been given to Hollace Reed (1992), Joan Webber Jones (1993), Rita Laferriere (1996) Ellen Leff (1998), Iris MacDonald (1999), and Holly Shaner (2000). The Excellence in Education award has been given to Dennis Ross (1992), Edith Deck (1992), Judith Cohen (1996), Marie McGrath (1997), Katie Geran (1998), Liz Laferriere (1999), and Ellen Ceppetelli (2000).

The Program Committee, from its inception, created a structure for scholarly presentations. The induction ceremony in the fall and the annual meeting in the spring focus on scholarly presentations. Nursing leaders from the State are invited to speak at the induction ceremony. Nursing leaders with national and international perspectives, available through the Sigma Theta Tau International Distinguished Lecturer Program, are invited as keynote speakers for the Annual Meeting. Kappa Tau has supported and cosponsored (with Fletcher Allen Health Care and the Nightingale Foundation) presentations by distinguished speakers at local meetings.

The Research Committee, in concert with the Program Committee, organizes two programs each year dedicated to research activities of members within the State. The Research Committee has used a variety of venues to disseminate knowledge, including a half-day research program, poster presentations at Vermont State Nurses' Association Conventions, and at the Annual Meetings of the Kappa Tau membership. Programs have also disseminated research at evening meetings held at various locations throughout the State. The Committee also invites Kappa Tau members to submit research proposals for funding. Funding is provided annually to those researchers whose proposals successfully navigate the review process. The Silent Auction held at the Annual Meeting has been a major source of funding to support scholarship. Research-based scholarship has grown over the past decade as members prepared at the masters' and doctoral level join the Chapter.

Active participation in the Chapter builds leadership. Once students and community leaders are inducted, the Board of Directors hold an orientation program for these new members. The newly inducted members learn about the Chapter and are invited to participate in its activities. Undergraduate members have described this orientation as very important, for it is the first time they become members of the larger body of professional nursing. Orientation is not only important for new members, but it is also a critical activity for leadership development of newly installed Chapter officers. The complexity of the Chapter with its local, regional, and international affiliations provides an endless array of leadership opportunities. Seeking ways to advance the leadership mission will be a continuous challenge to the Chapter. In the most recent history of the Chapter, the leadership of the Board of Directors expanded the group by adding the office of president-elect. The term of office for the president-elect will provide another opportunity for a leader to use their talents to actualize the strategic plan for the Chapter.

The Kappa Tau Newsletter made its debut in 1997. Editor Louise Moon Rosales came to Vermont and asked what she could do for the Chapter. President Mary Botter had known for some time that there was a need for a publication to keep the membership informed of Chapter activities. Louise's previous newsletter experience was evident as the first edition came from the presses.

Regional Activity

In addition to promoting excellence, scholarship, and leadership at the local level, Chapter activities extend to the regional arena. Kappa Tau is a chapter in Region 5. All chapters in the Northeast United States are in

Region 5. A Regional Coordinating Committee carries out activities in the region. One such regional activity is the conference calls among Region 5 chapter presidents, which occur on a regular basis. The calls are fruitful sharing of the presidents' ideas and experiences in chapter development. This network of leaders also provides opportunities for chapters in the region to plan activities between chapters. An example of regional chapters working together was the 1992 Rural Health Conference sponsored by Eta Iota (University of New Hampshire), Epsilon Tau (St. Anselm's College), and Kappa Tau (The University of Vermont). Twenty-one scholars from the region addressed the unique challenges faced by nurses in rural areas.

Communications among the chapters in the region provided the stimulus for chapter growth. The newsletter, *Region 5 Connections*, is an important communication link between chapters. Each chapter contributes news to this publication.

There is a second level of activity that connects regional to international efforts to promote nursing excellence, scholarship, and leadership. This is the Biennial Regional Assembly. Chapters compete to host the Regional Assembly. President Laurie Murray put in a chapter bid to host the 1994 Regional Assembly in Burlington, Vermont. She successfully campaigned for that honor. Laurie's move to Wiedner University in Pennsylvania precluded her fulfilling this chapter landmark accomplishment. President Lorri (Clarke) Welch picked up the challenge. She was very fortunate to have chapter members Holly Reed, Judy Cohen, Nancy Rainville, and Mary Botter join her on the Local Arrangements Committee to host the event. Advice and encouragement also came from the officers of the Regional Coordinating Committee and Sigma Theta Tau International staff. Kappa Tau members had a memorable experience working together on all the details of a very successful assembly. One highlight of the Regional Assembly was an address by Vermont Governor, Howard Dean. President of Sigma Theta Tau International Fay Bower and Executive Director Nancy Hazard were delighted by the Governor's address. They were also genuinely appreciative of the warm reception they received in Vermont.

Members of Kappa Tau also have served on Region 5 Committees. Brenda Hamel-Bissell, Peg Gagne, and Lorri Welch (chair) formed the Chapter Research Dissemination Award Committee for the 1996 Regional Assembly held in Rhode Island. The Chapter supported Lorri's attendance at the Assembly where she presented the award to Beta Zeta Chapter at the University of Massachusetts.

International Activity

The Kappa Tau Chapter has also developed connections to the international nursing community. Financial support for a student participating in a nursing educational exchange with Yuroslavo, Russia, was one of the first international initiatives undertaken by the Chapter. Kappa Tau inducted its first international member from England. Kappa Tau president Lorri Welch served as chair of the House of Delegates Committee for a Sigma Theta Tau International Biennium, and Mary Botter is serving on the Virginia Henderson Library Committee. Kappa Tau has also sponsored a keynote speaker for the Sigma Theta Tau International Convention. The Kappa Tau Chapter and individual members have contributed financial support for scholarship and for the building of Sigma Theta Tau International's new headquarters in Indiana.

In its short, twelve-year history, the Kappa Tau Chapter of Sigma Theta Tau International, Inc. can be proud of its many accomplishments. It has set its roots deep into a tradition of nursing excellence, scholarship, and leadership.

—Lorraine M. Welch, RN, EdD

Vermont Nursing Initiative

In 1989, a small group of nurse executives in rural Vermont ignored the harsh winter and mountainous roads and gathered to discuss issues of health care delivery. Three problems were identified:

1. limited resources
2. lack of continuing education opportunities for nurses
3. changing demands in clinical care

This discussion, which grew to include all fifteen of Vermont's acute care hospitals, was led by Ann Marchewka of Copley Hospital and eventually became known as the Vermont Nursing Initiative (VNI). In 1990, the Robert Wood Johnson Foundation recognized the work of the VNI with a $1 million grant aimed at strengthening hospital nursing and improving patient care. For administrative purposes, Copley Hospital was designated the grantee hospital and Toni Kaeding was named Project Director. Based on the notion that those who suffer from a lack of resources can benefit from working together, the VNI became a model for collaboration and a catalyst for change.

One of the main accomplishments of the VNI was the creation of an infrastructure which allowed hospitals to work together to meet needs. The VNI also offered nurses a voice, a platform for change, and the resources to make it happen. In response to the three problems identified, the VNI developed 3 programs.

Rural Resource Pool (RRP). In Vermont, where hospitals are isolated and resources are limited, the RRP was a registry that enabled hospitals to share staff in order to meet patient needs, prevent unnecessary transfers, and provide specialty services. The VNI brokered the Resource Pool and at project's end, the model was continued as a framework for staff-sharing by newly created hospital networks.

Network for Education. In a rural community, where educational opportunity is scarce, the task of keeping professional knowledge current is a particular challenge. Through the Network for Education, hospital nurse educators began working together to co-sponsor programs, as well as share learning. Affordable accessible continuing education for Vermont nurses was the result, and the project became a model for cooperatively

VNI People and Participants

Carolyn Roberts	Chair of VNI Board and President/CEO of Copley Hospital
Toni Kaeding	Project Director
Ellen Ceppetelli	Assistant Project Director
Norma Lang	Administrative Assistant
Cam Page	Director, Rural Resource Pool
Sally Sample	Co-Chair, Network for Education
Jane Hayward	Co-Chair, Network for Education

Brattleboro Memorial Hospital
Central Vermont Hospital
Copley Hospital
Fanny Allen Hospital
Gifford Medical Center
Grace Cottage Hospital
Medical Center Hospital of Vermont
Mt. Ascutney Hospital and Health Center
North Country Hospital
Northeastern Vermont Regional Hospital
Northwestern Medical Center
Porter Medical Center
Rutland Regional Medical Center
Southwestern Vermont Medical Center
Springfield Hospital

developed education programs and projects between hospitals. At project's end, The University of Vermont joined hospital educators in offering an ongoing subscription seminar series for nurses.

Hospital Restructuring Projects. It was during this period that two major dynamics were occurring in hospitals. The emphasis in health care was shifting from inpatient to outpatient, and managed care was gaining presence. Both of these influences called for changes in the delivery of care, and hospitals turned to the VNI for support in their restructuring efforts. "Bedside innovations" such as case management, cross-training, and shared governance were selected and managed by hospital-based multidisciplinary project teams. The VNI provided support to hospital projects through: planning assistance, expert consultation, research, networking, problem solving, evaluation, and some financial aid.

At the same time that Vermont nurses were rethinking the delivery of care, many external forces were also influencing change. In Washington, sky-rocketing health care costs became a major concern and in 1992 President Clinton was elected on a platform of health care reform. Concurrently in Vermont, the legislature adopted Act 160—health reform policy aimed at controlling costs, improving quality, and expanding access. Consumers, too, were pressing health care providers for change and managed care began to penetrate Vermont.

This cacophony of reform surely worked both for and against efforts of the VNI. On one hand, the VNI was well positioned to take advantage of this new mood of change and encountered relatively few obstacles in program implementation. On the other hand, the durability of innovations was constantly challenged by changing leadership, realigned relationships, new incentives, and organizations in turmoil.

At the days end, however, the work of the VNI contributed to change in the way that patient care is given. New and improved systems of care within hospitals emerged, as did new models of collaboration between hospitals. Vermont nurses were recognized for their work nationally and several articles were published describing the experiences of this project. Although the VNI officially closed its doors in 1995, it left Vermont nurses with a legacy of accomplishment and recognition and perhaps, most importantly, the knowledge of what can be achieved through the strength of working together.

—Toni H. Kaeding, MS, RN
Project Director, Vermont Nursing Initiative

FOUR

Vermont State Board of Nursing

Vermont State Board of Nursing

THE VERMONT State Board of Nursing is the people's agency, created by Title 26 V.S.A. Chapter 28, to safeguard the health and safety of the people of the State of Vermont. The law is administered and implemented by the Vermont State Board of Nursing, whose members are appointed by the governor of Vermont. The Board is currently mandated by law to approve all nursing education programs in Vermont, examine the graduates of state-approved educational programs, register and license successful examinees, register and license qualified applicants licensed by other states, relicense qualified applicants periodically, endorse advanced practice nurses, regulate the practice of nursing, publish interpretive statements, discipline licensees for cause, and regulate the proceedings of the Vermont State Board of Nursing in accordance with law and administrative rules.[1]

Since the passage of the earliest nurse registration law in 1911—credited to the efforts of a physician, Dr. Donley C. Hawley[2]—there have been many changes in the law and the public's expectation of the members of the Board of Nursing. *We Who Serve: A Story of Nursing in Vermont* records the development of the Board of Nursing from its earliest days through 1940. The impact of world events and societal change is nowhere more apparent than in the decade of the 1940s. World War II created a shortage of nurses which demanded the attention of the Board of Nursing, the State Legislature, the state's hospitals, and all of the citizens of Vermont throughout the forties and well into the succeeding decades.

In 1940, the Board of Registration of Nurses (so designated until 1961 when a revision of the nursing law changed the name to the State Board of Nursing) granted registration and licensure to 145 applicants by examination, one by waiver (a 1910 graduate), and fifty-nine by reciprocity.[3] At the February 26, 1941, meeting, the Board created an "inactive list" consisting of nurses practicing out-of-state and other nurses not in active practice. The Board members voted that these nurses "may retain their status as registered nurses by so signifying to the Board, and by payment of the one dollar fee when active practice in Vermont is resumed."[4] The three-member Board consisted of Dr. Charles Goyette of Barre, president; Helen L. Little, RN, of St. Albans, secretary; and Sister Mary

Bisson, RN, of Winooski, treasurer. Sometimes referred to as the Board of Examiners, these professionals developed and administered the examinations for the new graduate nurse. Subject assignments for the May 8 and 9, 1941, examinations were:

Thursday AM – Surgical Nursing and First Aid – Dr. Goyette
Anatomy and Physiology – Helen Little
Thursday PM – Dietetics and Nutrition – Sister Bisson
Hygiene and Sanitation, Microbiology and Communicable Disease – Helen Little
Friday AM – Obstetrics and Pediatrics – Dr. Goyette
Medical Nursing, Urinalysis and Psychiatry – Sister Bisson
Friday PM – Materia Medica – Helen Little[5]

The Board of Registration ruled that a hospital must maintain a daily average of 50 or more patients to have an accredited training school. It must also have "segregated services in obstetrics, pediatrics, and medical cases or a daily average of 50 or over without segregated services in above departments but [with] proper affiliation to make up the deficiency."[6] The status of Vermont nursing schools is described in the Board minutes of May 1941: "Vermont training schools are sadly in need of competently trained people to act as supervisors and instructors."[7] At that time, the Board voted scholarships of $400 per applicant with a requirement that upon completion of the advanced education, the recipient work for at least two years in Vermont nurse training schools, the title by which schools preparing nurses were known at the time. Some months later, November 1942, the Board lowered the applicant age to 17½ years, waived chemistry as a high school requirement, accelerated training courses, and accepted New York registrants without examination; all of this a result of the acute "nursing situation" brought about by war conditions.

Another impact of World War II was the employment of the first staff person for the Board of Registration of Nurses. At a joint meeting of the Board and the Student Recruitment Committee, chaired by Nellie Jones (Miss Jones was the first director of the Public Health Nursing Division, Vermont State Health Department), the Board determined that it was "in need of a paid worker to carry out and investigate problems and programs made necessary by the war and the part being played by the nursing profession."[8] In response to the Board's request, Governor Wills appointed Catherine Terrien, RN, for a period of one year, at an annual salary of $2,000 and an expense account of $800. The appointment was effective September 1, 1943.[9]

The Cadet Nurse Corps was an important and effective recruitment tool in attracting young female high school graduates to the local hospital nurse training programs. The Vermont diploma programs (with the exception of two) met the United States Public Health Service requirements for participation in the Cadet Nurse Corps.[10] In April 1944, The University of Vermont offered pre-clinical instruction for students enrolled in Vermont hospital training schools. The course was approved by the Board with the condition that the decision for participation be left to the local hospital boards of directors. Heaton Hospital in Montpelier and Barre City Hospital indicated that they would participate.[11]

Vermont continued to experience the countrywide shortage of nurses resulting from wartime demands for nursing personnel. In November 1945, the Board went on record in favor of introducing legislation to provide for licensure of practical nurses. Board minutes state: "There is a definite place for the practical nurse . . . licensing of this type of nurse would give her definite standing . . . standards [would] be set up for the licensing of such [a] nurse . . . this measure would also protect the public from incompetents calling themselves nurses."[12]

Board minutes of April 1946 reflect the Board's first use of the national test pool questions for registered nurses in examining the newly graduated nurses. National examinations in pharmacology and dietetics were utilized in 1946. Vermont's use of the test pool examinations increased gradually, and in February 1948, the Board voted to use test pool questions in all areas except psychiatry. In May 1949, Vermont examinees tested below the mean in every area. The Board of Registration of Nurses cited such major weaknesses as inadequately prepared faculties, as well as inadequate classrooms, libraries, and housing facilities.[13] In 1949, 107 nurses were licensed by examination; sixty were endorsed from other states.[14]

Board minutes of May 1949 cite the accreditation status of Vermont's schools of nursing; six hospital diploma programs and one college baccalaureate program were fully accredited by the Vermont Board of Registration of Nurses:

University of Vermont, Burlington
Mary Fletcher Hospital, Burlington
Fanny Allen Hospital, Winooski
Bishop DeGoesbriand Hospital, Burlington
Rutland City Hospital, Rutland
Heaton Hospital, Montpelier
Barre City Hospital, Barre

Provisionally accredited:
Gifford Memorial Hospital, Randolph
Brightlook Hospital, St. Johnsbury

On December 20, 1949, Brightlook Hospital officials advised the Board of Registration of Nurses of the pending closure of its nurse training program due to insufficient funds, the official closure date to be in 1951 to allow the senior students to complete the program. The St. Albans Hospital program closed September 13, 1949.

1950s

During the 1950s, the Vermont Board of Registration of Nurses continued to work with community and professional groups in resolving the shortage of nurses in the state. These years marked the closure of more hospital diploma schools of nursing, the licensure of the practical nurse, the development of approved schools to prepare the practical nurse, and financial incentives for registered nurses to secure preparation for teaching at both the registered nurse and practical nurse levels.

Minutes of the Board dated October 16, 1950, cite both Brightlook and Rutland Hospital Schools of Nursing as officially closed. The Gifford Memorial Hospital School of Nursing in Randolph ". . . remains conditionally approved in view of the building plans."[15] Board members continued to work supportively with the Gifford program until November 1958, when the Board moved to recommend to the Gifford Hospital trustees that the program be discontinued due to lack of faculty. It was further stated that the "best means of protecting the student body" (four students) was to terminate the program while it was still provisionally approved by the State Board.[16]

In 1953, the Fanny Allen and the Bishop DeGoesbriand Schools of Nursing requested permission from the State Board to "form a central school" to be known as the Jeanne Mance School of Nursing with the privilege of retaining the presently enrolled students in their respective schools. Permission was granted.[17] The national movement to develop college/university based two-year programs to prepare the registered nurse was implemented in Vermont after extensive preparation during the fifties and culminated in the Board's preliminary approval of the proposed associate degree program at Vermont College in Montpelier in June of 1960.[18]

House bill H.62, an Act to Provide for the Licensure of Practical Nurses, passed the Vermont State Legislature on March 21, 1951, and became effective on that date. This act also amended Section 6897 of the nursing law by increasing Board membership to five: one physician who should be in active practice and have experience instructing nurses in the state; two registered nurse graduates of approved schools with at least 5 years active practice and two years in supervision or teaching in an approved school of nursing; two practical nurse graduates of an approved school with at least 5 years active practice.[19] By appointment of the governor, the Board now consisted of the following members: Chester A. Newhall, MD, Burlington; Eleanor M. Dyke, RN, Barre; Dorothy M. Allen, RN, Newfane; Dorothy P. Howard, PN, Barre; Clara A. Roitero, PN, Brattleboro.

On July 10, 1951, Board members met to plan for the licensure of practical nurses. Three rules were established: 1) Graduates of approved schools of practical nursing would have a choice as to licensure by waiver or by examination, 2) Evaluation of the two schools of practical nursing (Henry W. Putnam in Bennington and Thompson School in Brattleboro) would be made as soon as minimum standards were established, and 3) The numerical series for practical nurse licensure would begin with 1A; the letter A would be used for all practical nurse license numbers.

Board members Dorothy Allen and Clara Roitero were assigned the task of developing minimum standards for evaluating the practical nursing schools. The proposed standards were presented to the Board in September and adopted temporarily. At the same time, rule 3 was rescinded and the Board voted to adopt the letters LPN after all practical nurse licensure numbers, including the yearly renewals.

The 1953 Board minutes cited some specific problems facing the Vermont Board of Registration of Nurses, including limitations on Board activities due to serious financial constraints, a great need for scholarship assistance for graduate nurses preparing for faculty positions, and faculty shortages in Vermont's nursing schools. The Board secretary addressed the Board's acute financial situation in the January 1953 minutes:

> . . . the board is facing a very serious situation in that it will be impossible to carry on even limited activities for the entire year because of depleted funds (with) which this board now has to function. Plans are being made to close the board office for one to three months in the year of 1954 to stay within the limited budget.[20]

Apparently the financial dilemma continued, because in the years 1954, 1955, and 1956, a direct appeal was made to members of the Vermont State Nurses' Association (VSNA) for each nurse to make a small contribution to help finance the Board of Registration of Nurses.

> The total amount given to the Board was $624.56. Of this amount, $127 was paid directly to the Board and went into the general funds of Board revenue; $497.56 was paid to the Board by the State Nurses' Association, and this was put into a separate account in the Chittenden Trust Company.[21]

Expenses were as follows:

Chittenden Trust Company checking account		$497.56
Postage stamps	$345.00	
Office cleaning	2.75	
Office pen	15.50	
Stencil cutting	75.98	
Northeastern Conference—Board worker	53.90	
Bank charges	2.50	
	$495.63	$495.63
Balance in Chittenden Trust Co. 1/26/56		$1.93

The acute need for prepared nurses in Vermont continued through the fifties. Three hospitals in northern Vermont—St. Albans, St. Johnsbury, and Morrisville—approached the Board of Registration of Nurses relative to exploring the development of additional resources for the preparation of practical nurses. In 1958, Brightlook Hospital in St. Johnsbury was approved by the Board to provide a medical-surgical affiliation for students from the Fanny Allen School of Practical Nursing in Winooski.[22] Fanny Allen Memorial Hospital School of Practical Nursing was fully approved by the Board in 1957.

In September 1957, the Vermont State Hospital welcomed the first group of nursing students to its newly established affiliate program in psychiatric nursing. Students came from the Mary Fletcher Hospital and Jeanne Mance Schools of Nursing, both in Burlington, and from the Heaton Hospital School of Nursing in Montpelier.[23] A review of the Vermont State Hospital affiliate program by Lena Oakley and Jean Milligan, faculty members of The University of Vermont's School of Nursing, resulted in the program's being fully approved by the State Board of Registration of Nurses as an affiliation program in psychiatric nursing for registered nurse students. Full approval was voted at the December 16, 1958, meeting of the Board.

In March 1957, the Vermont Conference on Nursing was developing and planning to submit bills to the Vermont Legislature supportive of nursing education. One of these bills would provide scholarships for "graduates of a state-approved hospital school of nursing to obtain additional educational preparation leading to the baccalaureate degree in nursing to more adequately prepare them for faculty or nursing service positions in the state."[24] This bill came up without a legislative sponsor and was withdrawn. Prior to this and effective June 3, 1953, was an Act of the Legislature providing for nursing scholarships and appropriating $10,000 to provide financial assistance for enrollees "in schools of nursing in this state for a three year course of study leading to a diploma." Eligibility requirements: a Vermont resident for two years; must agree to work in Vermont for one year for each year of assistance received; must contract with the State Board of Registration of Nurses. Funding available: first year, $250; second year, $150; third year, $100. The funding would be provided annually for the ensuing biennium.[25]

1960s

The 1960s were turbulent years for the Vermont State Board of Nursing. There were major changes in nursing and in the administration of state government. In reviewing Board minutes and in consultation with people who served as Board members during those years, it became clear that the 1960s was a decade of transition in which the national professional nurse organizations were encouraging upgrading nursing education programs to prepare graduates to participate constructively in providing care to patients in an increasingly complex health care system. The educational programs for all health professionals were facing the challenge to prepare graduates to apply the burgeoning scientific knowledge to patient care. As in other health professions, the response to suggested changes were marked with conflicting philosophies among the members of the Board at that time. The transition from diploma programs into academic programs presented a radical departure from hospital base to university/college base instruction. Gaining acceptance of this obvious reduction in hands-on experience presented many challenges, as the public, some health professionals, and patients and families looked upon the clinical experience as being greatly jeopardized by more theory and less practice.[26]

Early in the 1960s, the Legislative Committee of the Vermont State Nurses' Association, under the leadership of Norma Woodruff, chairman of the Department of Nursing at The University of Vermont School of Nursing, prepared and submitted for Board review and comment a proposed mandatory nurse licensing law, consistent with a national trend to upgrade nursing care. This proposal, to be presented to the 46th Biennial Session of the State Legislature, included a complete revision of the Nurse Practice Act in Vermont. It updated the definition of both professional and practical nursing, provided for an all-nurse board, and increased Board member terms from three to five years; examinations would be required for waivered practicing RNs; practical nurse candidates must have graduated from high school or its equivalent; and the Board of Registration of Nurses would now be named the Vermont State Board of Nursing.[27]

Senate bill S.72 was passed by the legislature and approved June 28, 1961; it became effective at the time of passage.[28] With the passage of this law, Wilmer W. Angell, MD, retired from the Board of Nursing. At the August meeting of the Board, the members formally extended to Dr. Angell their appreciation for his service and for his understanding and support of nursing as a profession.

Members of the first all-nurse Board of Nursing were Ruby C. Carr, RN (president), Fairlee; Grace M. Buttolph, RN (secretary-treasurer), Burlington; Eleanor M. Diack, RN, Barre; Esther L. Martinson, RN, Burlington; Dorothy Patterson, LPN, Montpelier; and Clara A. Roitero, LPN, Vernon. Board members would serve five-year terms and their compensation would be $10 per day plus "necessary expenses." The Board was attached to the office of Secretary of State Howard E. Armstrong; administrative and secretarial services would be provided by Secretary Armstrong's office. Catherine Terrien, RN, continued to serve as administrative secretary.[29]

The possibility of securing the services of a part-time executive secretary was considered by the Board members at this time. Miss Terrien, the first professional nurse employed by the Board, submitted her resignation after serving the Board as administrative secretary for twenty years. A formal resolution of the Board of Nursing commended Terrien for "putting the interests of nurses and nursing always in the forefront; . . . her work intimately touched the lives of all registered professional nurses and licensed practical nurses and, indirectly, the patients they serve; . . . she has capably served the Board through a period which has seen many changes in nursing education and practice in this state"[30] Shortly after Terrien's resignation, Eleanor J. Smith, RN, MA, assumed the position of executive secretary at an annual salary of $7,300.[31]

Two associate degree nursing programs, one at Vermont College in Montpelier and the other at Castleton State College in Rutland County, were granted full approval by the Board of Nursing on May 22, 1963. Board minutes of the early sixties reflect turbulent years for the developing Castleton associate degree program: the program received initial approval from the Board on June 22, 1962; all nursing faculty resigned in 1965. An August 24, 1965, visit by Board representatives reported the college president's concern that the program would be phased out. However, hard work, perseverance, and statewide support was rewarded when again, in May 1966, Castleton received "reasonable assurance" of accreditation and recovered the Board's full approval on July 15, 1969.

In October 1967, The University of Vermont advised the Board of plans to establish a two-year associate degree nursing program, planned to coincide with the closing of the last two three-year nursing programs, the Jeanne Mance School of Nursing and the Mary Fletcher School of Nursing.[32] The University received initial approval of its associate degree nursing program in January 1969.

Board minutes of January 9, 1962, cite a communication from Alice Robinson, President of the Vermont League for Nursing (VLN), relative to a need for refresher courses for graduate professional nurses. Board discussion supported this need and Board Secretary Grace Buttolph, in a letter of January 17th to the VSNA-VLN Coordinating Council, assured that there was a continuing need for this kind of educational program. Additionally, 84% of nurse respondents to a statewide survey indicated their interest in refresher courses.[33] President Robinson's report of May 24, 1962, to the VLN membership stated that a refresher course entitled, "The Emotional Aspects of Illness" was currently in progress in St. Albans, and would be repeated in July in Rutland. A refresher course in obstetrical nursing was being planned for the Burlington area for July 1962.[34] According to the VLN Advisory Council minutes of May 1, 1963 meeting, tentative plans for a refresher course in medical-surgical nursing were under way.[35]

Passage of Public Law P.L.89-97 and the federal rules and regulations creating Medicare were impacting Vermonters and their nurses. In 1966, the Board approved, in principle, a plan proposed by the Vermont State Health Department's Public Health Nursing Division for the training and employment of home health aides. Home Health Aide Service was an extension of the federally certified nursing services offered by visiting nurse services and newly organized home health agencies.[36]

Two nurse practice issues were brought to the attention of the Board: intravenous procedures performed by registered nurses, and the assignment of nursing responsibilities to variously prepared levels of nursing personnel. Discussion of the legality of intravenous techniques was first dealt with in the Board minutes of November 14, 1964; it was referred to the Nursing Practice Committee of the VSNA. Queried by Board Executive Secretary Louise P. Alcott, Attorney General Charles E. Gibson and Deputy Chester S. Ketcham responded on December 7, 1964, with Opinion No. 19 relative to "Registered Nurses, Venipuncture." They quoted and concurred with a New York attorney general opinion dated 1961 that "the responsibility for the direction of the administration of each specific intravenous procedure must rest solely upon the physician ordering its performance."[37] Since the nurse must be qualified and competent through training and experience, and physicians may not know the skills of the registered nurse who will perform the venipuncture, the hospital should assume responsibility for training and supervision of nurses qualified to perform venipuncture under physicians' orders. Both the New York and the Vermont attorney generals recommended that the venipuncture procedure be included in the curriculum of schools preparing registered nurses. On February 23, 1965, the Board met with thirty-six directors of nursing schools and service agencies to review and discuss new Board regulations and these two practice issues. The attorney general's opinion regarding the intravenous issue "was discussed at length with many opposing points of view from directors of nursing services. There was a general belief that nurses were performing this function as a necessity. The scope of performance should be regulated by well-defined hospital policy."[38] A statement to assist in assigning patient care responsibilities to nonRN nursing personnel was presented by the VSNA executive secretary, and it was the feeling of the group that newspaper publicity should be utilized to provide the public with an understanding of the assignment of nursing functions to various levels of personnel.[39]

In 1960, the Vermont State Legislature passed two major bills providing for the reorganization of state government, a reorganization which would dislocate, relocate, and generally challenge the ability of the Board of Nursing to carry out its mandated functions for the next two decades and beyond. Responding to nationwide trends to save money, these laws were developed in response to legislative concern and the report of the Commission to Study State Government. Created in 1957 and frequently referred to as the "Little Hoover Commission," the creating act stated:

> Declaration of policy. It is hereby declared to be the policy of Vermont to increase economy, promote maximum efficiency, and improve services, with wisest use of the taxpayers' money in the transaction of public business in the departments, bureaus, agencies, boards, commissions, offices, independent establishments, and all instrumentalities of the state government . . .[40]

Centralization and coordination were basic to the reorganization that took place, but slowly. Subsection 112 of Title 3 V.S.A. established in the office of the secretary of state a Division of Registration, Licensing, and Secretarial Services to which eighteen boards, including the Board of Nursing were to be assigned.[41] In November 1960, the Board received notice of the centralization of licensure renewals in the office of the secretary of state. This plan, endorsed by the American Nurses' Association Council of State Boards of Nursing, marked the beginning of many changes. On February 28, 1962, a letter from Finance Director William K. Marsh advised transfer of Board monies to the Division of Licensing and Registration; this being "necessary to hasten employment of an executive secretary"[42] for the Board. A few months later, Morton Stillings, director of the Division, approached Board members about the possibility of moving the Board of Nursing office from Burlington to Montpelier.[43] The

Board did move, in January 1963, from 323 Pearl Street in Burlington to Riverside Annex in Montpelier.

In October 1964, there was discussion with Mr. Stillings regarding Board financial "support of the Division of Licensing and getting little (postage) or nothing in return." Board members agreed that the only way to change the situation was through a change in the law.[44] Executive Secretary Eleanor Smith, submitted her resignation July 2, 1965, because of "conflicting philosophy of the Board and that of the Division of Licensing and Registration."[45] Smith later rescinded her resignation; but she did actually resign and leave the position in 1967.[46] She was replaced October 25, 1967, by Board member and former director of the State Health Department's Division of Public Health Nursing, Esther Martinson.

A law establishing the Vermont Student Assistance Corporation (VSAC) was passed in 1965. This nonprofit corporation would provide opportunity for Vermont residents to attend colleges and other institutions of higher education by awarding grants and guaranteeing loans to eligible Vermont students. This law repealed a number of appropriations supporting Vermont students, including the scholarship funds awarded to nursing students through the Board of Nursing since 1953.[47]

1970s

Issues of the 1970s included the licensure of attendants at the Vermont State Hospital in Waterbury, closure of Vermont's remaining hospital diploma schools of nursing, continuing fallout from the ongoing reorganization within state government, revision of the Nurse Practice Act, responses to inquiries from legislators, and creation of the National Council of State Boards of Nursing (NCSBN).

Over a period of eight years, licensure of psychiatric attendants at the Vermont State Hospital (VSH) became a controversial consideration for both the Board and VSH. The controversy stemmed from the continued inclusion in revisions of the Nurse Practice Act, by legislators, of psychiatric attendants at VSH and the Brandon Training School under exemptions from licensure under the Nurse Practice Act. These attendants were obviously carrying out some nursing responsibilities with no regulatory provisions except those of the employing institutions. An attendant training program was developed at VSH in the early 1950s by Vera Hanks, RN. As a requirement of employment, VSH aides were required to take an in-house two year psychiatric aide training program; in 1954, 180 aides were trained in the program.[48] Upon successful completion of the two-year program, selected aides/attendants might enroll for an additional two years in a program preparing them to become psychiatric technicians. The latter program, supported by a grant from the National Institutes of Mental Health (NIMH), graduated sixty-five psychiatric technicians in 1968, and seventy in the spring of 1969.[49] It was at this time that VSH Superintendent George Brooks, MD, sought licensure for the psychiatric technicians from the Vermont State Board of Nursing. Marsha Kincheloe presents specific details of the VSH effort in Section Two of this volume.

Members of the Vermont State Board of Nursing studied and explored ways and means of licensing psychiatric technicians in Vermont. Board President Mary Thompson, RN, and Executive Secretary Grace Buttolph, RN, attended and convened numerous meetings on the issue. Attendees and conferees represented VSH, Vermont Association of Psychiatric Technicians, Vermont State Nurses' Association (VSNA), Practical Nurses Association of Vermont (PNAV), and other concerned agencies. At a December 1970 meeting at the Board office in Montpelier, consideration was given to similar laws already enacted in California, Colorado, and Arkansas.[50] Dr. Brooks and Pauline Martin of the Vermont Association of Psychiatric Technicians disagreed as to the functions of the proposed licensee: Brooks explained that the work of psychiatric technicians was not primarily nursing, while Martin maintained that their duties were nursing and they wished to identify with nursing.[51] Various possibilities were advanced including the proposal that VSH work with the Division of Allied Health Sciences at The University of Vermont and/or Vermont College on curriculum development toward the goal of legitimizing the program through affiliation with an accredited educational institution rather than a service institution. In January 1971, the Board of Nursing was informed that the American Nurses' Association and the American Medical Association had officially taken the position of declaring a moratorium on further licensure of new health personnel. These positions lessened the urgency for action on the controversy.

In 1972, the VSH Psychiatric Technician Program became affiliated with the Community College of Vermont, which awarded thirty-three credits for the VSH program toward a sixty-credit curriculum for an associate degree in mental health technology. Completion of the CCV program qualified many of the VSH program graduates for jobs in the community mental health centers.[52] In 1975, the Vermont Psychiatric Technicians applied to the State Legislature for licensure under their own board. This was not acted upon; and again in 1976 their bill was stalled by legislative evaluation of all licensing boards including the Board of Nursing.

In an effort to assure that the nurse licensing law meet the needs of practicing nurses and provide for the public's health and safety, the Board of Nursing, the VSNA, and the PNAV formed a committee to address

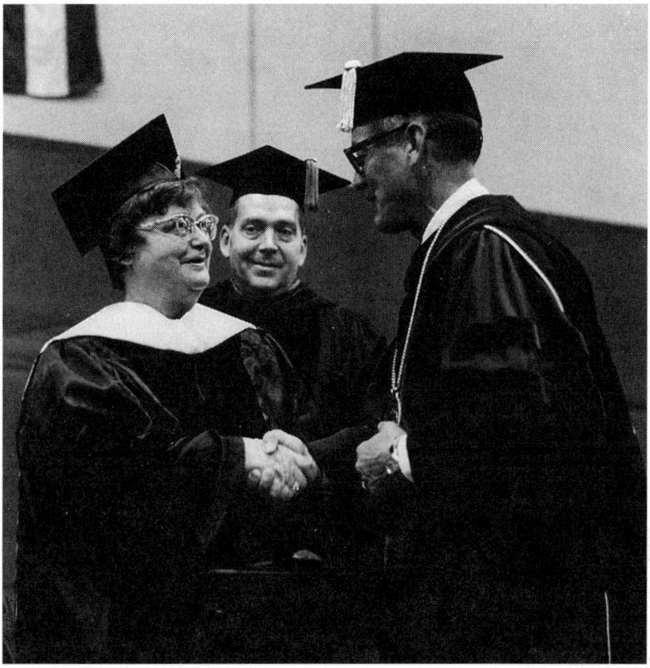

Grace M. Buttolph, executive secretary of the Vermont State Board of Nursing from 1970 to 1975, receiving honorary degree from The University of Vermont President Edward Andrews, May 1975.

revisions of the law. Minutes of the Board from 1972 report that the joint committee had met twice to discuss:

1. Updating the definitions of professional and practical nursing,
2. Adding a public member to the Board,
3. A PNAV proposal that one of the four RN members should be a faculty member from a school of practical nursing,
4. Opening new nursing education programs preparing individuals to be registered nurses in a post-secondary educational institution,
5. Limiting the inactive status of a licensee to five years and requiring completion of a refresher course for any practicing nurse who had been inactive for five or more years, and
6. No longer exempting employees of state agencies—including VSH at Waterbury and the Brandon Training School at Brandon—from the law.[53]

Months of intensive work ensued before the proposed legislation was introduced by Washington County Senator Dorothy Shea as S.181. The

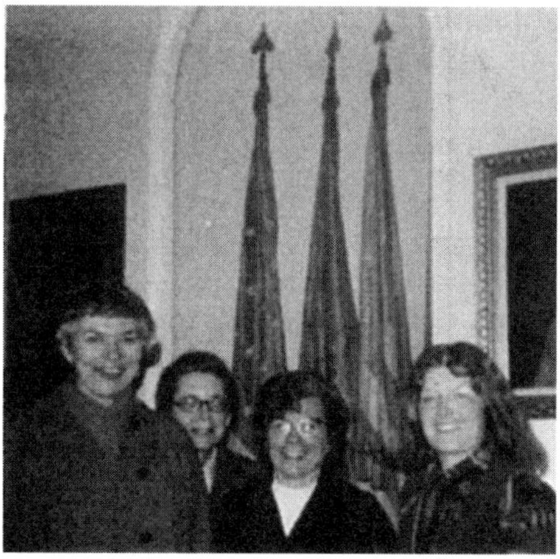

At the Statehouse celebrating the March 1974 revision of the Nurse Practice Act
Left to right: Faith Emerson, Vermont State Board of Nursing;
Ann Janney, executive secretary, VSNA; Pat Allen, legislative aide, VSNA;
Karen Estey, chair, VSNA Legislative Committee

bill did pass the legislature, was signed by Governor Thomas Salmon, and became effective July 1, 1974.[54]

Members of the Vermont State Legislature were very responsive, as they should be, to inquiries from the public. One communication from a constituent to his/her representative was often seen as a mandate to pursue a complaint about a Board of Nursing rule or regulation and to question why an exception could not be made. A particular concern arose as the result of numerous medics and corpsmen returning from military service who sought to become licensed by waiver as practical nurses. Many of the legislators were veterans themselves, and were very sympathetic to these requests—not understanding that, though these medics and corpsmen could have been outstanding in providing emergency care or another care specialty, their training and experience did not cover the scope of education, training, and practice of practical nurses. Not unlike the general public, many legislators had limited knowledge and appreciation of the educational preparation and responsibilities of both professional and practical nurses.[55] Interpretation of the role and functions of nurses, as well as the Board of Nursing, was an important responsibility of every member of the Board and many practicing RNs and LPNs; this became especially important during the legislative sessions.

The Board of Nursing convened a special meeting in February 1971 to discuss and respond to the stated plan of the Vermont State Colleges to close the associate degree nursing program at Castleton State College.

Nurse Graduates from Vermont Schools[56]

School	1966	1967	1968	1969	1970	Estimated[1] 1971	1972
University of Vermont (BS)	29	28	46	38	50	42	44
University of Vermont (AD)	—	—	—	—	—	35	32
Castleton State College	11	13	9	19	22	14	15
Vermont College	18	13	18	17	19	25	26
Mary Fletcher[2]	28	34	42	42	42	34	—
Jeanne Mance[2]	29	32	54	35	35	39	—
Total	115	120	169	151	168	189	117

[1]1972 figure is adjusted to allow for 10 fewer students graduating than were enrolled on 15 October 1970

[2]Closing June 1971 2/18/71

This was also the year that the last two hospital diploma schools of nursing in Vermont, Mary Fletcher Hospital and Jeanne Mance Schools of Nursing, would close. Closure of these schools was based upon assurance that the State of Vermont would provide educational opportunities for students to major in nursing in its general educational system, which presumed the need for two state-supported associate degree programs, one at The University of Vermont and the other at Castleton State College. In fact, closure of the two hospital-based diploma programs in Burlington had, as previously mentioned, been planned to coincide with The University of Vermont School of Nursing's opening an associate degree program to accommodate qualified candidates who would have applied to the three-year diploma programs. Board President Mary Thompson sent a letter of protest to the chairman of the Vermont State Colleges Board of Trustees (VSC), William Moeser, urging reconsideration and continuance of the Castleton program in the interests of the health needs of the citizens of Vermont. Accompanying this letter was graphic presentation of the number of nurses graduated from Vermont schools, with estimates for 1971 and 1972 (see table). Strong public and legislative support of the associate degree nursing program in southern Vermont resulted in a VSC trustees' decision for continuance of the nursing program at Castleton State College.

The once free-standing, autonomous Board of Nursing continued to be challenged by administrative controls from state government which frequently hampered the ability of the Board in carrying out the requirements of the Nurse Practice Act, Title 26 V.S.A. Chapter 28. Throughout the 1970s and the 1980s, Board of Nursing minutes reflect the ever-present struggle for money and power waged between the Board members and representatives of the newly created Division of Professional Registration and Licensure (DPRL) based in the office of the Vermont Secretary of State. Frequent personnel changes in the DPRL only added to the difficulties. Conflicts between the nursing law and the administrative mandates of Title 3 V.S.A. Chapter 5 were the source of frequent intervention from various committees of the state legislature. Following are excerpts from Board minutes which illustrate some of the concerns, not only of Board members, but also of various state agencies and associations:

> *June 1972.* Proposed that the executive secretary of the Board of Nursing would no longer be responsible to the Board but rather to DPRL; she would handle Medical Board technical problems in addition to having major Board of Nursing responsibilities. Longtime secretarial employee, Hilda Webster, would no longer work for the Board of Nursing's executive officer; she would be under the direct supervision of the administrative assistant in DPRL.[57] One of the major problems was the perception of DPRL that the licensure renewal process involved merely the receipt of the renewal application and the check for the renewal fee and, as such, could be assigned to any secretary. Mrs. Webster's years of experience with the Board were essential in applicant review to determine that renewal requirements were met and questionable applications referred to the Board's executive secretary for follow-up.
>
> *February 22, 1972.* On February 15th, Board members Ruby Carr, Faith Emerson, and Joyce Fellows, with Executive Secretary Grace Buttolph, appeared at a hearing of the House Appropriations Committee to protest a lack of communication with the Agency of Human Services relative to the Agency's licensure proposal. Previously, the Board had sent a letter to the Appropriations Committee protesting the "taking of Board funds for other purposes."
>
> *July 11, 1973.* The Board treasurer reports that Board money "is being taken in small amounts by the DPRL: $5,700 taken at the end of [the] fiscal year and given to WHEELS Program in Springfield; also, 2 non-coded items [were] taken."
>
> *March 4, 1976.* The State Board of Nursing is handicapped by lack of money to send representatives to attend the ANA Council of State Boards of Nursing—an experience important both in orientating new board members, as well as updating the executive secretaries of state boards of nursing on current issues and activities affecting the practice of nursing and licensing functions of the board. Executive Secretary Louise Alcott tells the Board that she will attend "at her own expense if necessary."

April 29, 1976. The fiscal year supplemental appropriation cites $15,000 for the Secretary of State for licensing boards requesting $40,000; $3,493 is allotted to the Board of Nursing; it had requested $7,678 (H.533). H.550 appropriated $42,713 to the Board of Nursing for FY1977. The Board reported an expected deficit and was advised to seek Emergency Board assistance in July or August. Board members Faith Emerson and Mabel Buley would assist in drafting a proposal to the state legislature that funds received by the Board of Nursing under Title 26 V.S.A. Chapter 27, now deposited in the General Fund, be placed in credit to the Board for administration and enforcement of Title 26 V.S.A. Chapter 27. Board revenues from licensee fees were estimated at $76,605; $42,713 was appropriated by the DPRL for Board use.[58] Clearly, the money generated by licensing and renewal fees for nurses exceeded the amount provided by the DPRL.

February 18, 1977. The Board's executive secretary, Louise Alcott, advises the Board members that "secretarial and clerical support for the Board of Nursing is inadequate to carry out the functions of the office."

June 22, 1977. At a special Board meeting, the members are advised that many complaints are being received about delays in the licensing process. Executive Secretary Alcott responds that there is a "great backlog" and insufficient staff to deal with it. In a letter to the director of DPRL, Miss Alcott complains that the nursing licensure situation "jeopardizes the legality of nursing practice for nurse and employer." According to a Finance Department report, the Board of Nursing has 1977 revenues of $80,601 from licensing fees and expenditures of $43,454.81: personal services, $31,246; operating expenses, $12,208.81.[59]

March 22, 1979. S.130 is introduced; this bill provides for the Medical Practice Board to be detached from the Secretary of State's office and its revenues dedicated to a special fund. The Board of Nursing acted to explore the possibility of an amendment to S.130 for the inclusion of the Nursing Board. All renewal licenses were mailed with an insert asking licensees to contact their legislators asking them to take action to appropriate the nurse license fees to the Board of Nursing rather than to the General Fund. Nursing schools, other agencies, and associations were contacted and the governor's office was kept advised.

July 19–20, 1979. The minutes of this annual meeting of the Board of Nursing are replete with problems related to the Secretary of State's administration of budgetary and personnel problems. Four pages of discussion resulted in Board members supporting the motion of Rosemary Hittle, public member, and Mary Edwards, LPN member, that "The Board in cooperation with the VSNA Legislative Committee initiate action to draft legislation to create an autonomous Vermont State Board of Nursing."

Two bills introduced into the 1979–80 sessions of the State Legislature were reflective of issues being addressed by the Board in the late 1970s and the early 1980s. S.230 was introduced by Senators Daniels and Niquette of Chittenden County and Hewitt of Bennington County and proposed to "expand certain powers of the Board, to enable it to retain fees collected for the purposes of regulating the practice of Nursing, to enable it to establish standards and qualifications for professional nursing specialties and for other purposes." S.230 passed as Act No. 192, a revision of the Nurse Practice Act; it repealed 26 V.S.A. Chapter 27 relating to nursing, and added 26 V.S.A. Chapter 28. Section 1574, sub-section (4) would allow the Board to provide standards and regulations for nurse practitioners and other nursing specialties. Section 1573 changed the way in which nurse appointees to the Board would be selected: they would no longer be nominated by the nursing associations but they must be representative of the various nursing education programs and nursing services. An additional public member was added to the Board for a total of two public members, and terms of Board members were changed from five to three years. Section 1580 provided that all fees received by the Board would be paid into the General Fund of the state, and that the Board should submit its proposed budget to the Secretary of State, to be submitted together with the Secretary of State's budget to the governor for review, amendment, and submission to the General Assembly.[60]

S.182 introduced by a state agency and classified as "administrative procedures–rulemaking" also passed into law. The effect of S.182 was to strongly advance the goals of the "Little Hoover Commission" of the late 1950s and 1960. A letter from Deputy Secretary of State Paul Gillies to the Board of Nursing relative to the implications of S.182 described this process as an "advanced consolidated sunset" which put the budgets of the licensing boards under the Secretary of State. Additionally, consideration would be given to moving the Board of Nursing to the building of the Medical Board, thus reducing the cost of photocopying and other materials and services, and possible sharing of secretaries and executive directors. Attorney Gillies referred to S.182 as a "forceful bill . . . which increases the power of the Secretary of State and decreases the power of the Boards with the resultant . . . centralizing of power."[61]

Board of Nursing President Faith Emerson and Executive Secretary Louise Alcott attended the 32nd Annual Meeting of the American Nurses' Association Council of State Boards of Nursing in Los Angeles, California, in June 1978. This was an historic meeting at which the representatives from fifty-two jurisdictions created the National Council of State Boards of Nursing (NCSBN), an independent, nonprofit organization comprised of sixty-one boards of nursing in the United States and its territories. There had been discussion at the national level for several years encouraging separation of the state boards' responsibilities from the ANA because of the potential for bias and conflict of interests. This was particularly relevant to the examination of candidates to become registered nurses by the professional organization for nurses, the ANA, which represented the standards and interests of professional nurses. Thus the NCSBN was established as a free-standing organization with no affiliation with any professional organization.

> The mission of the National Council of State Boards of Nursing is to lead in nursing regulation by assisting Member Boards, collectively and individually, to promote safe and effective nursing practice in the interest of protecting public health and welfare.[62]

Accomplishments of this first meeting of the NCSBN are cited in the minutes of the July 1978 Annual Meeting of the Vermont State Board of Nursing:

1. Accepted Articles of Incorporation which included name change to National Council of State Boards of Nursing;
2. Adopted by-laws changing the fiscal year from the calendar year to July 1–June 30;
3. Adopted standing rules;
4. Accepted contract formats as previously proposed;
5. Accepted membership contract of $1000 annually for each state board member for use of the State Board Test Pool Examination (SBTPE);
6. Proposed headquarters sites for study and selection by the board of directors: Chicago, St. Louis, Dallas, and Oklahoma City;
7. Elected officers and nominating committee members.[63]

At the end of the 1970s, issues of concern to the Vermont State Board of Nursing are reflected in agenda items submitted by the Board to the Northeast Council of State Boards of Nursing:

1. The current political climate in Quebec, Canada—is it causing a significant increase in Canadian applicants for licensure in other border states of the region?
2. The status of statutory and administrative rule regulation of nurse practitioners of the region,

3. The expanded role of the nurse in community health services and the status of third party payment for nursing services,
4. HEW Region I's current definition of professional nursing practice in the region.[64]

1980s

Of primary concern to the Board of Nursing throughout the decade of the eighties was employing and retaining a qualified executive director. This was no small task, and required an ever-increasing expenditure of time and effort on the part of Board members: there was the need for members to actually assist in the professionally related office work during times of vacancy in the position; the effort and time required in searching, interviewing, and negotiating with various state officials and agencies relative to position requirements and appropriate salary; orienting and re-orienting as executives came and went; the ever-increasing backlog of work. At this time, the Board staff consisted of one clerical-level person, employed by and responsible to a supervisor in the Division of Professional Registration and Licensure under the Secretary of State's jurisdiction.

Many serious practice issues were of concern to 1980s Board members. Discipline cases were becoming a larger part of the workload for Board members and staff; newer approaches to dealing with the disciplined licensees were being considered and tried by various other state boards around the country. P.L.100-203 had promulgated new regulations related to the training and evaluation of nurse aides—some state agency must assume responsibility for development and implementation of this program. The increasing mobility of nurses via "traveling nurse agencies" that provided registered nurses for hire in areas where there was a shortage of nurses impacted the Board's Rules and Regulations. The availability of refresher/re-entry programs currently approved by the Board of Nursing was again demanding attention. Many questions relative to the practice of Vermont's nurse practitioners (nurses in advanced practice) came before the Boards of Nursing, Medicine, and Pharmacy. Rapid advances in science and technology were reflected in the nursing problems brought before the Board of Nursing and often, eventually, to the State's Attorney General. A deputy attorney general was assigned to the Board, and met frequently with Board members and staff relative to the legal implications of problems brought before the Board.

During the 1980s, the Board of Nursing executive officer position was vacant, or filled by part-time employees; this was a direct result of budgeting by the DPRL that provided salaries inadequate to attract nurses whose education and experience met the criteria established by law. Full-time executive officer Louise P. Alcott left the position October 1, 1980, after serving nearly five-and-a-half years. She was followed by Dr. Barbara Boisse, professor of nursing at Norwich University, who filled the post in a part-time capacity from June 1, 1981 to June 1, 1982. Her successor, Dr. Francesca Faye, professor of nursing and pediatric nurse practitioner, was also employed part-time (Tuesday and Thursday 7:50 AM to 3:50 PM);[65] she terminated June 20, 1984.[66] After a vacancy of eight months in the position, Lynne B. Hardee, RN, MSN, MDiv, succeeded Faye on September 10, 1985, again part-time at a pay level of $15 an hour.[67] Hardee's resignation was accepted in May 1987, to be effective July 1, 1987. In July 1988, Priscilla (Pat) Allen, RN, MSN, immediate past president of the VSNA, became the first full-time executive officer since Alcott's resignation. As was the case with her predecessors, Allen's time was limited to one year, again due to disputes over a salary inconsistent with the demands of the position. Various groups, including the Vermont State Nurses' Association, the Practical Nurse Association of Vermont, and others were convinced that the goal of the state bureaucracy had been and continued to be to reduce the qualifications of the professional nurse executive officer to clerical level; this had been and would continue to be accomplished by means of financial constraints.[68]

In February 1990, Claire LeFrancois, RN, MPH, long-time maternal child health nursing consultant with the Vermont Health Department, transferred to the Board of Nursing position and for the first time in ten years the Board secured a full-time executive director with a salary almost commensurate with the position requirement. LeFrancois remained in the position until her untimely death in July 1994. She was succeeded by Anita Ristau, RN, MS, previously a Board of Nursing member for six years and director of the Division of Nursing at Norwich University; Ristau continues as executive director of the Vermont State Board of Nursing. From a position of weakness and disarray in the 1980s, the Board of Nursing came to a position of strength, rapid growth, and development in the 1990s.

On February 11, 1980, the Vermont Legislature's Joint Committee on Administrative Rules directed the Vermont Board of Nursing to "come up with a plan to make re-entry programs available statewide on a frequent recurring basis, at a low cost, and available to nurses who simply wish to hold a license, but not practice."[69] This legislative action was in response to a Vermont nurse who complained about the lack of refresher programs to meet the requirements of the Board of Nursing Administrative Rules N.05 and N.06 promulgated to carry out the requirements of Title 26 V.S.A. Chapter 28, Section 1579(c). Re-entry programs had been available since passage of the nursing law Title 26 V.S.A. Chapter 27, Section 1556(f) which required that the Board "make such regulations . . . as . . . necessary to assure itself that an applicant for renewal . . . is professionally qualified." In a later amendment, effective July 1, 1980, Section 1579(c) clarified the requirement:

> All applicants for renewal of a license to practice shall have practiced nursing within the last five years as defined in section 1572 of this title or comply with the requirements for updating knowledge and skills as defined by the Board rules.

In April 1980, the Board convened a conference of providers of re-entry programs. Attendees were representatives of programs at Castleton State College, Northwestern Medical Center Hospital, Putnam Memorial Hospital, Fanny Allen Hospital, Medical Center Hospital of Vermont, The University of Vermont School of Nursing, Vermont College/Norwich University Nursing Program, and the Fanny Allen School of Practical Nursing.[70] The purpose of the meeting was to plan for developing resources for nurses to update knowledge and skills. This group recommended that 1) The Board of Nursing needed to establish more specific guidelines for individually designed programs, and 2) Agencies and institutions planning to provide a "formal course" should try to coordinate with other providers to avoid duplication and to provide for a variety of offerings statewide throughout the year.[71] At its May 23, 1980, meeting the Board authorized the appointment of a task force, representative of each type of re-entry program, to develop guidelines for providers and attendees.

In the Fall of 1988, the task force concept was formalized and now titled Board of Nursing Advisory Committee on Re-entry Programs. This committee convened November 22, 1988, to revise and update the guidelines for providers of re-entry programs. Members of the Advisory Committee were Wendy Austin, Inservice Education, Porter Medical Center; Joanne Brickley, Director, Thompson School for Practical Nurses; Betsy Hartman, Inservice Director, North Country Hospital; Sharon Kartsimas, Director of Nursing, Springfield Hospital; Linda Phypers, Inservice Education, Burlington Convalescent Center; Carolyn Smith, Administrator, McKerley Health Care Center; and Kathy Watts, Inservice Education, Central Vermont Hospital.[72]

Board of Nursing review and approval was required prior to conducting any re-entry program whether it be individual or institutional. Board surveys of existing programs in 1983 and 1988 provided a baseline and an aid to the Board in monitoring the re-entry programs. On May 8, 1989, the Board approved completed guidelines for the development of re-entry programs for RNs and LPNs; these were distributed to providers of re-entry programs and to individual nurses affected by Board Rules N.05 and N.06. In 1988, forty nurses re-entered nursing practice through the Vermont Re-entry Programs.[73]

In the Spring of 1989, twelve Vermont institutions offered Board-approved re-entry programs to nurses. Five providers offered programs to both RNs and LPNs, one offered a program to LPNs only, and six provided programs limited to RNs.[74]

Institutions Offering Programs	*RN*	*LPN*	*Frequency of Offering*
Burlington Convalescent Center, Burlington	×	×	As needed
Castleton State College, Castleton	×		Spring and Fall
Central Vermont Medical Center, Berlin	×		March 1989
Dartmouth-Hitchcock Medical Center, Hanover	×		March 1989
McKerley Health Care Center, Morrisville	×	×	Continuing
Medical Center Hospital of Vermont, Burlington	×		Once yearly
North Country Hospital, Newport	×	×	As needed
Porter Medical Center, Middlebury	×	×	Ongoing
Southwestern Medical Center, Bennington	×		No schedule
Springfield Hospital, Springfield	×		PRN
Thompson School of Practical Nursing, Brattleboro		×	
Veterans Administration Hospital, White River Jct.	×	×	

In 1987, federal regulations promulgated under P.L.100-203 relative to the training and registry of nursing assistants presented the Board of Nursing with the need to decide what its involvement should be in the regulation of nursing assistants, commonly referred to as nurses' aides. Some states were already placing registration of these workers with the boards of nursing. Historically, Vermont's regulation of the nursing assistant was by the employer with accountability to the facility licensing agency, i.e., the State Health Department's Division of Medical Care Facilities. At that time, training of the nursing assistant occurred in several settings: on-the-job training within the employing health care facility, the Department of Education's Adult Education Program, and some vocational-level high school programs. P.L. 100-203 would require a minimum short-term training of seventy-five hours, with competence evaluation at the end of the training period. An accurate count of the nursing assistants employed in Vermont health care facilities was not available; however, it was generally accepted that nursing homes accounted for the greatest number. The Board assigned member Anita Ristau and Executive Director Pat Allen the responsibility for meeting with, and coordinating the efforts of, the various state agencies and representatives of the nursing home industry.[75]

Funding was a critical factor for all the agencies involved, and especially for the Board of Nursing now dependent upon the Secretary of State and various intra-agency managers for approval and funding. On October 13, 1988, Executive Director Allen reported to the Board: "It seems quite clear that the Department of Health will receive the monies for implementation of registry, training, and testing of nursing assistants in nursing homes, and at this time it appears that the State Health Department intends to assume full responsibility."[76] This situation soon changed with a "shake-up" in state government which transferred certain Health Department functions to a newly created Department of Aging and Disabilities—among them the responsibility for meeting federal requirements relative to nursing assistants under P.L.100-203.[77] This action added a new voice to the interagency committee which was already well along with fact-finding and planning. The new agency was ably represented by Patrick Flood, director of the Division of Licensing and Protection, and he assumed a leadership role. The Board of Nursing, with support from Secretary of State James Douglas, was now convinced that the responsibility for regulation of the nursing assistant belonged with the Board of Nursing. It would take an act of the Vermont Legislature to give this control, including adequate funding, to the Board of Nursing.[78]

During the 1980s, the Board of Nursing was confronted with steadily increasing numbers of disciplinary cases. Annual Reports on Licensing, published by the Office of the Secretary of State, provide numerical data about complaints received and action taken. Of the eight complaints against licensees in fiscal year 1986, the Board took action against four: one RN for incompetent practices related to medications; one RN for making a false statement on an application regarding a previous conviction for heroin possession; one LPN for lewd and lascivious behavior; and one RN for diversion of drugs for personal use.[79] Legal basis for Board action was provided in Section 1582 of Title 26 V.S.A. Chapter 28 of 1980, and detailed in the 1983 Board of Nursing Administrative Rules N 6.01 through N 6.06. Following the written complaint, in-depth investigation, and appropriate hearings with direction and advice from the assigned Deputy Attorney General, Board action frequently resulted in revocation or suspension of the nurse's license.

Year	*No. Complaints Received*	*No. Licenses Revoked/ Suspended*
1981	1	2
1982	2	2
1983	7	6
1984	8	5
1985	12	9
1986	8	4
1987	20	14
1988	13	9
1989	21	6

Based upon models developed in Kansas, New Mexico, and California in the mid-to-late eighties, the Vermont Board did modify its regulatory procedures as they related to the chemically dependent nurse. This new management process required that 1) the nurse leave practice and be admitted to a residential treatment facility for a minimum of one month; 2) the employer, treating professional, and a representative of the Board work together to monitor the licensee's return to the workplace with a conditioned license; and that 3) there must be monthly reporting to the Board by the subject, the treating professional, and the workplace monitor. This modified approach to disciplining the licensee avoided stigma for the nurse and preserved his/her job and the health care benefits tied to the workplace health insurance—a necessity for the nurse to receive treatment. The close monitoring assured patient safety. This less punitive, rehabilitatively oriented approach appeared to be well received by the employing agencies and the nursing community.

1990s

The decade of the nineties saw the resolution of many of the problems that faced the Board of Nursing in the previous decade. Licensing of nursing assistants came under the administrative regulation of the Board. As a result, licensees regulated by the Board increased as did the Board staff responsible for administering the law and regulations governing the practice of the newly licensed nursing assistants (LNAs). The definition of advanced practice registered nurse (APRN) was approved by the Vermont Legislature. Disciplinary issues continued to mount and to require increasing attention from Board members and staff as well as staff of the Office of Professional Regulation of the Secretary of State. The accreditation of nursing education programs extended from entry level to all nursing education programs within the state. The licensing examination of the National Council of State Boards of Nursing (NCSBN) responded to nineties technology and adopted computer testing. In response to issues of the times, nursing practice changed to encompass additional legally authorized responsibilities.

In October 1991, the Board of Nursing contracted with the Agency of Aging and Disabilities to assume responsibility for approving nurse assistant educational programs and for monitoring the written and clinical testing contracted through the Psychological Corporation. This national testing service was awarded a contract to provide competency evaluations and to establish and maintain a registry. Testing began in the spring, and the registry commenced in October 1990. Brenda Chamberlin, RN, MHSA, was employed as the program coordinator.

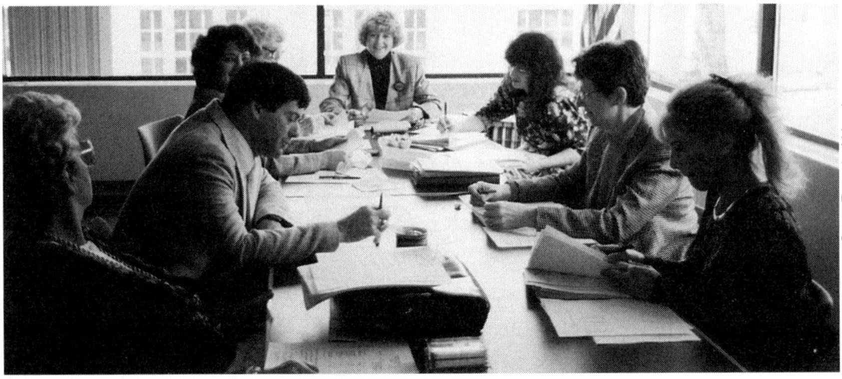

Courtesy Vermont State Board of Nursing

Vermont State Board of Nursing, 1991
Left to right: Bunny Beard, public member; William Butterfield, LPN; Anita Ristau, RN; Claire LeFrancois, RN, executive director; Kathleen Geran, RN, chair; Jackie Pierce, staff secretary; Ruth Walker Woodard, LPN; Brenda Smith, RN

A revision of the Nurse Practice Act and the Rules and Regulations was approved by the legislature in 1994, giving the Board of Nursing authority to license nurse assistants. The Board Rules and Regulations defined nursing assistant education standards, licensure and endorsement, examination, and discipline.[80] Vermont was the second state in the country to license nursing assistants; New Hampshire was the first.

The Board ruled in February 1995 that Level III and Level II care facilities and intermediate care facilities for the mentally disabled did not need to license their staff because the care was not assistive and not rendered under the supervision of a nurse.[81]

In 1944, the Nurse Practice Act was opened and the legislature approved the definition of APRN as a "licensed RN authorized to practice in this state who because of specialized education and experience is endorsed to perform acts of medical diagnosis and to prescribe medical, therapeutic or corrective measures under administrative rules adopted by the Board."[82] The legal definition emphasized Administrative Rule Chapter IV, Rule III D (2)a(i) that had been adopted in 1991 and stated:

> The Nurse Practitioner performs medical acts independently within approved protocols mutually agreed upon by the Nurse Practitioner and collaborating physician or pursuant to clinical privileges approved by the facility or facilities at which the Nurse Practitioner practices. Initial protocols or delineation of clinical privileges will be on file in the work place and the Board Office. The Board will be apprised of any changes in collaborating physician.

The law and rules in tandem made it clear to the Board of Nursing that all APRNs must submit practice guidelines that described clinical practice, including practice site(s), focus of care and general category of clients, and the name of at least one physician licensed in Vermont who practiced in the same specialty area and who would be routinely utilized for collaboration, consultation, and referral.

The Advanced Practice Committee was asked to study the Board of Nursing's ruling on APRNs who do not have prescriptive authority. Lorraine Impey, APRN, CS, represented the psychiatric clinical specialists who felt this ruling was very restrictive to those nurses engaged in psychotherapy. In a July 1995 letter to the Board of Nursing she wrote: "Changes are needed to allow psychiatric clinical nurse specialists to continue to practice independently of a psychiatrist if they have a psychotherapy practice and are not prescribing medication."[83] Impey elaborated on the scarcity of psychiatrists and on those psychiatrists willing to enter into collaborative agreements with a psychiatric clinical nurse specialist.

With the cooperation of Dr. John Mazzuzin, chair of the Medical Board, the Administrative Rule was changed in 1996 to allow psychiatric clinical nurse specialists without prescriptive authority to practice without a collaborating physician, as long as they had practice guidelines that delineated the process for consultation and referral, and methods of quality assurance.[84]

By 1996 there were 346 APRNs endorsed in Vermont. Prior to this time, those APRNs who did not have prescriptive authority were not required to follow the Administrative Rule regarding collaborative practice. Collaboration as it pertains to advance practice was not defined in the rules at this time.

In 1994, Mary Guyette requested that she be given advanced practice endorsement based upon her education and certification as a clinical nurse specialist in urological nursing. This request prompted the Board of Nursing to convene the Ad Hoc Advanced Practice Committee to study the issue and to make recommendations to the Board. The Committee, chaired by Kathleen Keleher, APRN, CNM, received conflicting opinions on APRN endorsement of clinical specialists, particularly from nurse practitioners. Nurse practitioners were concerned about the difference in education (physical assessment, pharmacology, and the use of prescriptive medications) and felt that the quality and standards set by the nurse practitioners would be weakened. After months of study, the ad hoc committee presented the following recommendation to the Board and it was adopted by the Board of Nursing in July 1995:

> In addition to the educational requirements (Chapter 4, Rule VIII A.2) the CNS [Clinical Nurse Specialist] will fulfill the following criteria:

The APRN formal educational program shall:

1. Be a formal academic/educational didactic program within an accredited educational institution: a clinical component is part of the program and is specific to the scope of practice in the area of the CNS' specialty
   The clinical component is a supervised, clinical "hands-on" preceptorship
   The preceptor must be a licensed APRN or MD in the CNS' area of specialty
2. Include advanced physical assessment (or psycho-social assessment) and differential diagnosis as it applies to the CNS' area of specialty
3. Advanced pathophysiology as defined by the educational program's curriculum and transcript
4. Pharmacology—specifically clinically focused and geared toward the nurse prescriber with a clinical management component.[85]

Mary Guyette became the first APRN clinical specialist in medical-surgical nursing in Vermont on February 13, 1995.

In the summer of 1989, the Vermont Legislature enacted a law (Title 3, subsection 128 Chapter 5) requiring that all unprofessional conduct be reported to the Board of Nursing:

> Subsection 128. Unprofessional conduct to be reported to [the] board
> a) Any hospital, clinic or other health care institution in which a licensee performs professional services shall report to the appropriate board, along with supporting information and evidence, any disciplinary action taken by it or its staff which significantly limits the licensee's privilege to practice or leads to suspension or expulsion from the institution. The report shall be made within ten days of the date such disciplinary action was taken. This section shall not apply to cases of resignation or separation from service for reasons unrelated to disciplinary action

As a result of this law and the licensure of nursing assistants in 1994, there was a dramatic increase in the number of complaints brought against licensees regulated by the Board of Nursing, as illustrated in the following:[86]

	1990	*1991*	*1992*	*1993*	*1994*	*1995*	*1996*
Complaint received	27	31	24	39	56	70	126
Action taken	13	21	17	21	22	63	108

A profile of the complaints received in 1996 indicated that reports of physical abuse occurred most frequently against LNAs. Incompetence was the complaint most often brought against the APRN-RN-LPN licensees, with medication errors in second place; drug abuse and physical abuse tied in third place for frequency of complaint against the APRN-RN-LPN group.

> As of September 1, 1996, 123 licensees were under investigation due to a complaint by a colleague, a facility or an agency administrator or a member of the public. Following is a breakdown of the investigations:

RNs	42	APRNs	3
LPNs	22	Applicants	6
LNAs	49	Unlicensed	1[87]

The decade of the nineties brought a radical change in the way nursing applicants would take the "State Board Examination." Early in the eighties, the national testing service of state boards of nursing, working through the NCSBN, began to study and conduct research to develop examinations that more nearly met NCSBN standards for safety, reliability, validity, and security. (Previously a single break in security somewhere in the country could affect every examinee throughout the country!) Vermont's Board has been directly involved in this study and the development of new methods of testing through the efforts of Executive Directors Claire LeFrancois and Anita Ristau. In 1993, Vermont participated in Beta Testing for the proposed computer adaptive testing (CAT) for RNs and LPNs that was adopted and implemented in 1994. This test replaced the paper and pencil examination. Executive Director Ristau currently serves as a member of the NCSBN Examination Committee.

In 1994, the Board of Nursing was granted authority by the Vermont Legislature (H.619 Act 201) to approve all nursing education programs in the state of Vermont. Prior to this, Board review and approval was limited to those programs which prepared the individual for entry level nursing practice. With the growth of upper division baccalaureate programs at Southern Vermont College and Norwich University, the Board determined that it was necessary to set standards for all nursing education programs.

In August 1995, the Board of Nursing gave provisional approval to Vermont Technical College (VTC) for the implementation of an associate degree program based upon a one-plus-one model. Students who graduated from the LPN program would be able to exit after one year and receive their LPN certificate and sit for the NCLEX PN examination; or they could continue for another year and earn an associate degree in nursing. In February 1996, the Board approved the Upper Division Baccalaureate Program at Southern Vermont College in Bennington.

On September 22, 1990, the Vermont State Medical Society's House of Delegates, in concurrence with the Board of Nursing, adopted a resolution that RNs may determine the death of a patient when that death is anticipated. This resolution demonstrates the supportive efforts of the Medical Society and the Medical Board. This was followed, on June 5, 1991, by a joint statement of the two boards, Medical and Nursing, regarding the administration of nonprescriptive medicines by RNs. It was determined and approved that "while providing nursing care, the utilization of non-prescription medications is within the scope of practice of the registered nurse."[88] These two opinions placed the extended scope of practice of Vermont nurses well ahead of their counterparts in the other states.

In the early nineties, the Board of Nursing was faced with reductions in nursing staff and the concomitant increase in numbers of unlicensed personnel. An Ad HOC Practice Committee convened in 1993 at the request of the Board to study the issue of delegation of nursing tasks. The Committee, chaired by Kathleen Geran, RN, MSN, issued a recommendation that was adopted by the Board to study the issue of delegation of nursing tasks. The recommendation defined delegation and unlicensed personnel, and delineated the provisions that must be met prior to delegation. A decision-making grid was also produced by the Committee. In 1995, the Board adopted the NCSBN's delegation concept paper that defined appropriate tasks to be delegated to assistive personnel.

Nurses continued to need clarification regarding delegation of nursing tasks, particularly with the administration of medications in schools. Claire LeFrancois, Executive Director of the Board of Nursing, wrote to the president of the Vermont State School Nurses Association (VSSNA) expressing the opinion of the Board that the school nurse may delegate appropriate tasks, including the administration of medications, to unlicensed personnel under designated guidelines. This opinion extended the delegation responsibility to the nurse who was not present in the building, or even employed by the agency on that particular day.[89]

Other issues, including abandonment, also surfaced due to the shortage of nurses. Nurses were being required to work double shifts and/or extend their shifts with the threat that, if they did not cooperate, they would be subject to Board of Nursing discipline for abandonment. An advisory opinion was issued March 1996 relative to "patient abandonment." The opinion defined and differentiated between patient abandonment and employer abandonment. Nurses guilty of patient abandonment (i.e., leaving a person without care after accepting an assignment to provide care), are subject to discipline under 26 V.S.A., Section 1595 (5) and Administrative Rule IV B 4 (f). Licensees are not subject to discipline for employer abandonment (i.e., leaving the employing agency without giving sufficient notice).

In December 1996, the Fifteenth Annual Report on Professional Licensing reported

> The Board of Nursing has the largest single regulatory program under this Office, the most complaints, the most investigations, the most disciplinary actions and the most oversight of professionals working in nursing homes. With 14,610 licensees, the Board of Nursing can justify a 10 member board. The Board of Nursing now regulates nursing assistants, a program with 4,924 licensees.[90]

It is apparent from this historical review of the trials and tribulations and accomplishments of the Vermont State Board of Nursing from 1940 through the mid nineties, that the nurse leaders of Vermont were committed and conscientious in attempting to maintain the quality of nursing care. The Board of Nursing monitored trends in practice as well as educational programs across the nation, and submitted legislation to insure the continuance of high standards for nursing practice in Vermont.[91]

—PRISCILLA (PAT) ALLEN, RN, MSN
with contributions from
ANITA F. RISTAU, RN, MS
and edited by
FAITH G. EMERSON, RN, BS, MA

Vermont State Board of Nursing

Administrative Secretary	Catherine Terrien, RN	1943–1963
Executive Secretary	Eleanor J. Smith, RN, MA	1963–1967
	Esther L. Martinson, RN, MA	1967–1970
	Grace M. Buttolph, RN, MA	1970–1975
	Louise P. Alcott, RN, MA	1975–1980
Executive Director	Barbara Boisse, RN, PhD	1981–1982
	Francesca C. Fay, RN, EdD, PNP	1983–1984
	Lynne B. Hardee, RN, MSN, M.Div	1985–1987
	Priscilla (Pat) Allen, RN, MSN	1988–1989
	Claire T. LeFrancois, RN, MPH	1990–1994
	Anita F. Ristau, RN, MS	1995–

Members of the Board[92]

1940s

Sister Marie Anne Bisson, RN, *Colchester*
Rita A. Cleveland, RN, *Huntington Center*
*Eleanor M. Dyke, RN, *Barre*
Charles H. Goyette, MD, *Barre*
Caroline C. Hatch, RN, *Montpelier*
Helen L. Little, RN, *St. Albans*
*Chester A. Newhall, MD, *Burlington*

1950s

Dorothy M. Allen, RN, *Newfane*
Wilmer W. Angell, MD, *Randolph*
Dorothy S. Brown, RN, *Williamstown*
*Grace M. Buttolph, RN, *Burlington*
Claire Chaffee, RN, *Poultney*
Myrlee E. Clark, RN, *Brattleboro*
Dorothy P. Howard, LPN, *Barre*
Lena R. Oakley, RN, *Burlington*
*Clara A. Roitero, LPN, *Brattleboro*

1960s

*Mabel M. Buley, LPN, *Vernon*
*Sister Irene Duchesneau, RN, *Burlington*
Ruby C. Carr, RN, *Fairlee*
Eleanor M. Diack, RN, *Barre*
Joyce C. Fellows, RN, *Morrisville*
Marion Gorham, RN, *Montpelier*
Esther L. Martinson, RN, *Burlington*
Dorothy C. Patterson, LPN, *Montpelier*
*Mary E. Thompson, RN, *Burlington*
Ethel Vallencourt Waite, LPN, *Bennington*

1970s

Hilda Packard, RN, *Brattleboro*
*Faith G. Emerson, RN, *Williston*
*Rolande Irvine, RN, *Essex Junction*
*Mary Edwards, LPN, *Jeffersonville*
*Stella Skibniowsky, RN, *Vernon*
*Effie Chamberlin, LPN, *Townshend*
*Rosemary Hittle, Public Member, *Montpelier*

1980s

Carol Elmendorf, RN, *Johnson*
Susan Bruce, Public Member, *St. Albans*
Lucy Frasier, LPN, *Colchester*
Mary Goodwin, Public Member, *Rutland*
Barbara King, RN, *Barre*
Joan Smidutz, RN, *Westminster*
Jean Milligan, RN, *Burlington*
Dennis Ross, RN, *Bomoseen*
*William Butterfield, LPN, *Essex Junction*
Carolyn Chase, Public Member
*Kathleen Geran, RN, *Burlington*
*Jane Campbell, RN, *So. Burlington*
Esther Sorrell, Public Member, *Burlington*
*Jeanette Sachse, RN, *St. Johnsbury*
*Bunny Beard, Public Member, *St. Albans*
Clare Dyer, Public Member
Jeanne Kay, LPN, *Brattleboro*
*Anita Ristau, RN, *Barre*
Ronald LaTour, Public Member

1990s

Ruth Walker Woodard, LPN, *Jericho*
Marjorie Allard, RN, *Burlington*
Ingrid Brodin, RN, *Manchester*
Catherine C. McGee, Public Member, *Norwich*
Raymond Phillips, Public Member, *Burlington*
Brenda Smith, RN, *Lyndon Center*
Kim Keaton, RN, *Barre*
Marjorie Kerr Allen, LNA, *Springfield*
Margaret Luce, RN, *Waterbury Center*
Effie Chamberlin, LPN, *Townshend*
Diane Dowgiewicz, LPN, *Bennington*

---

* Indicates that these board members' terms extended into the next decade.

NOTES

1. State of Vermont, Vermont State Board of Nursing, *Title 26 V.S.A. Chapter 28 and Administrative Rules*, 1995, 1.
2. Vermont State Nurses' Association, *We Who Serve: A Story of Nursing in Vermont* (Winooski, Vt.: Vermont State Nurses' Association, 1941), 25.
3. Vermont Board of Registration of Nurses, Minutes of the meeting of 26 February 1941. Vermont State Archives, Office of the Secretary of State, Montpelier, (hereafter cited as VBRN Minutes).
4. Ibid.
5. VBRN Minutes, 7 May 1941, 15.
6. VBRN Minutes, 3 November 1941, 15.
7. VBRN Minutes, 7 May 1941, 15.
8. VBRN Minutes, 12 April 1943, 66.
9. VBRN Minutes, 1 September 1943, 66.
10. VBRN Minutes, 7 January 1944, 73.
11. VBRN Minutes, 12 April 1944, 73.
12. VBRN Minutes, 8 November 1945, 92.
13. VBRN Minutes, 11 May 1949, 176.
14. VBRN Minutes, 20 December 1949, 171–73.
15. VBRN Minutes, 16 October, 1950, 191–92.
16. VBRN Minutes, 4 November 1958, 5.
17. VBRN Minutes, 1 January 1953, 244.
18. VBRN Minutes, 29 June 1960, 2.
19. State of Vermont, *Public Acts, 1951 Session*, 164–67.
20. VBRN Minutes, 1 January 1953, 223.
21. VBRN Minutes, attachment to minutes, 6 March 1956.
22. VBRN Minutes, 18 June 1958, 2.
23. Marsha Kincheloe and Herbert G. Hunt, Jr., *Empty Beds: A History of Vermont State Hospital* (Barre, Vt.: author, 1988), 75.
24. VBRN Minutes, 1 March 1957, 1.
25. State of Vermont, *Acts and Resolves: General Assembly of the State of Vermont, 42nd Biennial Session, 1953*, 273.
26. Sister Irene Duchesneau, RTSJ, personal communication, 14 September 1999.
27. Vermont State Board of Nursing, Minutes of the meeting of 28 June 1960, 3; 15 November 1960, 4. Vermont State Archives, Office of the Secretary of State, Montpelier (hereafter cited as VSBON Minutes).
28. State of Vermont, *Acts & Resolves: General Assembly of the State of Vermont, 46th Biennial Session, 1961*, 213–25.
29. State of Vermont, *Vermont Legislative Directory and State Manual, 1961*, 663.
30. VSBON Minutes, attached resolution, 27 March 1963.
31. VSBON Minutes, 16 October 1962, 1.
32. VSBON Minutes, 25 October 1967, 3.
33. Vermont State Nurses' Association, VSNA–VLN Coordinating Committee Minutes, February 1962, 3. Vermont State Nurses' Association Special Collection, Library Research Annex, The University of Vermont, Burlington, VLN box I (hereafter cited as VLN Collection).
34. Alice Robinson, President's Report, *VLN Newsletter* IX, no. 1 (August 1962). VLN Collection.

35. Vermont League for Nursing, Advisory Council Minutes, 1 May 1963. VLN Collection.
36. VSBON Minutes, 13 May 1966, 1.
37. Charles E. Gibson, *Opinion No. 19*, Biennial Report of the Attorney General, State of Vermont, 30 June 1966, 208–11.
38. VSBON Minutes, 23 February 1965, 1.
39. VSBON Minutes, 19 May 1965, 1.
40. Andrew Nuquist and Edith Nuquist, *Vermont State Government and Administration* (Burington, Vt.: The University of Vermont, 1966), 145–46.
41. Vermont Statutes Annotated, *1960 Law Pamphlet: Acts of the Adjourned Session of the 45th Biennial Legislature, January 12–February 9, 1960*, 6. Vermont State Archives, Office of the Secretary of State, Montpelier.
42. William K. Marsh, letter to VSBON, 28 February 1962.
43. VSBON Minutes, 2 May 1962, 5; 16 October 1962, 2.
44. VSBON Minutes, 29 October 1964.
45. VSBON minutes, 2 July 1965, 1.
46. VSBON Minutes, 9 June 1967, 1.
47. VSBON Minutes, 13 May 1966, 1.
48. Kincheloe and Hunt, *Empty Beds*, 143–45.
49. Ibid., 143.
50. VSBON Minutes, 4 December 1970.
51. Ibid., Report of Conference on Psychiatric Technicians, attached to minutes.
52. Kincheloe and Hunt, *Empty Beds*, 147.
53. VSBON Minutes, 30 August 1972, 3–4.
54. Vermont Statutes Annotated, Title 26 Chapter 24, 1974.
55. Faith G. Emerson, personal communication to the author, August 1999.
56. Mary Thompson, letter to William Moeser, 18 February 1971.
57. VSBON Minutes: Addendum, 1 July 1972.
58. VSBON Minutes, 8 July 1976, 2.
59. VSBON Minutes, 18 August 1977, 2.
60. State of Vermont, *Acts and Resolves, 55th Biennial Session of Vermont Legislature, 1979–1980*, 408–23.
61. VSBON Minutes, 4 June 1981, 2.
62. National Council of State Boards of Nursing, *20th Anniversary Meeting Brochure*, 4–8 August 1998, Albuquerque, New Mexico.
63. VSBON Minutes, 19 July 1978, 3–4.
64. Ibid., 5–6.
65. VSBON Minutes, 21 June 1983, 2.
66. VSBON Minutes, 19 March 1984, 1.
67. VSBON Minutes, 10 September 1985, 1.
68. VSBON Minutes, 17 November 1981, 1.
69. VSBON Minutes, 13 March 1980, 5.
70. VSBON Minutes, 17 April 1980, 3.
71. Ibid., 4.
72. Vermont State Board of Nursing, *Board of Nursing Newsletter*, Spring 1989, 3–4.
73. Ibid., 4.
74. Ibid.
75. VSBON Minutes, 25 July 1988, 4; 12 September 1988, 6.
76. Vermont State Board of Nursing Report of Executive Director, 13 October 1988, 3.

77. VSBON Minutes, 12 December 1988, 3.
78. Ibid., 3.
79. James Douglas, *Secretary of State: Annual Report on Licensing, 1986.* Office of the Secretary of State, Montpelier.
80. Vermont State Board of Nursing, Title 26 V.S.A. Chapter 28 and Administrative Rules, Chapter 5, 1994.
81. VSBON Minutes, February 1995, 3.
82. State of Vermont, *Acts and Resolves, 62nd Biennial Session, Adjourned Session of the Vermont Legislature*, H.616, Act 201, 426, 1994.
83. Lorraine Impey, letter to VSBON, 11 July 1995.
84. Vermont State Board of Nursing, *Administrative Rules*, Chapter IV, Rule 6, 3D 4, 1996.
85. Vermont State Board of Nursing. Ad Hoc Committee on Advanced Practice, July 1995.
86. Vermont State Board of Nursing, *Board of Nursing Newsletter*, Fall 1996.
87. Ibid.
88. Vermont State Board of Nursing, Joint Statement of the Vermont Boards of Medical Practice and Nursing regarding the Administration of non-prescription medications by registered nurses, 8 July 1991.
89. Vermont State Board of Nursing, Letter to Martha Ide, 15 April 1993.
90. Vermont Secretary of State, Office of Professional Regulation, "15th Annual Report on Professional Licensing," December 1996, 7.
91. Faith G. Emerson, personal communication, 2 January 2000.
92. State of Vermont, *Vermont Legislative Directory and State Manual*, 1961.

Nurse Practitioners in Vermont

THE NURSE PRACTITIONER movement began in 1965 at the University of Colorado with the establishment of the first program for pediatric nurse practitioners. The program was started by Loretta Ford, RN, PhD, and Henry Silver, MD.

In 1971, Idaho became the first state to authorize in their Nurse Practice Act an expanded role for registered nurses. Vermont amended its Nurse Practice Act to allow the expanded practice, July 1, 1974. The terminology that began the process for allowing the expanded role of nurses was added to Section 1552E and stated: "Performance of such additional acts requiring education and training and which are recognized jointly by the Medical and Nursing professions as proper to be performed by registered professional nurses."

The Vermont State Nurses' Association (VSNA) and the Vermont Medical Society (VMS) developed a Joint Practice Committee in 1971 to look at the issues that were appearing nationally with regard to the expanded role of nurses. Both associations sent representatives to a national conference of Joint Practice Committees in 1972, held in Itaska, Illinois. Paul Young, MD (VMS), Kathryn Lambert, RN, and Elizabeth Morgan, RN (VSNA), reported on the meeting and made joint recommendations to their organizations. In 1975, the Vermont Joint Practice Committee was revitalized to address the problems identified by the VSNA to be inherent in nursing and medical joint practice: writing of prescriptions by nurse practitioners, performance of minor surgery, and intravenous (IV) chemotherapy. The Vermont Joint Practice Committee was composed of equal numbers of nurses appointed by VSNA and physicians appointed by the VMS.

An Attorney General's opinion (1/25/75) regarding nurse practitioners writing prescriptions stated that as long as there are written protocols with the physician and professional nurse, "performance of these tasks, including the prescription of specified medications, are well within the scope of the licensed professional nurse under the present state of the law." As these issues were being dealt with by the professional associations, the Vermont Nurse Practice Act was again opened in 1980 and gave the power and duty to regulate the nurse practitioners to the Vermont State Board of Nursing. In 1980, Governor Snelling appointed Joan

Smidutz, Westminster, Vermont, as the first nurse practitioner to the Vermont State Board of Nursing.

In 1983, the Board of Nursing promulgated the rules governing the nurse practitioners in Vermont. Public hearings were held and these rules were adopted; they became effective August 4, 1983, and included prescriptive practice. An ad hoc Nurse Practitioner Advisory Committee representing the various advanced practice areas was instrumental in the formation of the rules adopted by the Board of Nursing. The Advisory Committee continues to advise the Board when requested. The rules were again revised in 1994.

The first nurse practitioners in the state of Vermont were pediatric nurse practitioners (PNP). They initially organized in 1973, and formally became the Vermont Pediatric Nurse Practitioner Group in 1976. They have been meeting sporadically ever since. At the present time, the Board of Nursing lists thirty pediatric nurse parctitioners. In 1976, other nurse practitioners organized as the Vermont Nurse Practitioner Interest Group and later broke into a Northern Group and Southern Group. A professional and clinical conference sponsored by the group is held annually, and they publish a newsletter several times a year. The Vermont State Board of Nursing lists more than 350 nurses in advanced practice. Nurse practitioners have become viable, primary health care providers with prescriptive authority in the state of Vermont.

—JOAN SMIDUTZ, BS, RN, CS-FNP

Contributors

Elizabeth R. Allen, RN, BSN, is a graduate of Adelphi School of Social Work and Duke University School of Nursing. She has extensive experience in maternal child health nursing and program administration. She is presently director of the Maternal Child Health Division of the Visiting Nurse Association of Burlington, Vermont.

Priscilla (Pat) Wood Allen RN, MSN, a graduate of Brightlook Hospital School of Nursing, St. Johnsbury, Vermont, Simmons College, Boston, Massachusetts, and Boston University, is experienced in public health nursing, teaching, and administration. She served as executive officer of the Vermont State Board of Nursing just prior to retirement from forty-five years of nursing in Vermont.

Faith Brothers, MS, RN, CRRN, is a graduate of St. Peter's School of Nursing, New Brunswick, New Jersey, Glassboro State College School of Nursing, Glassboro, New Jersey, Cedarcrest College, Allentown, Pennsylvania, and Russell Sage Graduate School in Troy, New York. She is a Certified Rehabilitation Nurse who has worked in a variety of settings, acute and chronic, institutional and community based. Currently, she is executive director of the Vermont State Nurses' Association, based in Winooski, Vermont.

Dr. Janet Brown-Wolff taught Community Health Nursing at Boston University and Boston College prior to coming to The University of Vermont. She had been active in community/public health nursing as a staff nurse, an administrator, and educational director. She was nurse coordinator of the first nurse practitioner program offered in the state of Vermont, and later became coordinator of continuing education programs for nurses at the School of Nursing, The University of Vermont.

Jane Packard Bryant, RN, PNP, CHTP, was with the Burlington Visiting Nurse Association for nearly thirty years. She then devoted herself to her healing touch private practice, seeing patients in hospital, homes, and her Shelburne office, where she continues her love of nursing.

JANE CAMPBELL, RN, CFNP, MEd, is retired from the position of director of Health Services of St. Michael's College. She currently practices part time as a family nurse practitioner at the Free Clinic, Fanny Allen campus, Fletcher Allen Health Care. She was a member of the Vermont State Board of Nursing and served as chair from 1987–1992. Jane is the mother of seven and the grandmother of twelve.

JUDY COHEN, PhD, RN, a native of Burlington, Vermont, is an associate professor of nursing in The University of Vermont School of Nursing. She is a captain in the U.S. Naval Reserve, Navy Nurse Corps, having served twenty-seven years, including three years of active duty (1975–78). She has served two terms as president of the Vermont State Nurses' Association (1994–96 and 1998–2000).

TRESSA CONDON, RN, BSPA, NHA, is currently owner and co-administrator of Holiday House in St. Albans, Vermont, and has worked for thirty years in geriatric nursing. She is also the vice-chair of the Nursing Home Licensure Board and vice-chair of the Advisory Board of the Fanny Allen School of Practical Nursing.

JOAN COTA, RN, BA, BS, CCRN, has worked as a staff nurse in medicine and surgery at Heaton Hospital, Montpelier, Vermont, and Rutland Hospital, and in the intensive care unit at Rutland Hospital for almost twenty years. She is currently office manager for Dr. David Austin of Rutland, Vermont.

LYNNE ANN DAPICE, MS, RN, was executive director of the Vermont State Nurses' Association from 1991 to 1999. She is currently coordinator of the diabetes program for the Vermont Department of Health. She has been an emergency nurse, a nursing educator, a pulmonary nurse specialist, a faculty member of the School of Nursing, The University of Vermont, and associate director of the Professional Nurses Service, Inc.

ELIZABETH J. DAVIS, RN, MPH, LLD (HON.) has worked in the field of home health and hospice care in Vermont for over thirty-five years. She served as staff nurse and then executive director of the VNA of Chittenden/Grand Isle Counties for twenty years, and she was vice president of operations for the Visiting Nurse Service of New York for five years. Currently, she is the president and CEO of the Visiting Nurse Alliance of Vermont and New Hampshire, Inc. She is an adjunct assistant professor at the University of Vermont, and received an honorary degree from UVM in 1998 for outstanding public service.

FAITH G. EMERSON, RN, BS, MA, was a staff nurse for seven years in public health, and was on the faculty of the School of Nursing, The University of Vermont, with major responsibility for teaching community health nursing. She served two terms on the Vermont State Board of Nursing (1971–81) including five years as president.

SUSAN O. FARRELL, RN, MA ED, MS, is a graduate of Castleton State College (1969 and 1977), The University of Vermont (1974), and Russell Sage College (1989). She is chairperson of the Vermont State Board of Nursing, president of the Vermont Council of Associate Degree Nursing Programs and is a member of Sigma Theta Tau Nursing Honor Society. Currently, she is chairperson of the Nursing Department at Castleton State College.

KATHLEEN R. GERAN, RN, BS, MS, a graduate of the University of Vermont and Texas Women's University Schools of Nursing, is an expert in maternal child health nursing with many years of experience in administration. She served six years on the Vermont State Board of Nursing as member, vice-chair and chairperson. Currently, she is nurse administrator for women's and children's services and staff development coordinator at Fletcher Allen Health Care, as well as adjunct professor, School of Nursing, The University of Vermont.

EILEEN GIRLING, RN, MPH, COHN, is co-founder of the Vermont Association of Occupational Health Nurses and has practiced in the specialty since 1983. She developed the first hospital-based occupational health program in the area at the Fanny Allen Hospital. This program now operates as the Fletcher Allen Health Care Occupational Health Services. Currently, she is employed by the State Department of Health and is a Visiting Scholar in Occupational and Environmental Health at Harvard School of Public Health.

MARTHA D. GRADY, RN, MSN, is a graduate of the University of Delaware and University of Texas (Austin) Schools of Nursing, with a major in maternal child nursing. She has extensive clinical experience in the care of new mothers and infants and in perinatal continuing education. She is currently education coordinator for the Vermont Regional Perinatal Program, Department of Pediatrics, UVM College of Medicine.

ROBERT E. GREEN, RN, AD, graduated in 1975 from The University of Vermont with an associate's degree in nursing. He has been employed at Central Vermont Medical Center for the past twenty-five years, most recently in the Surgical Services Department in the Operating Room. He is currently a senior at Trinity College, working toward a bachelor's degree in human resource development.

Virginia A. Incerpi, RN, BS, NCSN, Danville, Vermont, is presently employed Pre-K to 12 in the Danville school district. Member, past officer, and co-chair of the Professional Development Committee of the Vermont State School Nurses' Association, she was a member of the original Department of Education task force for the development of the Vermont Standards of Practice, School Health Services.

Toni H. Kaeding, MS, RN, was director of the Vermont Nursing Initiative from 1989 to 1995. She currently serves on Vermont's Blue Ribbon Nursing Commission and has a faculty appointment in the Department of Medicine at The University of Vermont College of Medicine.

Kathleen Keleher, CNM, MPH, FACNM, is currently employed at Fletcher Allen Health Care as the administrative director of nursing operations, where she has been a nurse-midwife since 1979. She is also an assistant clinical professor in The University of Vermont College of Medicine, Department of OB/GYN, and president-elect of the Vermont State Nurses' Association.

Marsha Kincheloe, RN, MS, MA, CS, received a master's degree in psychiatric nursing in 1969 from the University of Colorado, and a master's degree in psychology from the New School for Social Research in New York City. From 1985 to the present she has been nursing administrator of the Vermont State Hospital, Waterbury, Vermont.

Wendy L. LaFage, RN, MS, MA, CS, received a BSN from the University of Connecticut (1969), MSN from the University of Arizona (1974), and MA from Louisiana State University (1981). Areas of specialization are maternal child nursing, education, and counseling. Ms. LaFage served Southern Vermont College as director of the nursing program. Currently she is a doctoral candidate in health care education.

Audrey Larrow, RN, BS, MA, began work as a public health nurse for the Vermont Department of Health in 1971. She was assistant director and public health nursing supervisor from 1972 to 1978, district manager/director from 1978 to 1990, and public health nursing chief from 1990 to 1994. She is now retired.

Kathleen M. Ledo, MS, RN, CCRN, is an assistant professor and Health Sciences' Division's chairperson at Adirondack Community College in Queensbury, New York. She has a nursing background in education and critical care, and maintains a clinical practice in the Post Anesthesia Care Unit at the Rutland Regional Medical Center, Rutland, Vermont.

JEAN LERTOLA, RN, BSN, MA, graduated in January 1957 from The University of Vermont in Burlington, Vermont with a BS in nursing. She worked ten years as a staff nurse in various clinical areas. In 1968, she became an instructor of nursing at Castleton State College in Castleton, Vermont. She earned a master's in education from Castleton State College in 1980. She retired from CSC in 1990, but continues to work part-time at CSC, teaching clinical skills in the college lab and facilitating study sessions.

JOCELYN H. MACDONALD, BSN, RN, CPAN, is past president of the Vermont/New Hampshire Association of Peri Anesthesia Nurses, and currently communications chairperson of VT/NH APAN. Presently, she is a graduate student at the University of New England Master's of Nurse Anesthesia Program, Biddeford, Maine.

VIOLA ("RUSTY") CHASE MCGINN, RN, BS, now retired, was a hospital staff nurse in medicine and surgery, and worked for fifteen years at the Brattleboro Retreat, Brattleboro, Vermont, specializing in psychiatric nursing (1960–75). She was an instructor at the Thompson School for Practical Nursing, Brattleboro, and worked at the Beacon Detox and Beacon Clinic, Franklin Medical Center, Greenfield, Massachusetts.

MARY MCMAHON, MS, BSN, RN, is a graduate of Castleton State College and of Russell Sage College, Troy, New York. She is site director at Vermont Technical College Nursing Program, Putnam/Bennington Campus. She has practiced in medical-surgical settings and in nursing education at Southwestern Vermont Medical Center, Bennington, Vermont. She currently teaches basic nursing and medical-surgical nursing courses.

JEAN B. MILLIGAN, RN, EDD, came to Vermont after teaching nursing at Yale University and University of Michigan Schools of Nursing. She served as a faculty member and then dean at The University of Vermont School of Nursing, and is past president of the Vermont State Nurses' Association. She is also a recipient of the Distinguished Alumna Award from Yale University School of Nursing. She is currently retired and busy with many volunteer projects.

MARY QUINN O'BRIEN, RN, graduated from Fanny Allen Hospital School of Nursing, and has worked in Vermont, New York (medical-surgical nursing at Moses Ludington Hospital, Ticonderoga), and Massachusetts (obstetrical nursing at Mercy Hospital, Springfield, and St. Lukes in Pittsfield). Following the birth of the second of six children she retired from nursing to become a fulltime mother and homemaker.

MARY VAL PALUMBO, RN, MSN, GNP, is a gerontological nurse practitioner and certified continence care nurse. She has owned Continence Consultation Services since 1991 and sees clients in their homes, consults with long-term care staff, lectures around the country, and has an office practice with Women's Health Care Services in Williston, Vermont.

JANET C. PATTERSON, RN, BSN, was a nurse practitioner in Planned Parenthood (first in Planned Parenthood of Vermont, and then for Planned Parenthood of Northern New England) for fifteen years. After leaving PPNNE, she took courses in international development and health care in pursuit of a master's degree. Presently, she is working with elders through the Certificate in Gerontology Program at The University of Vermont.

NANCY PERRAULT, RN, MS, holistic nurse certified, certified healing touch practitioner has a holistic nursing practice providing integrative guided imagery, healing touch and other energetic therapies. She also mentors students of healing touch who are pursuing certification. She is employed part-time at The University of Vermont, where she teaches clinical nursing.

JOSEPH REILLY, BSN, CRNA, received his BSN from Fairleigh Dickinson University, Teaneck, New Jersey, attended the anesthesia program at Dartmouth-Hitchcock, Hanover, New Hampshire, and has been an anesthesia provider at Mt. Ascutney Hospital, Windsor, Vermont, since 1974.

MARILYN RINKER, RN, MSN, APN, OCN, is currently interim program chair for nursing at Norwich University, Northfield, Vermont. She was nurse administrator for medicine, which included oncology services at Fletcher Allen Health Care, Burlington, Vermont, oncology educator at Rhode Island Hospital, and clinic coordinator at the Vermont Regional Cancer Center.

ANITA FREGOSI RISTAU, RN, MS, is executive director of the Vermont State Board of Nursing. A graduate of The University of Vermont and St. Michael's College, with over twenty-five years' experience in nursing education, she served as chair of the Associate Degree Program and head of the Division of Nursing at Norwich University where she was promoted to rank of Professor of Nursing, granted tenure in 1992, and achieved Professor Emerita status in May 2000.

Dea Rotella, RN, is a 1945 graduate of Bishop DeGoesbriand Hospital School of Nursing, Burlington, Vermont. She did private duty and staff nursing prior to eight years as head nurse in the Intensive Care Unit. Following this, she continued staff nursing involving "progressive care," teaching patients, particularly diabetics, to care for themselves. She has been retired from active nursing since the early 1960s.

Marilyn (Lyn) Rothwell is a recently retired nurse practitioner at the Given Health Care center of Fletcher Allen Health Care and a clinical assistant professor of medicine, Primary Care Internal Medicine, The University of Vermont College of Medicine. A graduate in public health nursing at the University of Rochester, New York, she founded and directed the Visiting Nurse Association of Douglas County, Kansas, before coming to Vermont in 1970.

Sally A. Sample, DS (honorary), MN, RN, FAAN, was the first nursing director of the Medical Center Hospital of Vermont in the 1960s. She held nurse executive positions in three university hospitals before returning to Vermont as assistant professor of nursing at The University of Vermont, and director of MCHV's Center for Nursing in the 1990s. She currently serves in the first nurse-at-large position of the Joint Commission on Accreditation of Healthcare Organizations (JCAHO).

Diane Rich Sande, RN, MS, graduated from Albany Medical Center School of Nursing, Albany, New York in 1969. In 1972, she completed the requirements for the Bachelor of Science in nursing at Boston College, and in 1980 graduated from Russell Sage College in Troy, New York with a Master's of Science in nursing. Since graduation in 1969, Ms. Sande's area of clinical practice has focused on pediatric nursing. She has been employed at The University of Vermont School of Nursing since 1979, where she has been involved in teaching nursing students.

Hollie Shaner, RN, MSA, is president of the Nightingale Institute for Health and the Environment and is environmental health coordinator for Fletcher Allen Health Care. She is a Visiting Scientist at the Harvard School of Public Health, and has written and taught extensively on resource conservation and pollution prevention in health care.

Margaret Mahoney Sharpe, RN, BSN, a graduate of The University of Vermont School of Nursing, commenced her career in pediatric nursing at Children's Hospital, Boston, Massachusetts. She worked at Dartmouth-Hitchcock, taught pediatric nursing at Mary Hitchcock Hospital School of Nursing, Hanover, New Hampshire, and served thirteen years in the nurse manager role on the pediatric unit, Medical Center Hospital of Vermont. She is currently employed in the Patient Relations Department, Fletcher Allen Health Care, Burlington, Vermont.

JOHANNA SHEEHEY-JONES, RN, BSN, graduated from The University of Vermont in 1978. After working in rural Alaska and Washington state, she returned to Vermont and has been working at Fletcher Allen Health Care's Breast Care Center as a breast health specialist since 1995.

JOAN SMIDUTZ, BS, RN, CS-FNP, from Westminster, Vermont, is a graduate of St. Vincent Hospital School of Nursing, Worcester, Massachusetts, The University of Vermont Family Nurse Practitioner Program, and the University of New Hampshire. Ms. Smidutz has extensive experience in hospital, public health, and school health nursing. She served as chair of the Vermont State Board of Nursing for six years. She presently works as a family nurse practitioner for the Brattleboro (Vermont) Free Clinic.

BONNIE STRAND, RN, MA, CEN, is manager of Emergency/Endoscopy Services at Porter Hospital, Inc., Middlebury, Vermont. She is past president of the Vermont Emergency Nurses' Association, has served as a state delegate to ENA national conventions, and is currently state treasurer, newsletter editor, and webmaster (www.vermontena.com).

SUSAN CUCINELL SULLIVAN, RN, BSN, graduated from Villanova University in 1980 with a BSN. For the past twenty years she has been involved in nursing management and direct clinical nursing. She began her nursing career in Philadelphia, practicing at Graduate Hospital and the VA of Philadelphia. She has been a resource nurse, a critical care nurse, and a nurse manager for a Medical Intensive Care Unit at Fletcher Allen Health Care in Burlington, Vermont. Currently, Susan is raising a family and working part-time as staff nurse in an ambulatory care setting.

ROSE-MARIE TARBELL, RN, MED, has been involved with Thompson School for Practical Nurses since 1955. She has worked as a clinical instructor, then assistant director, and finally site director-instructor from 1982 to 1999. Historically, she was one of eight graduates from The University of Vermont in 1953 to earn a BSN in the new five-year program. In 1985, she earned a masters degree in education at Castleton State College. Since retiring in June of 1999 from Thompson School and Vermont

Technical College, she has worked as a volunteer parish nurse for Grace United Methodist Church in Aberdeen, Maryland.

MARY WAITE, RN, BSN, CSN, was an ICU/CCU nurse from 1965 to 1970, a family practice nurse from 1970 to 1987, and has been school nurse at the Fair Haven Grade School since 1987.

LORRAINE (LORRI) WELCH, RN, EDD, is currently an associate professor at The University of Vermont School of Nursing. She has been on the faculty for thirty years, serving under the leadership of most of the directors/deans of the School of Nursing. She was president of Kappa Tau Chapter of Sigma Theta Tau International, the Honor Society of Nursing from 1994 to 1996.

JANICE L. WIMMER, RN, BS, of Montpelier, Vermont, has been a school nurse since 1973, and is presently at U-32 Jr./Sr. High School, Washington Central Supervisory Union. She is a member of the Vermont State School Nurses' Association, co-chair of its Professional Development Committee, and member of the original Department of Education task force for preparation of the Vermont Standards of Practice, School Health Services.

MARY WRIGHT, RN, BA, has been an instructor of practical nursing students since 1965. She is currently the site director for Vermont Technical College Nursing Program at Fanny Allen/Colchester Campus.

JANET YANTACHKA, RN, BSN, COHNS, is a graduate of Wilkes-Barre General Hospital School of Nursing, Wilkes-Barre, Pennsylvania, and The University of Vermont School of Nursing, Burlington, Vermont. She is a certified occupational health nurse specialist. Her work experience includes staff nursing at Fanny Allen Hospital, Winooski, Vermont, occupational health nursing at Digital Equipment Corporation, South Burlington, Vermont, and presently she is with Employee Health Services at Fletcher Allen Health Care, Burlington.